Surgical Complications and Management of Kidney Transplantation

Surgical Complications and Management of Kidney Transplantation

Editor: Alice Foster

AMERICAN
MEDICAL PUBLISHERS
www.americanmedicalpublishers.com

AMERICAN
MEDICAL PUBLISHERS
www.americanmedicalpublishers.com

Cataloging-in-publication Data

Surgical complications and management of kidney transplantation / edited by Alice Foster.
p. cm.
Includes bibliographical references and index.
ISBN 979-8-88740-227-7
1. Kidneys--Transplantation. 2. Kidneys--Transplantation--Complications.
3. Kidneys--Surgery--Complications. 4. Kidneys--Diseases--Treatment.
5. Nephrology. I. Foster, Alice.
RD575 .S87 2023
617.461 059 2--dc23

American Medical Publishers,
41 Flatbush Avenue,
1st Floor, New York,
NY 11217, USA

ISBN 979-8-88740-227-7 (Hardback)

Contents

Preface

A kidney transplant is a surgical procedure that involves the replacement of a diseased kidney with a healthy kidney received from a donor. There are several surgical complications associated with kidney transplantation such as infection, bleeding, blockage of the blood vessels to the new kidney, lack of new kidney function at first, and leakage of urine or blockage of urine in the ureter. The post-operative management of a kidney transplant includes keeping the area of surgery dry and clean, since contact with water increases the risk for infection. Any activity or posture that places pressure on the operated area or the transplanted kidney should also be avoided. The blood pressure and weight of the operated patient should also be monitored regularly. Any signs or symptoms such as fever, increase in pain around location of incision, swelling, redness, or bleeding from the operated site must be reported to a doctor immediately. This book provides comprehensive insights into the surgical complications and medical management of kidney transplantation in detail. It is appropriate for students seeking detailed information in this area of medicine as well as for experts.

Various studies have approached the subject by analyzing it with a single perspective, but the present book provides diverse methodologies and techniques to address this field. This book contains theories and applications needed for understanding the subject from different perspectives. The aim is to keep the readers informed about the progresses in the field; therefore, the contributions were carefully examined to compile novel researches by specialists from across the globe.

Indeed, the job of the editor is the most crucial and challenging in compiling all chapters into a single book. In the end, I would extend my sincere thanks to the chapter authors for their profound work. I am also thankful for the support provided by my family and colleagues during the compilation of this book.

Editor

1

Donor Quality Scoring Systems and Early Renal Function Measurements in Kidney Transplantation

Quirino Lai et al.*
Department of General surgery and Organ transplantation,
Sapienza University of Rome, Rome
Italy

1. Introduction

Over the last years, an extensive improvement in the use of non-standard kidney allografts from deceased donors has been observed due to a chronic scarcity in the number of available donors. However, use of these donors seems to give worse results, higher delayed graft function (DGF) and rejection rates and briefer graft survivals.

Nevertheless, a standardized definition of non-standard donor is still under debate.

On these grounds, several studies have focalized on the importance of events immediately before or early post-transplant in determining allograft outcome: introduction of scores based on peri-operative features capable to predict graft function may yield huge implications for organ allocation policies, as well as for immediate and late clinical and immunological management of recipients. In fact, if pre-KT information could accurately predict suboptimal early graft function, the success of various mechanical, immunosuppressive and organ allocation strategies may be improved.

The aim of this review is to analyze the different pre- and post-transplant score systems, detecting their role in the clinical practice and comparing them in terms of prognostic ability.

2. Donor quality scoring systems

In the last decades, several different scoring systems based on donor, recipient and transplant parameters have been proposed with the intent to predict early and late post-KT graft function.

Despite several of these scores have been validated on large cohorts or have been adopted by national allocation systems, no one of them has been already internationally recognized as the best model for graft function prediction.

We analyzed these scores, stratifying them in three groups according to the different parameters by which they are composed: demographic and serological variables, histological graft variables, donor and histological graft variables.

---

* Francesco Nudo, Vincenzo Morabito, Giovanni Battista Levi Sandri, Fabio Melandro, Lucia Parlati, Nicola Guglielmo, Marco Di Laudo, Manuela Garofalo, Luca Poli, Renzo Pretagostini and Pasquale B Berloco

2.1 Demographic and serological variables

Several scores exclusively based on donor features or composed by a combination of parameters obtained by donor, transplant and donor-recipient match have been created. Some of these scores are commonly adopted in the care practice: we reported the most commonly used.

2.1.1 ECD

In March 2001, a consensus meeting who took place in Crystal City introduced a new definition of expanded criteria donor (ECD) (Rosengard et al, 2002). Under the work group's proposed plan, the Organ Procurement and Transplantation Network (OPTN), through its contract with the United Network for Organ Sharing (UNOS) developed a standard policy for national kidney allocation in the United States. In November 2001, the OPTN/UNOS Board of Directors adopted the new ECD definition and the new allocation system became operative in October 2002. The new definition of ECD derived from four different donor risk factors for graft failure: age, history of hypertension, cerebrovascular accident as a cause of death and final pre-procurement creatinine > 1.5 mg/dL.
Different combinations of these four parameters characterized each donor kidney and a relative risk of graft loss was determined for each donor profile (**Figure 1**).

	RR			
	Normal creatinine		High creatinine	
Age (years)	No HTN	HTN	No HTN	HTN
Cause of death was not cerebrovascular accident				
0–9	1.40**	1.59**	1.52**	–
10–39	1.00	1.14**	1.09*	1.24**
40–49	1.17**	1.33**	1.28**	1.45**
50–59	1.41**	1.60**	1.53**	**1.74****
60+	**1.90****	**2.16****	**2.07****	**2.36****
Cause of death was cerebrovascular accident				
0–9	1.60**	**1.82****	**1.74****	**1.98****
10–39	1.14**	1.30**	1.24**	1.41**
40–49	1.34**	1.52**	1.46**	1.66**
50–59	1.61**	**1.83****	**1.75****	**1.99****
60+	**2.17****	**2.47****	**2.37****	**2.69****

Source: SRTR data analyses as of August 1, 2002.
HTN = donor hypertension. Numbers in boldface indicate RR > 1.7.
$^{*}p < 0.05$, $^{**}p < 0.0005$.

Fig. 1. Relative risks (RR) of graft loss by four donor characteristics. Taken from Metzger et al., 2003.

The ECD kidney was then arbitrarily defined as any kidney whose relative risk of graft failure exceeded 1.7 when compared to a reference group of ideal donor kidneys (age 10–39 years, no hypertension, no cerebrovascular accident as cause of death and terminal predonation creatinine level < 1.5 mg/dL).

The definition of ECD status is the following (**Table 1**):

a. Donor age older than 59 years;
b. Donor age between 50 and 59 years with, additionally two of the following: death caused by cerebrovascular accident (CVA); terminal creatinine more than 1.5 mg/dL; history of hypertension.

	Donor age categories (years)				
Donor condition	**< 10**	**10-39**	**40-49**	**50-59**	**≥ 60**
CVA + HTN + Creat > 1.5				X	X
CVA + HTN				X	X
CVA + Creat > 1.5				X	X
HTN + Creat > 1.5				X	X
CVA					X
HTN					X
Creat > 1.5					X
None of the above					X

Source: OPTN.
CVA = cerebrovascular accident was cause of death.
HTN = history of hypertension.
Creat > 1.5 = Creatinine > 1,5 mg/dL.

Table 1. ECD for kidney donors. Taken from Rosengard et al., 2002 (with modifications).

A multicentre study (Metzger et al., 2003) based on OPTN/SRTR data showed a progressive increase in ECD utilization across the years, confirming the worse results obtained from these donors in terms of both patient and graft survivals.
Nevertheless, a more rational definition of ECD has given major opportunities to patients who had presented limited access to KT to be transplanted.
A monocentre analysis (Stratta et al., 2004) reported an effective increased volume of KTs within 1 year after the adoption of ECD policy; moreover, the authors observed similar results in terms of graft function and morbidity among recipients who received organs from standard or ECD. A systematic approach to ECD kidneys based on nephron mass matching and nephron sparing measures showed to provide optimal short-term outcomes and renal function comparable to standard kidneys.

2.1.2 DDS

Using ECD, a better allocation policy was obtained. On the other hand, the binary nature of the ECD definition may have underappreciated the variability of the quality of the organ.
On these grounds, (Nyberg et al., 2001) a more granulated scoring system (deceased donor score, DDS) was developed. DDS was based on seven different donor variables easily available at the moment of procurement. The end measure for the development of the score was the 6-month creatinine clearance value.
The variables analyzed were:
Cause of death (0-6 points), history of hypertension (0-6), renal creatinine clearance before procurement (0-6), age (0-6), history of diabetes mellitus (0-3), cold ischemia time (0-3) and severity of renal artery plaque (0-3).

The population enrolled for the study (241 cadaveric KT recipients) was stratified in four groups: grade A (0-5 points), grade B (6-10), grade C (11-15) and grade D (16-32).
Adoption of this score permitted an effective stratification of the population, showing that information available at the time of organ harvesting may estimate early graft function after cadaveric renal transplantation.
The same Authors (Nyberg et al., 2003) improved on their original scoring system studying the data 34.324 KT patients reported in the OPTN/SRTR registry. The five donor variables adopted were:
Age (0-25 points), history of hypertension (0-4), creatinine clearance before procurement (0-4), cause of death (0-3), HLA mismatch (0-3).
The entire population was stratified in four different grades according to the cumulative donor score: grade A (0-9 points), grade B (10-19), grade C (20-29) and grade D (30-39).
The influence of donor score on both graft function and survival was most severe above 20 points (**Figure 2**).

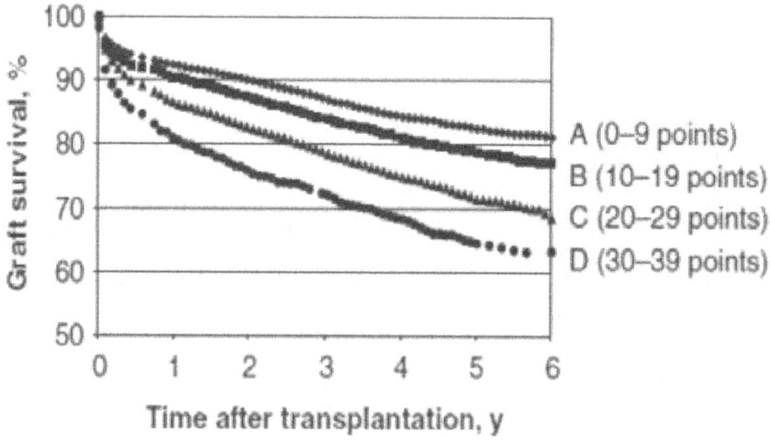

Fig. 2. Nyberg score grading significantly influences graft survival after transplantation. The greatest 6-year graft survival difference was observed between grades B and C, suggesting a cutoff for 'marginal' kidneys of approximately 20 points. Taken from Nyberg et al., 2003.

Afterwards, according to Nyberg score, this threshold value designates "marginal" kidneys.

2.1.3 DGF nomogram

According to the most commonly adopted definition, DGF is the need for dialysis in the first week after transplantation.
A multicentre study (Irish et al., 2003) analyzed data obtained from 13.846 patients reported in the United States Renal Data System (USRDS) registry from 1995 to 1998. Using a multivariable logistic regression analysis, factors contributing to DGF were analyzed.
The pre-KT donor and recipient factors analyzed were:
Donor: age, history of hypertension, terminal creatinine, donation after cardiac death, death caused by anoxia or CVA; cold ischemia time; HLA mismatch; combined organ transplantation.
Recipient: gender, race, diabetes, history of previous transplantation, history of transfusion, history of dialysis before transplantation, peak panel reactive anti-HLA antibodies.

A nomogram quantifying the relative contribution of each risk factor was created, providing a useful tool for developing a pretransplantation index of the likelihood of DGF occurrence (**Figure 3**).

Seven years later, a new analysis (Irish et al., 2010) was performed on 24.337 patients transplanted during the period 2003-2006. The authors developed a novel nomogram and a web-based calculator (http://www.transplantcalculator.com/DGF) as an easily accessible tool for predicting DGF.

Comparing risk factors in the modern (2003-2006) and in the earlier era (1995-1998), weight of immunological factors attenuated, while impact of donor renal function increased by 2-fold. The most significant factors associated with DGF were cold ischemia time, donor creatinine, body mass index, donation after cardiac death and donor age.

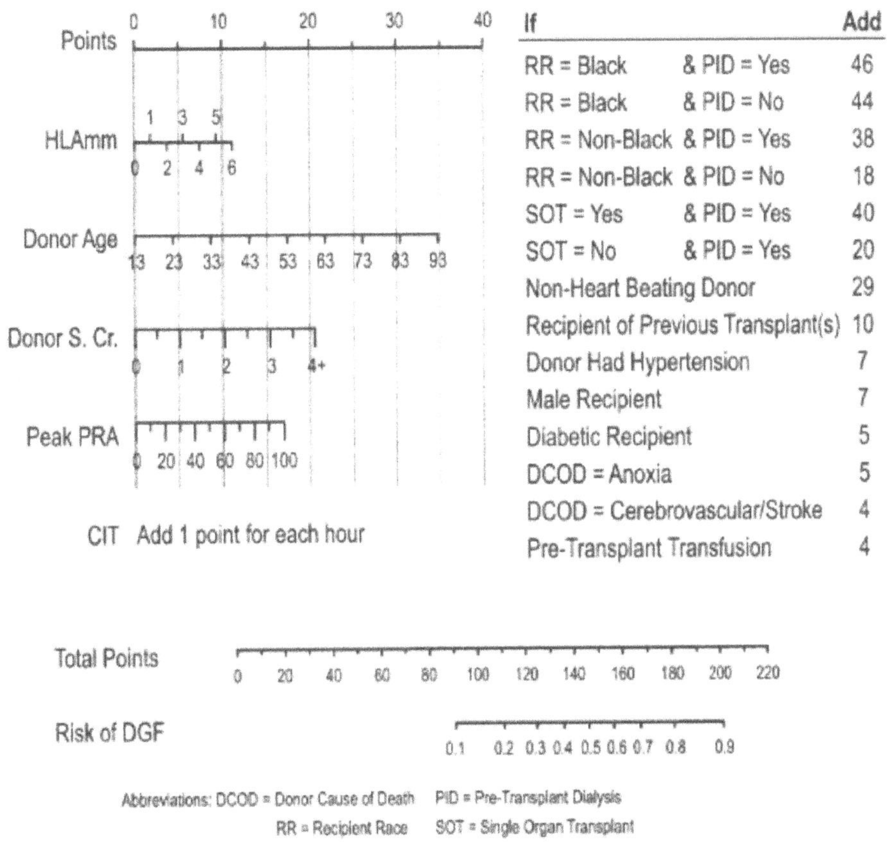

Fig. 3. Nomogram for estimating the risk of delayed graft function (DGF) in adult renal transplant recipients. HLAmm, HLA mismatch; S.Cr., serum creatinine; PRA, panel-reactive antibody; CIT, cold ischemia time; RR, recipient race; PID, pre-transplantation dialysis; DCOD, donor cause of death; SOT, single-organ transplant. Taken from Irish et al., 2003.

2.1.4 Pessione score

A retrospective analysis of a cohort of 7.209 deceased KT recipients transplanted in France from 1996 to 2000 was performed and a new scoring system (Pessione et al.. 2003) was ideated.

After multivariate analysis, only three parameters resulted as significant independent risk factors for graft failure:

Cerebrovascular cause of death, history of hypertension and elevated serum creatinine (> 150 micromol/L).

Donor age > 60 years was a statistically significant, but dependent, risk factor. The increased risk of graft loss in patients who presented the cumulative effect of donor risk factors was greater in recipients aged more than 60 years (one risk factor: RR = 1.8; two risk factors: RR = 2.7) (**Figure 4**).

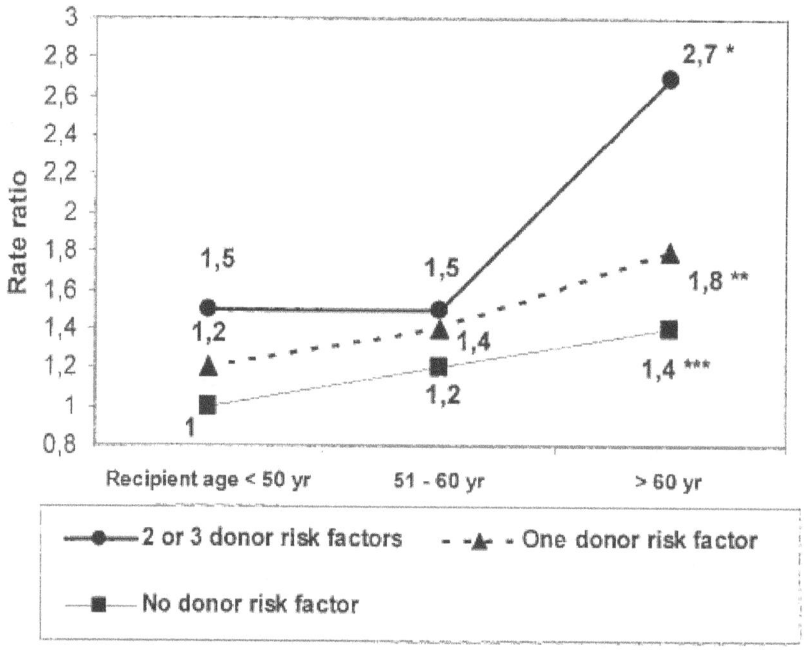

Fig. 4. Rate ratios of graft failure according to the absence or the presence of one or >2 significant donor risk factors in the different recipient age groups. *p-value = 0.008 (vs. patients <60 yr), ** p-value = 0.04 (vs. patients <60 yr), *** p-value = NS (vs. patients <60 yr). Taken from Pessione et al., 2003.

2.1.5 DRS

Donor risk score (DRS) (Schold et al., 2005) represents a model in which not only significant donor features, but also donor-recipient matches and cold ischemia time are adopted.

The variables used for the creation of the score were:

Donor race; donor history of hypertension; donor history of diabetes; donor death due to CVA; cold ischemia time; HLA mismatch; donor/ recipient cytomegalovirus (CMV) match.

The following grades based on accumulated "points" have been proposed: grade I (0-0.234), grade II (0.234-0.524), grade III (0.524-0.853), grade IV (0.853-1.17), and grade V (>1.17).

Adopting this model, the projected half-lives by donor grade, calculated utilizing data beyond 2-year posttransplant, were: grade I = 10.7 years; II = 10.0 years; III = 7.9 years; IV = 5.7 years; V = 4.5 years.
Comparing DRS with ECD and Nyberg score, the first one was the best model in graft loss stratification (**Figure 5**).

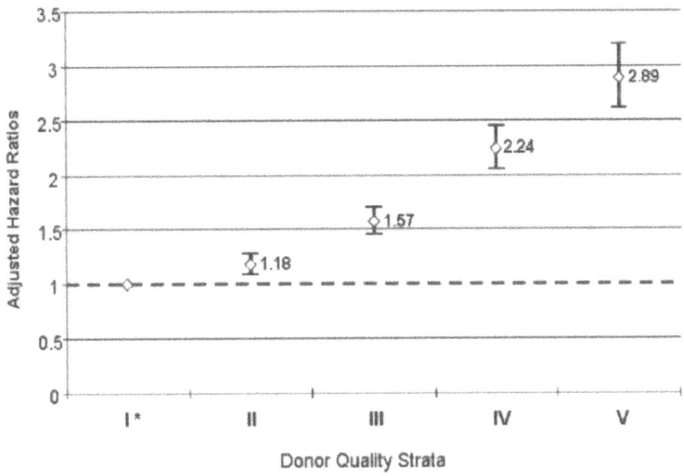

Fig. 5. Multivariate estimates for graft loss by donor grade. *Grade I donor serves as the reference group in the model. Taken from Schold et al., 2005.

2.1.6 KDRI

Kidney donor risk index (KDRI) (Rao et al., 2009) was proposed as a continuous combining donor and transplant variables to quantify graft failure risk. The authors analyzed 69.440 patients using national data from 1995 to 2005.
The fourteen proposed KDRI donor and transplant factors, each found to be independently associated with graft failure or death, were:
Donor: age, race, history of hypertension, history of diabetes, serum creatinine, cerebrovascular cause of death, height, weight, donation after cardiac death, hepatitis C virus status;
Transplant: human leukocyte antigen-B and DR mismatch, cold ischemia time, double or en bloc transplant.
The KDRI reflected the rate of graft failure relative to that of a healthy 40-year-old donor. Transplants of kidneys in the highest KDRI quintile (>1.45) had an adjusted 5-year graft survival of 63%, compared with 82% and 79% in the two lowest KDRI quintiles (<0.79 and 0.79-<0.96, respectively) (**Figure 6**).

2.1.7 DGF score

An analysis on a monocentre cohort of Italian KTs (Pretagostini et al., 2009) was performed with the intent to define the risk factors for the development of DGF.
The authors found five different donor and transplant parameters most commonly observed in non standard donors:
Donor age ≥ 60 years (P = 0.005), Creatinine Clearance < 40 mL/min (P = 0.025), history of diabetes mellitus (P = 0.026), history of hypertension (P = 0.017), and cold ischemia time > 15 hours (P < 0.0001).

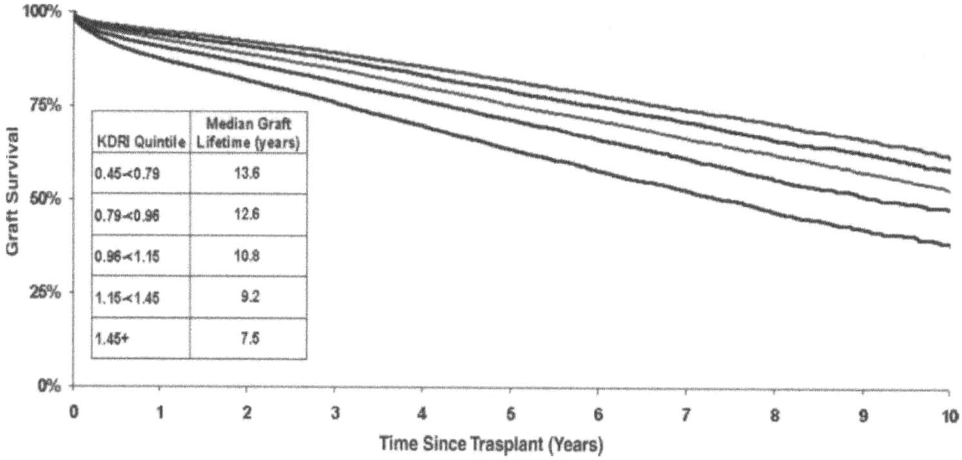

Fig. 6. Adjusted graft survival by KDRI quintile. Each survival pertains to a recipient who is aged 50 years, non-diabetic, and at the reference level of all other recipient factors. Extrapolation was used for the first and second quintile. Taken from Rao et al., 2009.

2.2 Histological graft variable

Above clinical features, another adopted approach fo4r the identification of high-risk kidneys is to use a pre-KT biopsy in order to characterize potential kidney grafts, help predict the graft outcome and provide a reference point for analysis of subsequent biopsies. Several different histological parameters have been correlated with poor outcomes (i.e. percentage of sclerotic glomerules, degree of tubulointerstitial and chronic vascular lesions). Starting from these considerations, all these histological changes were integrated into histological scoring systems with the intent to consent a better allocation of kidneys from elder donors. All the histological scores reported in literature in the last decades were based on the previously proposed semiquantitative analysis of renal histology (Pirani & Salinas-Madrigal, 1975).

2.2.1 Remuzzi score

The results of a consensus created by an international panel of pathologists (Remuzzi et al., 1999) consented the creation of a new score, This method was presented for the evaluation of kidneys procured from donors older than 60 years of age. This new method quantified the number of nephrons for each kidney with the intent to estimate if the grafts should be available for KT and whether single or dual transplantation should be used. This panel suggested a biopsy-based score ranging from a minimum of 0 (indicating the absence of renal lesions) to a maximum of 12 (indicating the presence of marked changes in the renal parenchyma) (**Table 2**).

The four different parameters considered in the scoring system were:

Glomerular global sclerosis (0-3), tubular atrophy (0-3), interstitial fibrosis (0-3) and arterial and arteriolar narrowing (0-3).

Kidneys with a score of 3 or lower were predicted to contain enough viable nephrons to be used as single transplants. Those with a score of 4, 5, or 6 could be used as dual transplants, on the assumption that the sum of the viable nephrons in the two kidneys approached the number in one ideal kidney. Kidneys with a score of 7 or greater were discarded, since it was assumed that they would deliver an insufficient dose of nephrons, even in a dual transplantation.

The validity of the score was tested (Remuzzi et al., 2006) analyzing a prospective cohort study of 62 patients who received one or two histologically evaluated kidneys from donors older than 60 years of age.

The outcomes of these grafts were compared with the outcomes among 248 matched recipients of single kidney grafts that had not been histologically evaluated and were either from 124 donors with age ≤ 60 years or from 124 donors older than 60 years.

Pretransplant biopsy protocol: semiquantitative method of evaluation of slides #
Glomerular global sclerosis Based on three sections (the first, middle, and last sections, if available); the number of globally sclerosed glomerules expressed as a percentage. 0 none globally sclerosed 1+ < 20% global glomerulosclerosis 2+ 20 to 50% global glomerulosclerosis 3+ > 50% global glomerulosclerosis
Tubular atrophy 0 absent 1+ < 20% of tubuli affected 2+ 20 to 50% of tubuli affected 3+ > 50% of tubuli affected
Interstitial fibrosis 0 absent 1+ < 20% of renal tissue replaced by fibrous connective tissue 2+ 20 to 50% of renal tissue replaced by fibrous connective tissue 3+ > 50% of renal tissue replaced by fibrous connective tissue
Arterial and arteriolar narrowing For the vascular lesions, if the changes are focal, the most severe lesion present gives the final grade. 0 absent 1+ increased wall thickness but to a degree that is less than the diameter of the lumen 2+ wall thickness that is equal or slightly greater to the diameter of the lumen 3+ wall thickness that far exceeds the diameter of the lumen with extreme luminal narrowing or occlusion
Final grade (range from 0 to a total of 12) 0 to 3 mild OK for single transplant 4 to 6 moderate OK for double transplant 7 to 12 severe should not be transplanted
Only biopsies with ≥ 25 glomerules considered for slide evaluation. Kidneys with evidence of acute tubular necrosis are not considered for the double transplant. Biopsies are graded as mild if they have 0 to 3 points in total provided they are less than 3 in any one category. Biopsies are graded as moderate if they have 4 to 6 points in total provided they do not have 3 points in more than one category.

Table 2. Histological score proposed by Remuzzi et al., 1999 (with modifications).

Analyzing long-term graft survival, excellent results were observed using the grafts previously selected by biopsy.
Graft survival in recipients of histologically evaluated kidneys did not differ significantly from that of grafts from younger donors previously evaluated with biopsy. On the other side, survivals were strongly superior to that of elder grafts not pre-operatively evaluated with biopsy.
Adopting this score, long-term survival of single or dual kidney grafts from donors older than 60 years of age were similarly excellent, showing that systematic hystological approach may help to expand the donor-organ pool for kidney transplantation without a contemporaneous lack of results .

2.2.2 Karpinski score

A New study based on histological aspects (Karpinski et al., 1999) was performed on 57 allografts procured by 34 elderly donors (age ≥ 60 years) with hypertension and/or vascular disease.
Graft survival of these patients was compared with the results of 57 control recipients selected to have similar baseline demographics but receiving transplants from younger donors.
Donor renal pathology was scored 0-3 (none to severe disease) in four areas (**Table 3**):
Glomerulosclerosis, tubular atrophy, interstitial fibrosis and vascular disease.
Vascular disease was composed by two different parameters (e.g. arteriolar narrowing and arterial sclerosis).
The number of sclerotic glomerules was expressed as a percent of the total number of glomerules available for evaluation.
For the vascular lesions, both arteries were evaluated separately. However, for the final vascular score, the most severe lesion of either arterioles or arteries determined the final grade. Each of the 4 compartments was given a score from 0 to 3; the total score was expressed out of 12.
A donor vessel score of 3/3 was associated with a 100% incidence of delayed graft function and poor 1-year graft function.

2.3 Donor and histological graft variables

A new model (Anglicheau et al., 2008) in which both histological and clinical variables were combined was developed in France. Before this study, in fact, a definitive role of pre-implantation biopsies versus clinical scores had not been extensively studied in marginal donors.
Pre-KT biopsies of 313 grafts from donors aged more than 50 years were analyzed.
Authors evaluated the ability in predicting 1-year poor graft function (estimated glomerular filtration rate [eGFR] < 25 mL/min/1.73 m2) of several donor clinical and histological features.
In multivariate analysis, the clinical and histological features that resulted statistically significant were:
Clinical parameters = donor hypertension and a serum Creatinine level ≥150 lmol/L before organ recovery.
Histological parameters: glomerulosclerosis, arteriolar hyalinosis, Pirani and CADI score.
However, the model who presented the highest performance in predicting low eGFR was achieved using a composite score that included donor serum creatinine (≥150 lmol/L or <150 lmol/L), donor hypertension and glomerulosclerosis (≥10% or <10%) (**Figure 7**).

Pretransplant biopsy protocol: semiquantitative method of evaluation of slides #
Glomerular wcore 0 none globally sclerosed 1+ < 20% global glomerulosclerosis 2+ 20 to 50% global glomerulosclerosis 3+ > 50% global glomerulosclerosis
Tubular score 0 absent 1+ < 20% of tubuli affected 2+ 20 to 50% of tubuli affected 3+ > 50% of tubuli affected
Interstitial score 0 absent 1+ < 20% of cortical parenchyma replaced by fibrous connective tissue 2+ 20 to 50% of cortical parenchyma replaced by fibrous connective tissue 3+ > 50% of cortical parenchyma replaced by fibrous connective tissue
Vascular score Arteriolar narrowing (or hyaline arteriolosclerosis)## 0 absent 1+ increased wall thickness but to a degree that is less than the diameter of the lumen 2+ wall thickness that is equal or slightly greater to the diameter of the lumen 3+ wall thickness that far exceeds the diameter of the lumen with extreme luminal narrowing or occlusion Arterial sclerosis (or intimal fibrous thickening-fibroplasia)## 0 absent 1+ increased wall thickness but to a degree that is less than the diameter of the lumen 2+ wall thickness that is equal or slightly greater to the diameter of the lumen 3+ wall thickness that far exceeds the diameter of the lumen with extreme luminal narrowing or occlusion
Only biopsies with at least 20 glomerules are considered for slide evaluation. ## For the vascular lesions, both arteries are evaluated separately. However, for the final vascular score, the most severe lesion of either arterioles or arterie determines the final grade.

Table 3. Scoring system proposed by Karpinski et al., 1999 (with modifications).

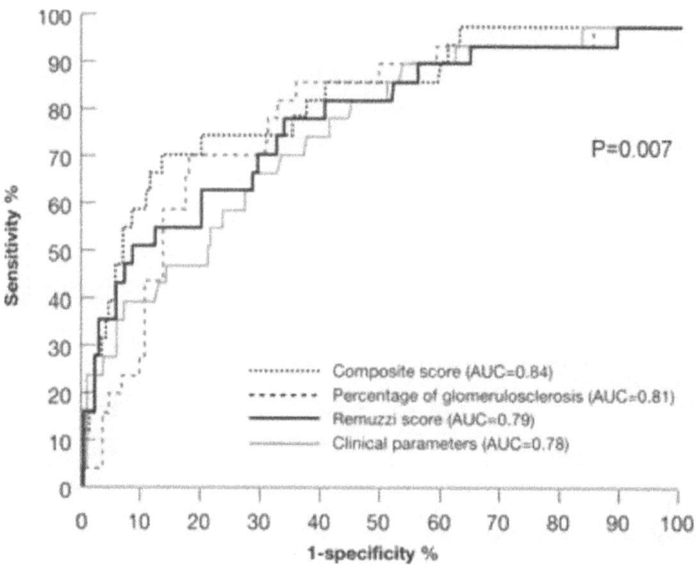

Fig. 7. Receiver operating characteristics (ROC) curves for clinical, histopathological and composite scoring systems as predictors of low eGFR at 1-year posttransplant. Global test: p-value = 0.007; composite score vs glomerulosclerosis: p-value = NS; composite score vs Pirani score: p-value = 0.001; composite score vs clinical parameters: p-value = 0.009). Taken from Anglicheau et al., 2008.

3. Measures of early graft function

Many measures of early graft function have been reported in Literature. Many of them were proposed with the intent to give a better definition of DGF. In fact, DGF is both an outcome and a predictor of the subsequent course of a renal transplant. Commonly adopted definition of DGF is the requirement for dialysis within the first week after KT (Daly et al., 2005). However, postoperative requirement of dialysis represents a very subjective and not standardized clinical decision. Recently, efforts have been made to quantify DGF more scientifically, adopting different scores based on urine output, serum creatinine levels, fluid overload and uremic status of the patient.
A comprehensive review of the literature (Yarlagadda et al., 2008) reported 18 different definitions for DGF (**Table 4**).

Definitions	No. of studies	No. of patients
Dialysis-based definitions		
Need for dialysis in the first week after transplant	41	259.251
Need for dialysis in the first week after transplant once hyperacute rejection, vascular and urinary tract complications were ruled out	2	760
Need for dialysis after transplant	2	737
Need for dialysis in the first 10 days after transplant	1	41
Absence of life-sustaining renal function that requires dialysis on two or more occasions within the first week after transplant	1	547

Definitions	No. of studies	No. of patients
Need for dialysis in the first 7 days after transplant with specific exclusion of single early post-operative dialysis performed for hyperkalemia	1	319
Return to maintenance hemodialysis within the first 4 days after transplantation	1	263
Creatinine-based definitions		
Serum creatinine increased or remained unchanged or decreased <10%/day during 3 consecutive days after the transplant	5	1471
Creatinine reduction ratio <30% and /or urine creatinine on Day 2 <1000 mg	2	401
Serum creatinine >2.5 mg/dL on Day 7 or the need for post-transplant hemodialysis	1	99
Time required for the kidney to reach Crcl>10 mL/min greater than 1 week.	1	843
Failure of creatinine to decline in the first 48 h in the absence of rejection	1	291
Combination		
Failure of serum creatinine to fall below pre-transplant levels, within 1 week regardless of the urine output	1	158
Patients with rise in serum Cr at 6–8 h post-operatively or <300 cc of urine despite adequate volume and diuretics	1	143
Dialysis requirement after transplant or a serum creatinine 150 μmol/L at Day 8	1	112
Urine output <1 L in 24 h and <25% fall in serum creatinine from baseline in first 24 h post-transplant	1	244
Urine output <75 mL/h in first 48 h or failure of serum Cr to decrease by 10% in the first 48 h	1	66
Need for dialysis in the first week after transplant or failure of serum creatinine to decrease within 24 h after transplant	1	104

Table 4. Different DGF definitions. Taken from Yarlagadda et al., 2008 (with modifications).

In the same study, 10 proposal of diagnostic technique to identify DGF were also proposed (**Figure 8**). Starting from these grounds, we have stratified the early measures of graft function in three different categories: creatinine-based definition, urine-based definition and combined definition.

3.1 Creatinine-based definition

a. Serum creatinine level of > 3 mg/dL on the fifth day after surgery (Humar et al., 2000).
b. CCR2 and 24-h UC2

This score was created (Govani et al., 2002) combining the creatinine reduction ratio between days 1 and 2 (CRR2) and the 24-h urinary creatinine levels at post-KT day 2 (UC2)

Equation: CRR2(%) = ([Cr1–Cr2]×100)/Cr1). (Cr1 = serum creatinine level at post-KT day 1; Cr2 = serum creatinine level at post-KT day 2).

The cut-off value for poor function corresponded to a CCR2 ≤ 30%.

c. CCR2

CCR2 was also adopted (Rodrigo et al., 2004; Salahudeen et al., 2004) as unique criterion for the definition of early graft function. The reported Authors used the same threshold value of 30%.

d. CCR7

Creatinine reduction ratio at day 7 (CCR7) (Johnston et al., 2007) was proposed as score of initial graft function.

Equation: CRR7(%) = ([Cr0–Cr7]×100)/Cr0). (Cr0 = serum creatinine levels immediately before KT and no later than 6 hours after last dialysis; Cr7 = serum creatinine levels at post-KT day 7).

The cut-off value for poor function corresponded to a CCR7 ≤ 70% (**Figure 9**).

e. Number of days to achieve a creatinine clearance of > 10 mL/min, calculated by the Gault-Cockroft formula (Giral-Classe et al., 1998).
f. Serum creatinine level increased, remained unchanged or decreased by less than 10% per day immediately after surgery during three consecutive days for > 1 week (Boom et al., 2000).

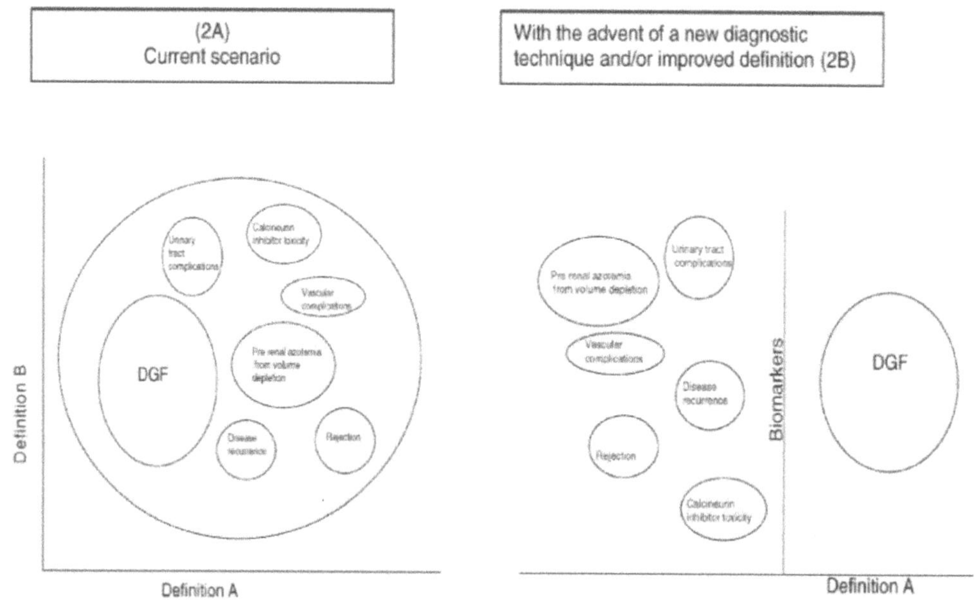

Fig. 8. Different clinical conditions that present as early graft dysfunction. (**A**) Current definitions do not allow us to distinguish DGF from other causes of graft dysfunction. (**B**) With an improved definition and/or diagnostic technique patients with DGF can be correctly classified. Taken from Yarlagadda et al., 2008.

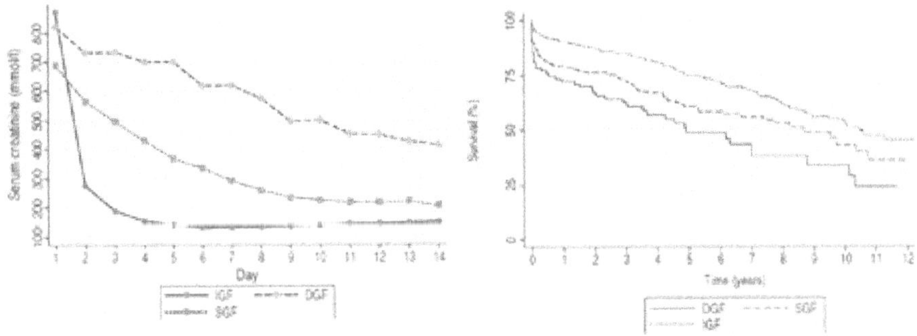

Fig. 9. *Left:* Decline in creatinine within 2 weeks post-KT. *Right:* graft survival curves. IGF: initial good function (CCR7 > 70%), DGF: delayed graft function (need for dialysis), SGF: scarce graft function (CCR7 ≤ 70% no dialysis). Taken from Johnston et al., 2007.

3.2 Urine-based definition

UO7

Urine output at post-KT day 7 (UO7) was recently proposed (Lai et al., 2010).
Equation: UO7 = total urine output on day 7 post-transplantation (mL)/weight (kg)/24 hours.
UO7 presented an elevated power for the prediction of 1-year graft function: at ROC analysis, UO7 presented an elevated area under the curve (0.811) (**Figure 10**). A cut-off value of 500 mL/24 h showed high sensitivity (98.5%).

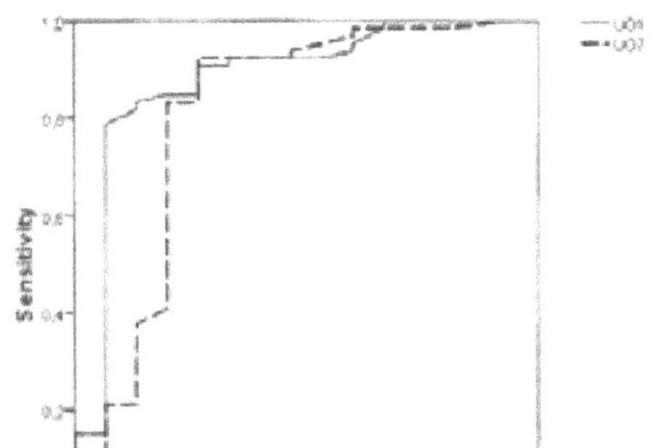

Fig. 10. ROC curves for post-KT day 1 urine output (UO1) and day 7 urine output (UO7) according to 1-year graft function (eGFR ≥ 30 mL/min/1.73 m2). Taken from Lai Q et al, 2009.

3.3 Combined definition

a. Cr7 and UO1

A score based on the combination of serum creatinine at post-KT day 7 (Cr7) and urine output at post-KT day 1(UO1) was proposed (Schnuelle et al., 2007).

Equation: UO1 = total 1st postoperative day urine output (mL)/weight (kg)/24 hours.

Kaplan-Maier survival estimates indicated a threshold effect of UO1 and Cr7, which could dissect the risk of graft failure. The thresholds referring to the 2nd quintile corresponded to a UO1 > 630 ml and a Cr7 <2.5 mg/dl. Combination of both of the parameters predicted a 5-year graft survival probability >90%, according to a hazard ratio of 0.21 (95% CI 0.09–0.46) (**Figure 11**).

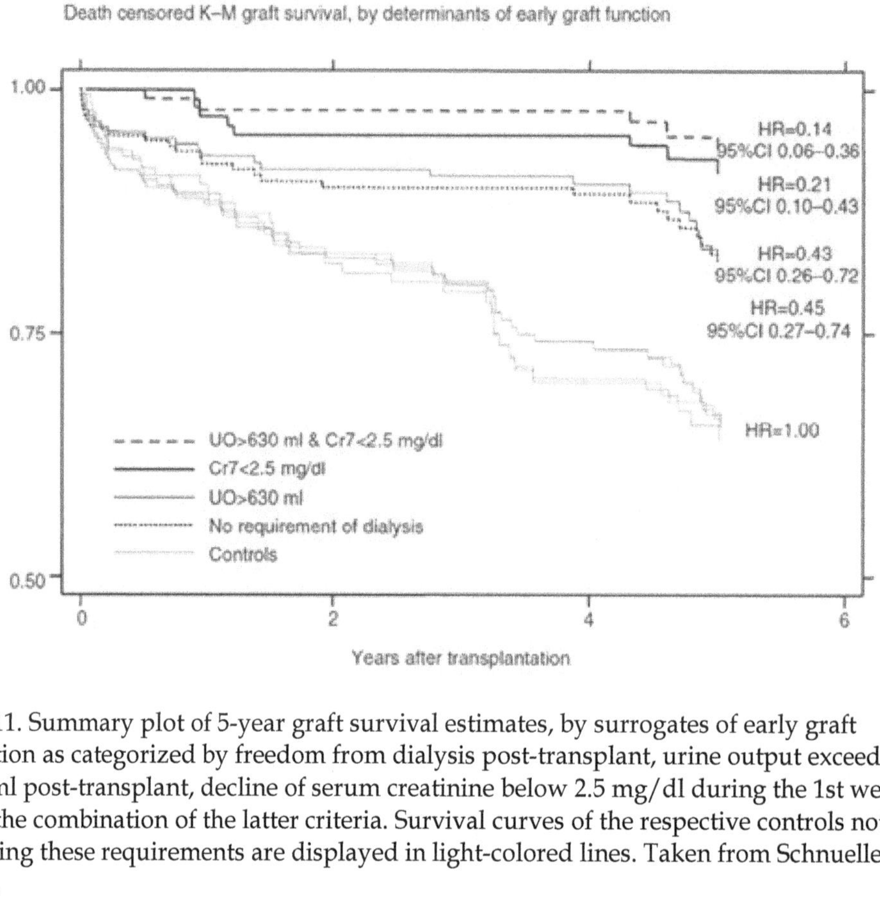

Fig. 11. Summary plot of 5-year graft survival estimates, by surrogates of early graft function as categorized by freedom from dialysis post-transplant, urine output exceeding 630 ml post-transplant, decline of serum creatinine below 2.5 mg/dl during the 1st week, and the combination of the latter criteria. Survival curves of the respective controls not meeting these requirements are displayed in light-colored lines. Taken from Schnuelle et al., 2007.

b. A definition of DGF obtainable within 6 hours after KT was proposed (Gonwa et al., 2002). It was based on a rising serum creatinine level above that before surgery or a urine output of < 300 mL within 6 h of transplantation, despite diuretics and adequate volume. Adoption of a very early definition of no-graft function was adopted with the intent to choose the correct immunosuppressive therapeutic approach to the patients.
c. A new model for the definition of DGF was created (Halloran & Hunsicker, 2001) by the combination of urine output of < 1 L in the first 24 h or a decrease in serum creatinine of < 20-30%.
d. DGF was recently defined (Lai et al., 2009) as the presence of one of the following conditions: at least 1-day persistent oligoanuria (≤ 500 mL/24 h) during the first week or an increased, unchanged, or decreased by ≤ 30% 7-day serum creatinine as compared with the pre-KT value.

4. Comparison among the scoring systems

Many researches have been performed on the identification of pre- or early post-operative clinical predictors of graft function; however, the great majority of them were based on isolated studies, usually in the populations from which they were initially derived. Moreover, only a small number of papers have focalized on their attention on the comparison among the different scoring systems.

For example, a previously reported study (Schold et al., 2005) compared preoperative scores (ECD, DDS and DRS), showing DRS was the best model for the prediction of graft survival at multivariable analysis. In the same period, another study (Nyberg et al., 2005) showed the superiority of DDS respect to ECD.

The first comparative analysis of preoperative and early post-operative scores (Moore et al., 2007) tested the ability of these clinical variables to predict suboptimal early function variably assessed by: DGF (dialysis requirement during the first week), DGF duration, slow graft function (creatinine > 3 mg/dl on day 5) and creatinine reduction ratio on day 2.

Multiple regression analysis was performed on 217 consecutive renal transplant recipients: DGF nomogram, DDS and ECD were compared. All scoring systems showed associations with early graft function, although only DGF nomogram remained statistically significant in the multiple regression model. However, the overall utility of the DGF nomogram in DGF prediction was moderate.

Two years later, a new comparative study (Moore et al., 2009) focalized on its attention on the role of pre- and post-KT models for the prediction of graft dysfunction: primary outcome measures were creatinine at 12 months and the development of chronic kidney disease stage 4T. The preoperative donor quality scores tested were: ECD, DDS, DRS and DGF nomogram: the postoperative early function measures were: dialysis requirement and duration; extended DGF according to Boom definition (Boom et al., 2000); Cr5, Cr7, CRR2, CRR7 and UO1.

Among the donor scoring systems, DRS was best associated with subsequent 6-month and 1-year allograft function. The study suggested a sort of "hierarchy": DRS > ECD > DDS > DGF nonogram.

These results could be explained by the different ways the scores were initially developed. For example, DGF nomogram was developed with regard to dialysis requiring DGF specifically, DDS was focalized on 6-month creatinine clearance, while DRS and ECD had graft failure as the end measure. The "granulated" complexity of DRS and DDS scores may explain their superiority above ECD.

Among the early function measures, extended definition of DGF, Cr5 and dialysis duration showed greatest predictive power in the patient population overall and in the subgroups of patients who not required or required dialysis, respectively. DGF resulted superior to the standard DGF definition: however, its importance lied in the simultaneous comparison of donor scores and early postoperative renal function to assess the best "baseline" indicator for later allograft dysfunction (**Figure 12**).

In another recent paper (Moore et al., 2010) dDGF (dialysis-based definition) and extDGF (extended; Boom et al., 2000) were compared (**Figure 13**). In the multivariable model, extDGF but not dDGF was significantly associated with graft failure (HR 1.47; p-value = 0.02). Similar results were observed for overall graft failure. The utility of extDGF as an early marker of late poor allograft outcomes suggested superiority over the traditional and often subjective dialysis-based definition.

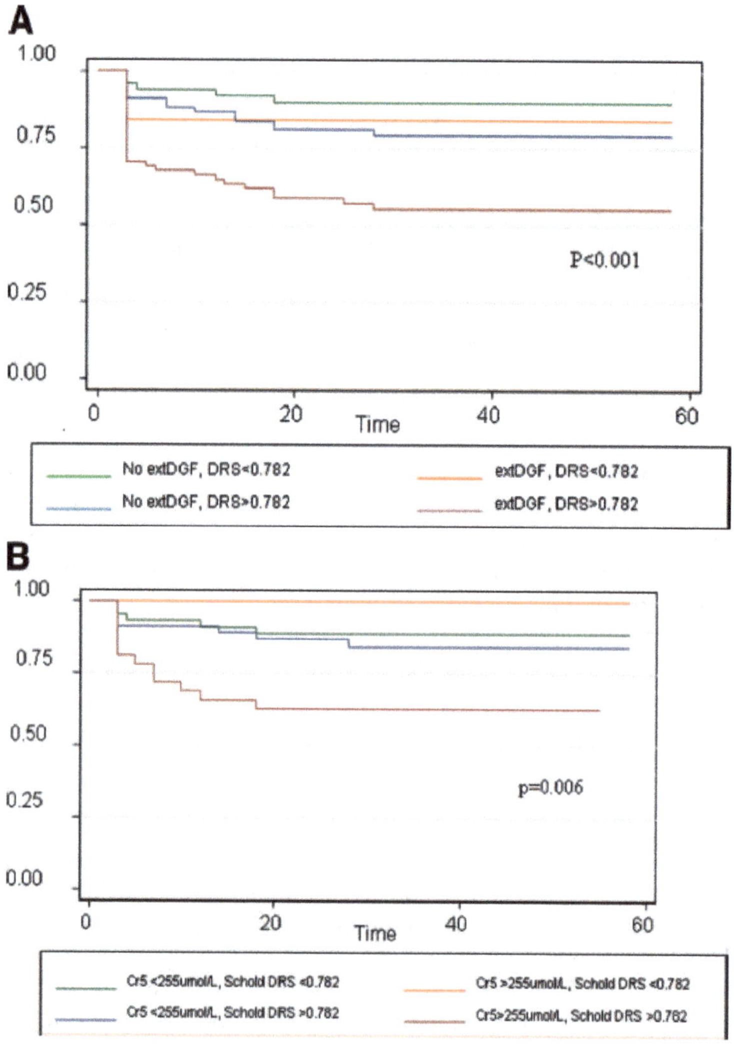

Fig. 12. (**A**) Kaplan-Meier survival curves for a combined variable of Donor Risk Score (DRS) and the extended definition of delayed graft function (extDGF) for time to stage 4T chronic kidney disease in all patients. (**B**) Kaplan-Meier survival curves for a combined variable of Donor Risk Score (DRS) and serum creatinine at day 5 (Cr5) for time to stage 4T chronic kidney disease in patients not requiring dialysis immediately postoperatively. Taken from Moore et al., 2009.

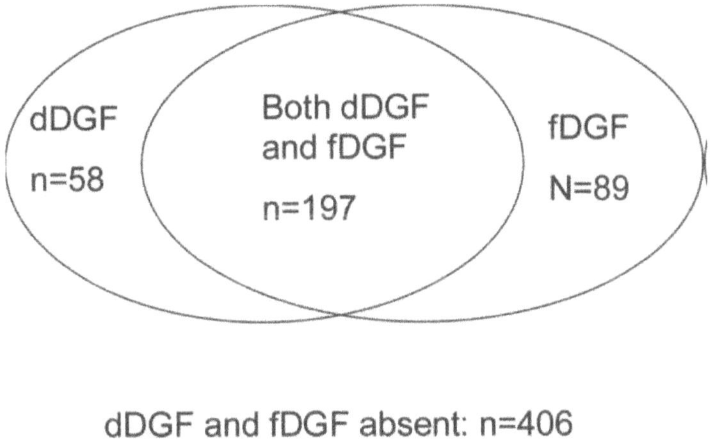

Fig. 13. Diagram shows distribution of early graft function. dDGF, dialysis-based definition of delayed graft function; fDGF (or extDGF), functional definition of delayed graft function. Taken from Moore et al., 2010.

Among creatinine-based models, Cr5 represented the "best" marker of early graft function in patients who didn't undergo a post-KT dialysis (Moore et al., 2009).

Indeed, the influence of pre- or post-KT dialysis on creatinine measurements independent of allograft excretory function was too great a confounder to allow meaningful interpretation of these parameters also in dialyzed patients.

Exclusive (Lai et al., 2010) or combined (Schnuelle et al., 2007) use of UO could be of some benefit in a better evaluation of these patients: however, more consistent large studies on this field are still required.

No comparative studies among clinical and histological scores have been reported. Studies are needed for a better understanding of the effective role of histological features and its comparison with pre- and immediately post-KT variables.

5. Conclusion

Donor scores, histological scores and early postoperative measures of renal allograft function may be of clinical utility in assessing the risk for subsequent renal dysfunction. This has relevance to organ allocation policy and also to the clinical management of individuals in the early postoperative period.

However, no one of the proposed criteria has still been internationally adopted.

Probably, a combined score based on pre- and post-operative clinical features and histological aspects may offer improved prognostication for graft outcome.

However, the first objective of a score must be its feasibility: its excessive "granulation" could transform it in a hardly adopted instrument in the care practice.

New studies focalized on the validation of previously proposed scores or for the development of new prognostication models are still required.

6. Acknowledgment

We thank the "Inter-University Consortium for Organ Transplantation".

We thank the "Kidney Transplant Group" of Sapienza University of Rome.

7. References

Anglicheau, D.; Loupy, A.; Lefaucheur, C.; Pessione, F.; Létourneau, I. & al. (2008). A simple clinico-histopathological composite scoring system is highly predictive of graft outcomes in marginal donors. *American Journal of Transplantation*, Vol.8, No.11, (November 2008), pp. 2325-2334.

Boom, H.; Mallat, MJ.; de Fijter, JW.; Zwinderman, AH. & Paul, LC. (2000). Delayed graft function influences renal function, but not survival. *Kidney International*, Vol.58, No.2, (August 2000), pp. 859-866.

Daly, PJ.; Power, RE.; Healy, DA.; Hickey, DP.; Fitzpatrick JM. & al. (2005). Delayed graft function: a dilemma in renal transplantation. *British Journal of Urology International*, Vol.96, No.4, (September 2005), pp. 498-501.

Giral-Classe, M.; Hourmant, M.; Cantarovich, D.; Dantal, J.; Blancho, G. & al. (1998). Delayed graft function of more than six days strongly decreases long-term survival of transplanted kidneys. *Kidney International*, Vol.54, No.3, (September 1998), pp. 972-978.

Gonwa, TA.; Mai, ML.; Smith, LB.; Levy, MF.; Goldstein, RM. & al. (2002). Immunosuppression for delayed or slow graft function in primary cadaveric renal transplantation. Use of low dose tacrolimus therapy with post-operative administration of anti-CD25 monoclonal antibody. *Clinical Transplantation*, Vol.16, No.2, (April 2002), pp. 144-149.

Govani, MV.; Kwon, O.; Batiuk, TD.; Milgrom, ML. & Filo RS. (2002). Creatinine reduction ratio and 24-hour creatinine excretion on posttransplant day two. Simple and objective tools to define graft function. *Journal of the American Society of Nephrology*, Vol.13, No.2, (June 2002), pp. 1645-1649.

Halloran, PF. & Hunsicker, LG. (2001) Delayed graft function. State of the art. Summit meeting, Scottsdale, Arizona, USA, November 10-11, 2000. *American Journal of Transplantation*, Vol.1, No.2, (July 2001), pp. 115-120.

Humar, A.; Payne, WD.; Sutherland, DE. & Matas, AJ. (2000). Clinical determinants of multiple acute rejection episodes in kidney transplant recipients. *Transplantation*, Vol.69, No.11, (June 2000), pp. 2357-2360.

Irish, WD.; McCollum, DA.; Tesi, RJ.; Owen, AB.; Brennan, DC. & al. (2003). Nomogram for predicting the likelihood of delayed graft function in adult cadaveric renal transplant recipients. *Journal of the American Society of Nephrology*, Vol.14, No.11, (November 2003), pp. 2967-2974.

Irish, WD.; Ilsley, JN.; Schnitzler, MA.; Feng, S. & Brennan, DC. (2010). A risk prediction model for delayed graft function in the current era of deceased donor renal transplantation. *American Journal of Transplantation*, Vol.10, No.10, (October 2010), pp. 2279-2286.

Johnston, O.; O'Kelly, P.; Spencer, S.; Donohoe, J.; Walshe, JJ. & al. (2006). Reduced graft function (with or without dialysis) vs immediate graft function – A comparison of longterm renal allograft survival. *Nephrology Dialysis Transplantation*, Vol.21, No.8, (August 2006), pp. 2270-2274.

Karpinski, J.; Lajoie, G.; Cattran, D.; Fenton, S.; Zaltzman, J. et al. (1999). Outcome of kidney transplantation from high-risk donors is determined by both structure and function. *Transplantation*, Vol.67, No.8, (April 1999), pp. 1162-1167.

Lai, Q.; Pretagostini, R.; Poli, L.; Melandro, F.; Ferretti, S. et al. (2009). Delayed graft function decreases early and intermediate graft outcomes after expanded criteria donor kidney transplants. *Transplantation Proceedings*, Vol.41, No.4, (May 2009), pp. 1145-1148.

Lai, Q.; Pretagostini, R.; Poli, L.; Levi Sandri, GB.; Melandro, F. et al. (2010). Early urine output predicts graft survival after kidney transplantation. *Transplantation Proceedings*, Vol.42, No.4, (May 2010), pp. 1090-1092.

Metzger, RA.; Delmonico, FL.; Feng, S.; Port, FK.; Wynn, JJ. & al. (2003). Expanded criteria donors for kidney transplantation. *American Journal of Transplantation*, Vol.3, Suppl.4, (2003), pp. 114-125.

Moore, J.; Tan, K.; Cockwell, P.; Krishnan, H.; McPake, D. & al. (2007). Predicting early renal allograft function using clinical variables. *Nephrology Dialysis Transplantation*, Vol.22, No.9, (September 2007), pp. 669-677.

Moore, J.; Ramakrishna, S.; Tan, K.; Cockwell, P.; Eardley, K. & al. (2009). Identification of the optimal donor quality scoring system and measure of early renal function in kidney transplantation. *Transplantation*, Vol.87, No.4, (February 2009), pp. 578-586.

Moore, J.; Shabir, S.; Chand, S.; Bentall, A.; McClean, A. & al. (2010). Assessing and comparing rival definitions of Delayed Renal Allograft Function for predicting subsequent graft failure. *Transplantation*, Vol.90, No.10, (September 2010), pp. 1113-1116.

Nyberg, SL.; Matas, AJ.; Rogers, M.; Harmsen, WS.; Velosa, JA. & al. (2001). Donor scoring system for cadaveric renal transplantation. *American Journal of Transplantation*, Vol.1, No.2, (July 2001), pp. 162-170.

Nyberg, SL.; Matas, AJ.; Kremers, WK.; Thostenson, JD.; Larson, TS. & al. (2003). Improved scoring system to assess adult donors for cadaver renal transplantation. *American Journal of Transplantation*, Vol.3, No.6, (June 2003), pp. 715-721.

Nyberg, SL.; Baskin-Bey, ES.; Kremers, W.; Prieto, M.; Henry, ML. & al. (2005). Improving the prediction of donor kidney quality: deceased donor score and resistive indices. *Transplantation*, Vol.80, No.7, (October 2005), pp. 925-929.

Pessione, F.; Cohen, S.; Durand, D.; Hourmant, M.; Kessler, M. & al. (2003). Multivariate analysis of donor risk factors for graft survival in kidney transplantation. *Transplantation*, Vol.75, No.3, (February 2003), pp. 361-367.

Pirani, CL. & Salinas-Madrigal L. (1975). Evaluation of percutaneous renal biopsy.; In: *Kidney pathology decentenial.; 1966-1975;* SC. Sommers; Norwalk CT (Ed.) ; Appleton-Century-Crofts: 1975.

Pretagostini, R.; Lai, Q.; Poli, L.; Levi Sandri, GB.; Travaglia, D. & al. (2009). Predictive characteristics of delayed graft function after expanded and standard criteria donor kidney transplantations. *Transplantation Proceedings*, Vol.41, No.4, (May 2009), pp. 1149-1151.

Rao, PS.; Schaubel, DE.; Guidinger, MK.; Andreoni, KA.; Wolfe, RA. & al. (2009). A comprehensive risk quantification score for deceased donor kidneys: the kidney donor risk index. *Transplantation*, Vol.88, No.2, (July 2009), pp. 231-236.

Remuzzi, G.; Grinyò, J.; Ruggenenti, P.; Beatini, M.; Cole, EH. & al. (1999). Early experience with dual kidney transplantation in adults using expanded donor criteria. Double Kidney Transplant Group (DKG). Journal of the *American Society of Nephrology*, Vol.10, No.12, (December 1999), pp. 2591-2598.

Remuzzi, G.; Cravedi, P.; Perna, A.; Dimitrov, BD.; Turturro, M. & al. (2006). Long-term outcome of renal transplantation from older donors. *New England Journal of Medicine*, Vol.354, No.4, (January 2006), pp. 343-352.

Rodrigo, E.; Ruiz, JC.; Piñera, C.; Fernández-Fresnedo, G.; Escallada, R. & al. (2004). Creatinine reduction ratio on post-transplant day two as criterion in defining delayed graft function. *American Journal of Transplantation*, Vol.4, No.7, (July 2004), pp. 1163-1169.

Rosengard, BR.; Feng, S.; Alfrey, EJ.; Zaroff, JG.; Emond, JC. & al. (2002). Report of the Crystal City meeting to maximize the use of organs recovered from the cadaver donor. *American Journal of Transplantation*, Vol.2, No.8, (September 2002), pp. 701-711.

Salahudeen, AK.; Haider, N. & May, W. (2004). Cold ischemia and the reduced long-term survival of cadaveric renal allografts. *Kidney International*, Vol.65, No.2, (February 2004), pp. 713-718.

Schnuelle, P.; Gottmann, U.; Köppel, H.; Brinkkoetter, PT.; Krzossok, S. & al. (2007). Comparison of early renal function parameters for the prediction of 5-year graft survival after kidney transplantation. *Nephrology Dialysis Transplantation*, Vol.22, No.1, (January 2007), pp. 235-245.

Schold, JD.; Kaplan, B.; Baliga, RS. & Meier-Kriesche, HU. (2005). The broad spectrum of quality in deceased donor kidneys. *American Journal of Transplantation*, Vol.5, No.4 Part.1, (April 2005), pp. 757-765.

Stratta, RJ.; Rohr, MS.; Sundberg, AK.; Armstrong, G.; Hairston, G. & al. (2005). Increased kidney transplantation utilizing expanded criteria deceased organ donors with results comparable to standard criteria donor transplant. *Annals of Surgery*, Vol.239, No.5, (May 2004), pp. 688-695.

Yarlagadda, SG.; Coca, SG.; Garg, AX.; Doshi, M.; Poggio, E. & al. (2008). Marked variation in the definition and diagnosis of delayed graft function: a systematic review. *Nephrology Dialysis Transplantation*, Vol.23, No.9, (September 2008), pp. 2995-3003.

2

ABO-Incompatible Kidney Transplantation

Mina Hur, Hee-Won Moon and Seog-Woon Kwon *Konkuk University and University of Ulsan Korea*

1. Introduction

ABO antigens are composed of sugar chains and exist not only on red cells but also on many other cells including endothelial cells and epithelial cells of various organs such as kidney, heart, bowel, lung, and pancreas (Marionneau et al., 2001). ABO antibodies, which have been called as isoagglutinins, are preformed antibodies directed against missing A or B antigens. The source of anti-A/B antibodies is thought to be gastrointestinal and environmental bacteria, such as the enterobacteriaceae, which possess ABO-like structures on their lipopolysaccharide coats (Yamamoto, 2004). These preformed ABO antibodies are clinically important in transfusion and organ transplantation medicine because they can cause acute hemolytic transfusion reaction in ABO-incompatible (ABO-I) blood transfusion and hyperacute rejection in ABO-I organ transplantation.

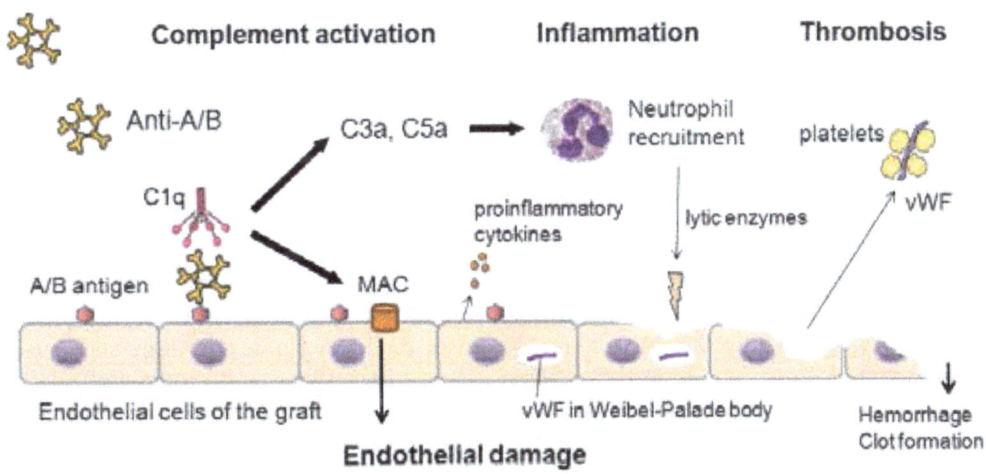

Fig. 1. Proposed mechanism of hyperacute rejection in ABO-incompatible organ transplantion.

Hyperacute rejection is induced by the binding of anti-A/B to antigens expressed on the endothelial cells of the ABO-I graft and activation of complement system (Fig. 1). Subsequently, endothelial damage, inflammation and platelet aggregation can be provoked, leading to vascular thrombosis, occlusion of blood supply and rejection.

ABO-I kidney transplantations were first reported in late 1950s and early 1960s (Hume et al., 1955; Murray et al., 1960; Starzl et al., 1964; Kissmeyer-Nielsen et al., 1966). These early experiences showed that hyperacute rejection could occur, and therefore, crossing the ABO barrier was excluded in the field of kidney transplantation.

In 1981, Slapak et al. first introduced the concept of depleting anti-A/B antibodies when they used modified plasmapheresis and successfully overcame the major donor-recipient blood group incompatibility in kidney transplant patient. Later, the same group reported on pre-transplantation immunoadsorption and plasmapheresis for ABO-I kidney transplantation, showing a high survival rate of 87% (Slapak et al., 1990).

Another group also started a living donor ABO-I kidney transplantation program in 1982, after this group inadvertently experienced an ABO-I cadaver kidney transplantation due to an error in donor ABO typing. In spite of the A_1 to O major ABO-incompatibility, the kidney graft from ABO-I cadaver functioned well with a basic immunusuppressive regimen including a short course of polyclonal antibody with azathioprine, and has been reported to be still functioning 22 years later (Squifflet et al., 2004). In this group, plasmapheresis was chosen to remove antibodies before transplantation and to prevent the occurrence of antibody-mediated hyperacute rejection. In addition, the immunosuppressive regimen was started 3 days prior to transplantation, and splenectomy was performed on the day of transplantation (Alexandre et al., 1985a, 1985b, 1986). Although the transplantation was successful, the return and persistence of anti-donor blood-group antibody was observed in spite of chronic immunosuppression. However, even with the continued presence of these antibodies and the persistence of the target antigen in the kidney, most of the graft continued to function well (Alexandre et al., 1991; Cardella et al., 1987; Reding et al., 1987). It was suggested that ABO blood group incompatibility need not be an absolute barrier to successful kidney transplantation.

2. Accommodation

It has been observed that ABO-I kidney grafts functioned well without rejection in recipients having high titers of anit-A/B antibodies. This phenomenon has been termed accommodation and regarded as an acquired resistance of an organ to immune-mediated damage (Bach et al., 1997; Lynch & Platt, 2008, 2010; Platt et al., 1990). In accommodation state, the graft is not pathologically injured despite the presence of circulating anti-donor antibodies.

The mechanism of accommodation is yet to be elucidated. It was postulated that accommodation might be involved in change in antibodies, change in antigen, modified control of complement, or acquired resistance to injury (Lynch & Platt, 2008). Complement regulation was thought to be essential for the survival of transplants over time and thus for accommodation to be manifested. C4d deposition without signs or symptoms of rejection can be observed in accommodated kidney (Lynch & Platt, 2010). The occurrence of complement activation means that antibody binding is intact in accommodated kidneys, and the lack of lysis means that some regulatory pathways are working for graft survival in the accommodation.

Three possible outcomes of the binding of complement-fixing alloantibody to endothelial cells have been postulated (Colvin & Smith, 2005). Hyperacute or acute rejection can be resulted, if the complement is fully activated. Accommodation can be achieved, if complement activation is completely inhibited. Incomplete inhibition of complement might be sufficient to prevent cell lysis but not to prevent complement activation, leading to endothelial cell activation and chronic antibody-mediated rejection (AMR).

Studies in mice showed that, in the absence of T-cell help, B cells that are exposed to incompatible carbohydrate antigens on allografts differentiate into cells that can produce non-complement-fixing antibody, and these B cells gradually become tolerant after prolonged exposure (Ogawa et al., 2004).

An acquired resistance to injury could reflect accommodation more comprehensively, but does not exclude other mechanisms. Actually, such resistance or protection could be appreciated, if some antibodies bind to graft and some complements are activated. Park et al. (2003) used microarrays, and compared five 1-year protocol ABO-compatible renal graft biopsies to four accommodated ABO-I graft biopsies. They identified significant alterations in gene expression in 440 probe sets, including SMADs, protein tyrosine kinases, TNF-alpha and Mucin 1. They concluded that accommodation is always present in well-functioning, long-surviving ABO-I kidney transplants. Regarding this self-protection against antibody-mediated damage, several novel mechanisms were suggested including the disruption of normal signal transduction, attenuation of cellular adhesion, and the prevention of apoptosis.

Accommodation is regarded as a good response to transplantation. It prevents acute antibody-mediated injury, thus allowing chronic process to ensue over time. Accommodation can be induced when antibodies that would cause rejection of a graft are removed from a recipient and then later return. In addition to this induced type, accommodation can occur spontaneously, without depleting antibodies. In this regard, the prevalence of accommodation would be higher than expected, and spontaneous accommodation may be the most common outcome of clinical organ transplantation (Tang & Platt, 2007). Accommodation still remains an evolving concept, and has a mixed support from experimental and clinical findings. The most important unanswered questions are how often and by which mechanisms accommodation occurs (Lynch & Platt, 2010). Accumulation of clinical evidences and research data would bring progress in understanding the biological implications of accommodation.

3. Current practice

The earlier works in the early 1980s were expanded greatly in Japan, where ABO-I kidney transplantation has been performed in more than 1,000 patients since 1989, and recently accounts for about 18% of all living donor kidney transplants (Takahashi, 2007). Later, a number of centers in USA and Europe have begun ABO-I kidney transplantations using similar protocols (Crew & Ratner, 2010).

The clinical outcome of ABO-I kidney transplantation improved remarkably in the last 10-15 years since the routine use of tacrolimus and mycophenolate. Clinical literatures repeatedly showed that ABO-I kidney transplantation has outcomes comparable to ABO-compatible kidney transplantation (Haidinger et al., 2009; Jeon et al., 2010; Kenmochi et al., 2008; Oettl et al., 2009; Thielke et al., 2007). One-year and five-year survival rates of ABO-I kidney transplants showed little difference from those of ABO-compatible kidney transplants, and their renal functions based on creatinine levels also showed no difference. Recently, the Japanese data on 851 ABO-I kidney transplantations was summarized (Tanabe, 2007a). According to this report, 1-, 3-, 5-, and 10-year patient survivals have been 95%, 92%, 90%, and 85%, respectively, whereas 1-, 3-, 5-, and 10-year graft survivals have been 89%, 85%,

79%, and 61%, respectively. These improved outcomes are attributed to a clearer understanding of the mechanisms underlying accommodation and acute AMR, permitting the development of new therapeutic strategies. There were significant differences in graft survival and the incidence of rejection before and after the introduction of tacrolimus/mycophenolate mofetil.

3.1 Induction therapies

Initial protocols for ABO-I kidney transplantation included splenectomy, which was performed in most recipients until 2004. Recently, a monoclonal antibody directed against CD20 on B cells, rituximab, has replaced splenectomy in most centers (Fig. 2). The use of rituximab eliminated the need for additional surgical intervention, and the outcomes with rituximab infusion alone were equal to those with splenectomy, providing more evidence that splenectomy is unnecessary (Crew & Ratner, 2010; Tanabe et al., 2009).

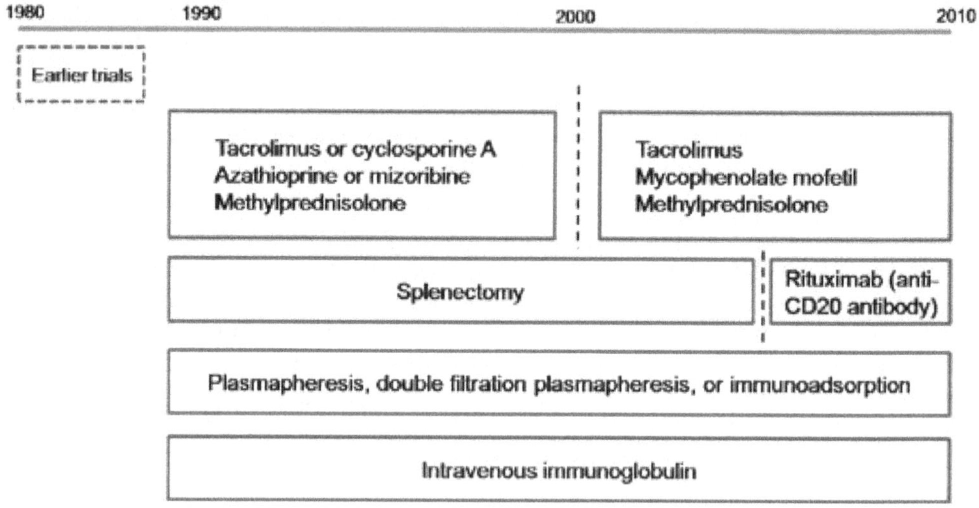

Fig. 2. Changes of preconditioning protocols for ABO-incompatible kidney transplantation. Between 1989 and 1999, a triplicate immunosuppressive regimen consisted of tacrolimus or cyclosporine A plus azathioprine or mizoribine plus methylprednisolone. Since 2000, tacrolimus, mycophenolate mofetil, and methylprednisolone have been used. Splenectomy was performed until 2004, and recently anti-CD20 antibody (rituximab) became an alternative to splenectomy. In most cases, 3-7 sessions of plasmapheresis or immunoadsorption have been performed before transplantation.

Rituximab as an alternative to splenectomy markedly reduced the incidence of AMR and greatly improved the results, becoming a clinically proven effective regimen for a successful ABO-I kidney transplantation. Interestingly, one recent study reported excellent outcomes without splenectomy or rituximab, questioning whether rituximab is indeed necessary (Segev et al., 2005). The authors suggested that rapid allograft accommodation may limit the need for long-term antibody suppression provided by splenectomy or anti-CD20, thereby eliminating the added infectious risk of these modalities and removing another disincentive to ABO-I transplantation.

Before 2000, a triplicate immunosuppressive regimen consisting of tacrolimus or cyclosporine A plus azathioprine or mizoribine plus methylprednisolone was mainly used. Thereafter, tacrolimus, mycophenolate mofetil, and methylprednisolone were used at most institutions. A greater incidence of acute rejection that was observed during the cyclosporine A era was markedly reduced in the tacrolimus era. In particular, the routine use of tacrolimus and mycophenolate mofetil significantly reduced acute rejection rates in patients with high-pretransplant isoagglutinin titers, and improved their outcomes to the levels comparable to those with low titers (Ishida et al., 2007).

3.2 Antibody reduction therapies

In all protocols, plasmapheresis to reduce and control anti-A or –B titers is a central feature. In most cases, ABO-I kidney transplantation recipients underwent 3-7 sessions of plasmapheresis (therapeutic plasma exchange) or double-filtration plasmapheresis before transplantation to reduce isoagglutinin titers. Plasmapheresis effectively removes anti-ABO antibodies, and approximately 20% of reduction is expected in each treatment. Its side effects, which are observed in approximately 5% of patients, are mainly hypocalcemia and pruritus/urticaria, and are usually mild and well tolerated (Tobian et al., 2008, 2009).

Plasmapheresis removes not only ABO antibodies but also the other protective antibodies or clotting factors, potentially increasing the risk of perioperative infection or bleeding. In contrast to plasmapheresis, immunoadsorption method can selectively remove anti-ABO antibodies, unaffecting the levels of the other plasma proteins. The blood type-specific columns can effectively remove anti-A or anti-B antibodies, and approximately 30% of anti-A/B IgM and 20% of anti-A/B IgG levels can be removed after a single treatment (Valli et al., 2009). In spite of its physiologic technique and successful clinical applications, the high cost of immunoadsorption column is a major limiting factor blocking its widespread use. The absence of randomized trials, which compared plasmapheresis and immunoadsorption, makes precise comparison of cost and outcomes impossible at the current point.

Plasmapheresis is a form of therapy to separate plasma from a person's circulating blood, removing pathogenic substances in plasma, and returning the remainder to the patient, usually with replacement fluids. The removal of a pathologic substance is affected by its concentration in circulating blood, the processing volume of blood and the degree of intravascular distribution. For example, IgM or fibrinogen are efficiently removed due to their predominantly intravascular distribution compared to IgG, which is predominantly extravascular. The alteration of immunoglobulin after single-plasma volume exchange was reported as about 63% decrease from baseline (Orlin & Berkman, 1980). An example of the changes of anti-A and anti-B antibody titers and creatinine levels before and after ABO-I kidney transplantation is shown in Fig. 3 (Moon et al., 2009). Efficiency of antibody removal is variable according to the patients. It is important that recipients or potential recipients of ABO-I kidneys should receive plasma that contains no ABO antibody against the graft for transfusion or plasmapheresis.

Plasmapheresis is indicated in various diseases such as thrombotic thrombocytopenic purpura, myasthenia gravis, or hyperviscosity in monoclonal gammopathy. Regarding indication for plasmapheresis, The American Society for Apheresis (ASFA) has published the guidelines and recommendations (Szczepiorkowski et al., 2010). According to this ASFA guideline, ABO-I kidney transplantation is classified as category II, in which plasmapheresis is generally accepted but considered to be supportive or adjunctive to other, more definite treatments, rather than a primary first-line therapy.

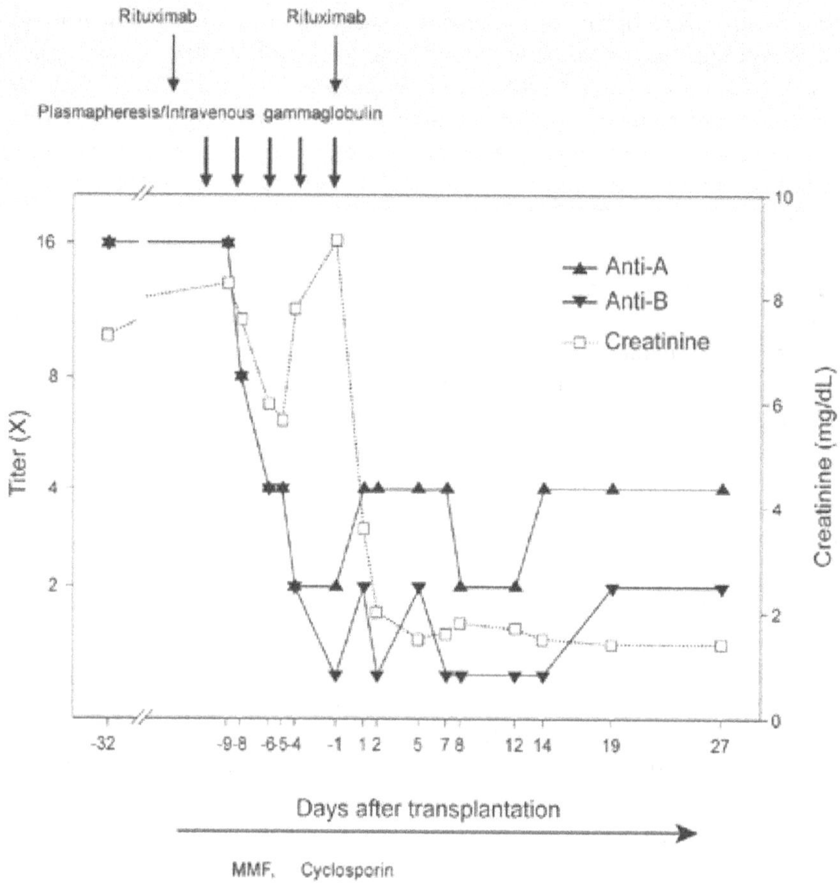

Fig. 3. An example of the changes of anti-A/anti-B antibody titers and creatinine levels before and after ABO-incompatible kidney transplantation. The patient's blood type was O, Rh+ and the donor's blood type was B, Rh+. A combination therapy with plasmapheresis, intravenous gammaglobulin, rituximab and potent immunosuppression was performed. Although the patient's baseline anti-A and anti-B titers were relatively low (1:16 for both anti-A and anti-B), titers were successfully decreased after each plasmapheresis procedure (average 1 fold), finally decreased to 1:1. The kidney transplantation was successful without any sign of hyperacute or acute rejection (modified from the refernece by Moon, et al (2009) with permission of Korean Journal of Laboratory Medicine).

Generally, plasmapheresis is performed using automated instruments. These instruments have specialized devices for blood withdrawal, anticoagulation, separation, return of blood, replacement and discard or collection of separated substances. The separation process is performed by centrifugation or filtration. In centrifugation method, blood components are separated by specific gravity and divided as plasma, platelets, leukocytes and red blood cells. In filtration method, blood is passed through a filter, and blood components are separated by their differences in particle size. Filtration and centrifugation can be combined by using rotating filter.

In conventional plasmapheresis, smaller proteins such as albumin are also removed in addition to pathogenic molecules, antibody or high molecular weight proteins. In general, plasma separated with a plasma separator is discarded and replaced with the same volume of replacement fluid such as fresh frozen plasma or albumin solution. There are several options of plasmapheresis, which separate blood components more selectively.

Double filtration plasmapheresis (DFPP) uses two filters which have different pore sizes. In the first filter, blood is separated as plasma and cell components, and plasma is further separated by the second filter. Large molecular-weight proteins including immunoglobulins such as anti-donor isoagglutinins are removed, while smaller molecular-weight substances such as albumin are returned to the patient's circulation. In this procedure, need of replacement is decreased compared with conventional plasmapheresis, thus adverse effects related to the replacement fluid can be reduced (Fig. 4) (Genberg et al., 2010; Tanabe, 2007b).

In the immunoadsorption, specialized adsorption column selectively adsorbs a specific substance such as immunoglobulin or low-density lipoprotein. This process removes the element of interest specifically and the remaining elements are returned to the patients. Many kinds of immunoadsorption devices for the removal of various types of components are commercially available but generally expensive. For the removal of anti-A and -B antibody, AB antigen-specific carbohydrate columns (Glycosorb AB, Glycorex Transplantation AB, Lund, Sweden) were developed (Tyden et al., 2005) and have been widely used in more than 400 cases of ABO-I kidney transplantation (Genberg et al., 2010; Tyden et al., 2005; Winters et al., 2004). This procedure could decrease the complications associated with plasma exchange such as coagulopathy and transfusion reactions.

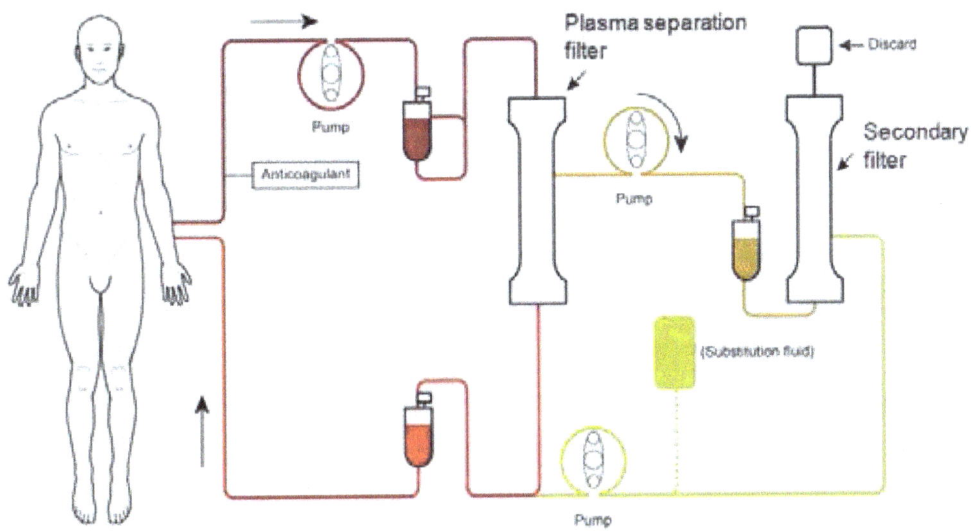

Fig. 4. Schematic presentation of double filtration plasmapheresis (DFPP). In DFPP, plasma separated with a plasma separator (1st filter) passes through the plasma component separator with a small pore size (2nd filter). Molecules that are larger than the pore size such as immunoglobulins are removed, and smaller molecules such as albumin are returned to the patient.

4. Determination of isoagglutinin titer

To reduce isoagglutinin titers prior to ABO-I kidney transplantation, preparative regimens including plasmapheresis, DFPP, or immunoadsorption and immunosuppressive therapy have been used. The clinical significance of isoagglutinin titer in ABO-I kidney transplantation is not entirely clear (Tobian et al., 2011). The goal of isoagglutinin titer to prevent hyperacute rejection is variable across transplantation centers, ranging from ≤ 1:8 to ≤ 1:32 before transplantation (Crew & Ratner, 2010). However, minimal research has been performed to determine the optimal pretransplant titer. The possibility of AMR would decrease as anti-donor antibody titer decreases. In our institution, the titer is lowered to ≤ 1:4 before transplantation. The measurement of isoagglutinin is known to be essential in the assessment of the efficacy of antibody removal, and the prediction of AMR (Kobayashi & Saito, 2006). Although most recipients with AMR had an elevated titer, the positive predictive value of a high titer for AMR was poor (Tobian et al., 2010). Thus, posttransplant titers should be monitored, but must be combined with the other factors assessing AMR.

Accurate measurement of isoagglutinin titer is an important aspect for successful ABO-I kidney transplantation. If the isoagglutinin titer is underestimated compared to the actual titer of patient, we could consider a patient as safe for transplantation and it could lead to rejection or short duration of allograft survival (Crew & Ratner, 2010). IgM antibody mediates complement activation and endothelial damage in AMR, and it is more rapidly removed by plasmapheresis than IgG. However, IgG titers are more emphasized for patient eligibility, rejection risk, and plasmapheresis guidance. Reporting both IgM and IgG titers has been recommended by a working group from US centers (Montgomery et al., 2004). Importantly, measured titers are method-dependent and considerably variable according to assays.

	Tube method	Column agglutination	Flow cytometry
A column ingredient	Not needed	Sephadex gel or glass bead	Not needed
Use of RBC	Yes	Yes	Yes
Antihuman globulin	Yes	Yes	No
Secondary antibody	No	No	Yes
Deletion of IgM	DTT or 2ME	DTT or 2ME	Not needed
Interpretation	Agglutination	Agglutination	Fluorescence detection
Result	Titer	Titer	MFIR or titer
Instrument	Not needed	Not needed	Needed
Cost	Low	Intermediate	Relatively high
Assay time	30 - 60 min	30 - 60 min	1- 2 hours

DTT, dithiothreitol; 2ME, 2-mercaptoethanol; MFIR, mean fluorescence intensity ratio.

Table 1. Various assays for measurement of isoagglutinin titer

There are several options for the measurement of isoagglutinin titers: conventional tube method, gel or bead column agglutination method, and flow cytometry (Krishnan et al., 2008; Stussi et al., 2005). These three methods are summarized in Table 1. In addition, enzyme-linked immunosorbent assay technique (Lindberg et al., 2011; Rieben et al., 1991), surface plasmon resonance (Kimura et al., 2005; Yurugi et al., 2007), and KODE technology (Frame et al., 2007) were developed, although these methods are not routinely available in most institutions.

4.1 Conventional tube method

The conventional tube method has been used in most institutions for the semiquantitative measurement of isoagglutinin titers. IgG and IgM can be measured together, and if dithiothreitol or antiglobulin reagents are used, they can be measured separately. In general, recipient serum is serially diluted and incubated with RBC aliquots of the appropriate blood type in a test tube for about 10 minutes at room temperature. After the mixture is centrifuged, macroscopic agglutinations of RBCs are checked for IgM detection. For IgG detection, additional testing with antihuman globulin is performed to check the agglutination. Titers are determined as the highest dilution that produces 1+ macroscopic agglutination. However, technical variables greatly affect the results, and care should be taken to achieve the most uniform practice (Roback, 2008). Considerable inter-examiner variability may occur, because the titer is determined mainly by visual observation of agglutinated RBCs in tubes. Inter-institutional difference can also occur possibly due to variations in procedures and lack of assay standardizations.

A recent study reported the results of isoagglutinin titers from 26 different labs using sera from six patients of different blood groups (Kobayashi & Saito, 2006). In this report, inter-institutional variation between maximum and minimum value reached as much as 32-fold in IgM and 256-fold in IgG. These variations seemed to be due to different techniques between laboratories, but considerable variation was still noted after standardization of techniques. Another report also showed a large variation of isoagglutinin titers (a median three-fold difference) among three centers performing ABO-I kidney transplants in Germany and Sweden (Kumlien et al., 2007). In this report, gel hemagglutination technique significantly decreased inter-center difference (a median one titer difference) compared with tube methods.

4.2 Gel or bead column agglutination

In gel or bead column agglutination method, a cassette (or card) containing gels or beads is used. Commercially available assays include DiaMed ID Micro Typing system (Bio-Rad, Hercules, CA, USA), BioVue System (Ortho Clinical Diagnosis, Raritan, NJ, USA), or Olympus ID-Micro Typing System (Olympus Co., Tokyo, Japan). In these assays, plasma from the patient is stepwise diluted 1:2 with normal saline or phosphate buffered saline and packed RBCs are used to make a suspension with cell stabilization solution. In each incubation well, recommended cell suspension is mixed with diluted plasma. After incubation and centrifugation, agglutination is observed in card or cassette. In column agglutination method, negative (unagglutinated) test cells pellet to the bottom of the column, and positive (agglutinated) cells are captured at the top of or within the body of column (Fig. 5). The gel or bead particles trap the RBC agglutinates as a filter during centrifugation. The agglutination is graded from 0 to 4 +, and inverted value of the highest plasma dilution that gives a 1+ agglutination reaction is interpreted as the titer (Kumlien et al., 2007).

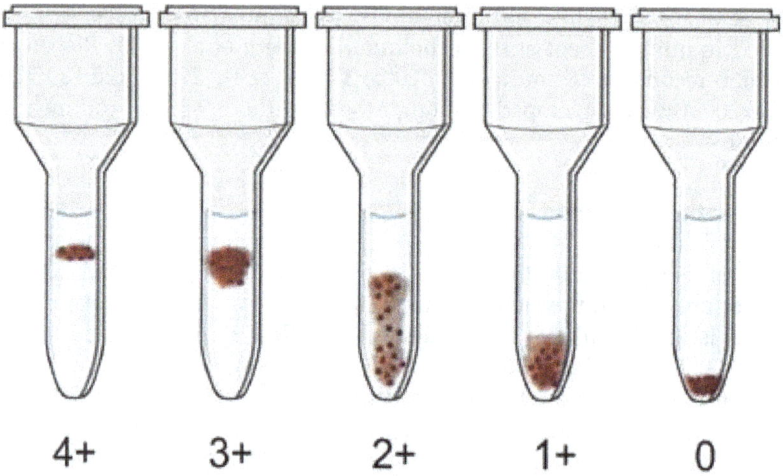

Fig. 5. Interpretation of column agglutination method. The agglutination is graded from 0 to 4+.

4.3 Flow cytometry

In flow cytometry method, quantifications of anti-A/B IgG and IgM are performed using fluorescence conjugated, anti-human IgG and IgM as secondary antibodies. A mixture of RBC suspension and recipient serum is transferred into the test tube and incubated (at 37°C in a CO_2 incubator for IgG antibody; and at room temperature, for IgM antibodies). After washing, fluorescence conjugated, anti-human IgG and IgM secondary antibodies are added in test tube. After incubation and washing steps, binding of anti-A/B antibody is measured by flow cytometry. Human AB serum, which is further depleted by incubation with highly concentrated A and B RBCs, can be used as a negative control, and human serum of blood group O is used as a positive control. Commercially available O RBCs with information of antigen expression are also helpful for the detection of irregular antibodies (Stussi et al., 2005).

Using undiluted serum, quantification of anti-A/B antibody can be determined by calculation of the geometric mean fluorescence intensity ratio (MFIR). This value is calculated by dividing the geometric mean fluorescence intensity of test sera with that of negative control. One study reported that the correlation coefficient between MFIR using flow cytometry and isoagglutinin titer was 0.870 for IgM and 0.783 for IgG (Stussi et al, 2005). For determination of titer using flow cytometry, recipient serum is serially diluted with normal saline solution (2% bovine serum albumin, 0.1% azide). After incubation and washing, secondary antibody is added. After reaction, binding of antibody is determined by flow cytometry. A gated value above assigned cut-off (5% for example) is regarded as positive serum dilution. In a study comparing the reproducibility of the results performed by various assays, flow cytometry showed excellent reproducibility and no measurement deviation was noted, whereas gel column agglutinin assay and tube technique showed two-fold and four-fold differences, respectively (Tanabe, 2007b). However, flow cytometry assay needs the flow cytometry instrument, and the reagents are relatively expensive.

5. Conclusion

The ABO blood group barrier is now being crossed in the field of transplantation, and ABO-I kidney transplantation is becoming more common worldwide. Removing the ABO barrier can expand the donor pool and increase the availability of organs for transplantation. Moreover, it can decrease the time on the organ waiting list, and eventually facilitate the timely transplantation before comorbid conditions develop in the patients. Currently observed long-term results of ABO-I kidney transplantation are similar to those of ABO-compatible kidney transplantation. With the application of adequate antibody reducing strategies, future results would be more promising. To promote accomodation and to prevent acute complement-mediated graft injury, methods for preventing and treating AMR are still needed. Researches for the insights into the mechanism of accomodation will provide us a scientific basis for the development of innovative approaches for the better outcome of ABO-I kidney transplantation.

As the number of ABO-I transplantation increases, there is a need of the optimal methods for ABO isoagglutinin titer for the effective monitoring of ABO-I transplanted patients. Compared with the conventional test tube method, gel card or flow cytometric measurement can provide more accurate and objective results. However, reproducibility, interpretation, and standardization of isoagglutinin titration methods are still unsatisfactory, and further researches should be performed to determine the optimal method for ABO antibody titer assessment. There are also several promising techniques under development, focused on the endothelium, enzymes, or blocking antibodies. Ongoing improvement of promising modalities could make more successful transplantation outcomes in this field.

6. Acknowledgment

The authors appreciate Professor Jin Q Kim, The President of Konkuk University, Korea, for his critical review and valuable comments on this work.

7. References

Alexandre, G.P.J.; De Bruyere, M.; Squifflet, J.P.; Moriau, M.; Latinne, D. & Pirson, Y. (1985). Human ABO-incompatible living donor renal homografts. *The Netherlands Journal of Medicine*, Vol. 28, No. 6, (August 1985), pp. 231-234, ISSN 0300-2977

Alexandre, G.P.J.; Squifflet, J.P.; De Bruyere, M.; Latinne, D.; Moriau, M.; Carlier, M.; Pirson, Y. & Lecomte, C. (1986). ABO-incompatible related and unrelated living donor renal allografts. *Transplantation Proceedings*, Vol. 18, No. 3, (May-June 1986), pp. 452-455, ISSN 0041-1345

Alexandre, G.P.J.; Squifflet, J.P.; De Bruyere, M.; Latinne, D.; Moriau, M. & Ikabu, N. (1985). Splenectomy as a prerequisite for successful human ABO-incompatible renal transplantation. *Transplantation Proceedings*, Vol. 17, No. 1 Pt. I, (January-February 1985), pp. 138-143, ISSN 0041-1345

Alexandre, G.P.J.; Latinne, D.; Gianello, P. & Squifflet, J.P. (1991). Preformed cytotoxic antibodies and ABO-incompatible grafts. *Clinical Transplantation*, Vol. 5, No. 6 Pt. II, (December 1991), pp. 583-594, ISSN 0902-0063

Bach, F.H.; Ferran, C.; Hechenleitner, P.; Mark, W.; Koyamada, N.; Miyatake, T.; Winkler, H.; Badrichani, A.; Candinas, D. & Hancock, W.W. (1997). Accommodation of vascularized xenografts: expression of "protective genes" by donor endothelial cells in a host Th2 cytokine environment. *Nature Medicine*, Vol. 3, No. 2, (February 1997), pp. 196-204, ISSN 1078-8956

Cardella, C.J.; Pei, Y. & Brady, H.R. (1987). ABO blood group incompatible kidney transplantation: a case report and review of the literature. *Clinical Nephrology*, Vol. 28, No. 6, (December 1987), pp. 295-299, ISSN 0301-0430

Colvin R. B. & Smith R.N. (2005). Antibody mediated organ allograft rejection. *Nature Review Immunology*, Vol. 5, No. 10, (October 2005), pp. 807-817, ISSN 1474-1733

Crew, R.J. & Ratner, L.E. (2010). ABO-incompatible kidney transplantation: current practice and the decade ahead. *Current Opinion in Organ Transplantation*, Vol. 15, No. 4, (August 2010), pp. 526-530, ISSN 1531-7013

Frame, T.; Carroll, T.; Korchagina, E.; Bovin, N. & Henry, S. (2007). Synthetic glycolipid modification of red blood cell membranes. *Transfusion*, Vol. 47, No. 5, (May 2007), pp. 876-882, ISSN 0041-1132

Genberg, H.; Kumlien, G.; Wennberg, L. & Tyden, G. (2010). Isoagglutinin adsorption in ABO-incompatible transplantation. *Transfusion and Apheresis Science*, Vol. 43, No. 2, (October 2010) pp. 231-235, ISSN 1473-0502

Haidinger, M.; Schmaldienst, S.; Körmöczi, G.; Regele, H.; Soleiman, A.; Schwartz, D.; Derfler, K.; Steininger, R.; Mühlbacher, F. & Böhmig, G.A. (2009). Vienna experience of ABO-incompatible living-donor kidney transplantation. *Wiener klinische Wochenschrift*, Vol. 121, No. 7-8, (June 2009), pp. 247-255, ISSN 0043-5325

Hume, D.L.; Merrill, J.P.; Miller, B.F. & Thorn, G.W. (1955). Experiences with renal homotransplantation in the human: report of nine cases. *The Journal of Clinical Investigation*, Vol. 34, No. 2, (February 1955), pp. 327-382, ISSN 0021-9738

Ishida, H.; Miyamoto, N.; Shirakawa, H.; Shimizu, T.; Tokumoto, T.; Ishikawa, N.; Shimmura, H.; Setoguchi, K.; Toki, D.; Iida, S.; Teraoka, S.; Takahashi, K.; Toma, H.; Yamaguchi, Y. & Tanabe, K. (2007). Evaluation of immunosuppressive regimens in ABO-incompatible living kidney transplantation--single center analysis. *American Journal of Transplantation*, Vol. 7, No. 4, (April 2007), pp. 825-831, ISSN 1600-6135

Jeon, B.J.; Kim, I.G.; Seong, Y.K. & Han, B.H. (2010). Analysis of the results of ABO-incompatible kidney transplantation: in comparison with ABO-compatible kidney transplantation. *Korean Journal of Urology*, Vol. 51, No. 12, (December 2010), pp. 863-869, ISSN 2005-6745

Kenmochi, T.; Saigo, K.; Maruyama, M.; Akutsu, N.; Iwashita, C.; Otsuki, K.; Ito, T.; Suzuki, A. & Miyazaki, M. (2008). Results of kidney transplantation from ABO-incompatible living donors in a single institution. *Transplantation Proceedings*, Vol. 40, No. 7, (September 2008), pp. 2289-2291, ISSN 0041-1345

Kimura, S.; Yurugi, K.; Segawa, H.; Kuroda, J.; Sato, K.; Nogawa, M.; Yuasa, T.; Egawa, H.; Tanaka, K. & Maekawa, T. (2005). Rapid quantitation of immunoglobulin G antibodies specific for blood group antigens A and B by surface plasmon resonance. *Transfusion*, Vol. 45, No. 1, (January 2005), pp. 56-62, ISSN 0041-1132

Kissmeyer-Nielsen, F.; Olsen, S.; Petersen, V.P. & Fjeldborg, O. (1966). Hyperacute rejection of kidney allografts associated with pre-existing humoral antibodies against donor cells. *Lancet*, Vol. 2, No. 7465, (September 1966), pp. 662-665, ISSN 0140-6736

Kobayashi, T. & Saito, K. (2006). A series of surveys on assay for anti-A/B antibody by Japanese ABO-incompatible Transplantation Committee. *Xenotransplantation*, Vol. 13, No. 2, (March 2006), pp. 136-140, ISSN 0908-665X

Krishnan, N. S.; Fleetwood, P.; Higgins, R. M.; Hathaway, M.; Zehnder, D.; Mitchell, D.; Hamer, R.; Fletcher, S.; Lam, F. T.; Kashi, H.; Tan, L. C.; Imray, C. & Briggs, D. (2008). Application of flow cytometry to monitor antibody levels in ABO incompatible kidney transplantation. *Transplantation*, Vol. 86, No. 3, (August 2008), pp. 474-477, ISSN 0041-1337

Kumlien, G.; Wilpert, J.; Safwenberg, J. & Tyden, G. (2007). Comparing the tube and gel techniques for ABO antibody titration, as performed in three European centers. *Transplantation*, Vol. 84, No. 12 Suppl, (December 2007), pp. S17-S19, ISSN 0041-1337

Lindberg, L.; Johansson, S.M.; Liu, J.; Grufman, P. & Holgersson, J. (2011). Is there a clinical need for a diagnostic test allowing detection of chain type-specific anti-A and anti-B. *Transfusion*, Vol. 51, No. 3, (March 2011), pp. 494-503, ISSN 1537-2995

Lynch, R.J. & Platt, J.L. (2008). Accommodation in organ transplantation. *Current Opinion in Organ Transplantation*, Vol. 13, No. 2, (April 2008), pp. 165-170, ISSN 1531-7013

Lynch, R.J. & Platt, J.L. (2010). Accommodation in renal transplantation: unanswered questions. *Current Opinion in Organ Transplantation*, Vol. 15, No. 4, (August 2010), pp. 481-485, ISSN 1531-7013

Marionneau, S.; Cailleau-Thomas, A.; Rocher, J.; Le Moullac-Vaidye, B.; Ruvoën, N.; Clément, M. & Le Pendu, J. (2001). ABH and Lewis histo-blood group antigens, a model for the meaning of oligosaccharide diversity in the face of a changing world. *Biochimie*, Vol. 83, No. 7, (July 2001), pp. 565-573, ISSN 0300-9084

Montgomery, R.A.; Hardy, M.A.; Jordan, S.C.; Racusen, L.C.; Ratner, L.E.; Tyan, D.B.; Zachary, A.A. & Antibody Working Group on the diagnosis, reporting, and risk assessment for antibody-mediated rejection and desensitization protocols. (2004). Consensus opinion from the antibody working group on the diagnosis, reporting, and risk assessment for antibody-mediated rejection and desensitization protocols. *Transplantation*, Vol. 78, No. 2, (July 2004), pp. 181-185, ISSN 0041-1337

Moon, H.W.; Yun, Y.M.; Hur, M.; Park, J.H.; Lee, H.W.; Chang, S.H. & Yun, I.J. (2009). An experience of ABO-incompatible kidney transplantation using plasmapheresis and anti-CD20 monoclonal antibody. *Korean Journal of Laboratory Medicine*, Vol. 29, No. 6, (December 2009), pp. 585-588, ISSN 1598-6535

Murray, J.E.; Merrill, J.P.; Dammin, G.J.; Dealy, J.B. Jr.; Walter, C.W.; Brooke, M.S. & Wilson, R.E. (1960). Study on transplantation immunity after total body irradiation: clinical and experimental investigation. *Surgery*, Vol. 48, (July 1960), pp. 272-284, ISSN 0039-6060

Oettl, T.; Halter, J.; Bachmann, A.; Guerke, L.; Infanti, L.; Oertli, D.; Mihatsch, M.; Gratwohl, A.; Steiger, J. & Dickenmann, M. (2009). ABO blood group-incompatible living donor kidney transplantation: a prospective, single-centre analysis including serial protocol biopsies. *Nephrology, Dialysis, Transplantation*, Vol. 24, No. 1, (January 2009), pp. 298-303, ISSN 1460-2385

Ogawa, H.; Mohiuddin, M.M.; Yin, D.P.; Shen, J.; Chong, A.S. & Galili, U (2004). Mouse-heart grafts expressing an incompatible carbohydrate antigen. II. Transition from accommodation to tolerance. *Transplantation*, Vol. 77, No. 3, (February 2004), pp. 366–373, ISSN 0041-1337

Orlin, J.B. & Berkman, E.M. (1980). Partial plasma exchange using albumin replacement: removal and recovery of normal plasma constituents. *Blood*, Vol. 56, No.6, (December 1980), pp. 1055-1059, ISSN 0006-4971

Park, W.D.; Grande, J.P.; Ninova, D.; Nath, K.A.; Platt, J.L.; Gloor, J.M. & Stegall, M.D. (2003). Accommodation in ABO-incompatible kidney allografts, a novel mechanism of self-protection against antibody-mediated injury. *American Journal of Transplantation*, Vol. 3, No. 8, (August 2003), pp. 952-960, ISSN 1600-6135

Platt, J.L.; Vercellotti, G.M.; Dalmasso, A.P., Matas, A.J., Bolman R.M., Najarian, J.S. & Bach, F.H. (1990). Transplantation of discordant xenografts: a review of progress. *Immunology Today*, Vol. 11, No. 12, (December 1990), pp. 450-456, ISSN 0167-5699

Reding, R.; Squifflet, J.P.; Latinne, D.; de Bruyere, M.; Pirson, Y. & Alexandre, G.P.J. (1987). Early postoperative monitoring of natural anti-A and anti-B isoantibodies in ABO-incompatible living donor renal allografts. *Transplantation Proceedings*, Vol. 19, No. 1 Pt 3, (Febrary 1987), pp. 1989-1990, ISSN 0041-1345

Rieben, R.; Buchs, J. P.; Fluckiger, E. & Nydegger, U. E. (1991) Antibodies to histo-blood group substances A and B: agglutination titers, Ig class, and IgG subclasses in healthy persons of different age categories. *Transfusion*, Vol. 31, No. 7, (September 1991), pp. 607-615, ISSN 0041-1132

Roback, J. D. (Ed.). (2008). *Technical Manual*. 16th ed. American Association of Blood Banks, ISBN 978-1563952609 (1563952602), Bethesda, USA.

Segev, D.L.; Simpkins, C.E.; Warren, D.S.; King, K.E.; Shirey, R.S.; Maley, W.R.; Melancon, J.K.; Cooper, M.; Kozlowski, T. & Montgomery, R.A. (2005). ABO incompatible high-titer renal transplantation without splenectomy or anti-CD20 treatment. *American Journal of Transplantation*, Vol. 5, No. 10, (October 2005), pp. 2570-2575, ISSN 1600-6135

Squifflet, J.P.; De Meyer, M.; Malaise, J.; Latinne, D.; Pirson, Y. & Alexandre, G.P. (2004). Lessons learned from ABO-incompatible living donor kidney transplantation: 20 years later. *Experimental and Clinical Transplantation*, Vol. 2, No. 1, (June 2004), pp. 208-213, ISSN 1304-0855

Slapak, M.; Naik, R.B. & Lee, H.A. (1981). Renal transplant in a patient with major donor-recipient blood group incompatibility: reversal of acute rejection by the use of modified plasmapheresis. *Transplantation*, Vol. 31, No. 1, (January 1981), pp. 4-7, ISSN 0041-1337

Slapak, M.; Digard, N.; Ahmed, M.; Shell, T. & Thompson, F. (1990). Renal transplantation across the ABO barrier - a 9 year experience. *Transplantation Proceedings*, Vol. 22, No. 4, (August 1990), pp. 1425-1428, ISSN 0041-1345

Starzl, T.E.; Marchioro, T.L.; Holmes, J.H.; Hermann, G.; Brittain, R.S.; Stonington, O.H., Talmage, D.W. & Waddell, W.R. (1964). Renal homografts in patients with major donor-recipient blood group incompatibilities. *Surgery*, Vol. 55, (Febrary 1964), pp. 195-200, ISSN 0039-6060

Stussi, G.; Huggel, K.; Lutz, H.U.; Schanz, U.; Rieben, R. & Seebach, J.D. (2005). Isotype-specific detection of ABO blood group antibodies using a novel flow cytometric method. *British Journal of Haematology*, Vol. 130, No. 6, (September 2005), pp. 954-963, ISSN 0007-1048

Szczepiorkowski, Z.M.; Winters, J.L.; Bandarenko, N.; Kim, H.C.; Linenberger, M.L.; Marques, M.B. ; Sarode, R.; Schwartz, J.; Weinstein, R. & Shaz, B.H. (2010). Guidelines on the use of therapeutic apheresis in clinical practice--evidence-based approach from the Apheresis Applications Committee of the American Society for Apheresis. *Journal of Clinical Apheresis*, Vol. 25, No.3, (June 2010), pp. 83-1217, ISSN 0733-2459

Takahashi, K. (2007). Recent findings in ABO-incompatible kidney transplantation: classification and therapeutic strategy for acute antibody-mediated rejection due to ABO-blood-group-related antigens during the critical period preceding the establishment of accommodation. *Clinical and Experimental Nephrology*, Vol. 11, No. 2, (June 2007), pp. 128-141, ISSN 1342-1751

Tanabe, K. (2007). Japanese experience of ABO-incompatible living kidney transplantation. *Transplantation*, Vol. 84, No. 12 Suppl, (December 2007), pp. S4-S7, ISSN 0041-1337

Tanabe, K. (2007). Interinstitutional variation in the measurement of anti-A/B antibodies: the Japanese ABO-Incompatible Transplantation Committee survey. *Transplantation*, Vol. 84, No. 12 Suppl, (December 2007), pp. S13-S16, ISSN 0041-1337

Tanabe, K.; Ishida, H.; Shimizu, T.; Omoto, K.; Shirakawa, H. & Tokumoto, T. (2009). Evaluation of two different preconditioning regimens for ABO-incompatible living kidney donor transplantation. A comparison of splenectomy vs. rituximab-treated non-splenectomy preconditioning regimens. *Contributions to Nephrology*, Vol. 162, (Febrary 2009), pp. 61-74, ISSN 0302-5144

Tang, A.H. & Platt, J.L. (2007). Accommodation of grafts: implications for health and disease. *Human Immunology*, Vol. 68, No. 8, (August 2007), pp. 645-651, ISSN 0198-8859

Thielke, J.; Kaplan, B. & Benedetti, E. (2007). The role of ABO-incompatible living donors in kidney transplantation: state of the art. *Seminars in Nephrology*, Vol. 27, No. 4, (July 2007), pp. 408-413, ISSN 0270-9295

Tobian, A.A.; Shirey, R.S. & King, K.E. (2011) ABO antibody titer monitoring for incompatible renal transplantation. *Transfusion*, Vol. 51, No. 3, (March 2011), pp. 454-457, ISSN 1537-2995

Tobian, A.A.; Shirey, R.S.; Montgomery, R.A.; Cai, W.; Haas, M.; Ness, P.M. & King, K.E. (2010). ABO antibody titer and risk of antibody-mediated rejection in ABO-incompatible renal transplantation. *American Journal of Transplantation*, Vol. 10, No. 5, (May 2010), pp. 1247-1253, ISSN 1600-6143

Tobian, A.A.; Shirey, R.S.; Montgomery, R.A.; Ness, P.M. & King, K.E. (2008). The critical role of plasmapheresis in ABO-incompatible renal transplantation. *Transfusion*, Vol. 48, No. 11, (November 2008), pp. 2453-2460, ISSN 1537-2995

Tobian, A.A.; Shirey, R.S.; Montgomery, R.A.; Tisch, D.J.; Ness, P.M. & King, K.E. (2009). Therapeutic plasma exchange reduces ABO titers to permit ABO-incompatible renal transplantation. *Transfusion*, Vol. 49, No. 6, (June 2009), pp. 1248-1254, ISSN 1537-2995

Tyden, G.; Kumlien, G.; Genberg, H.; Sandberg, J.; Lundgren, T. & Fehrman, I. (2005). ABO incompatible kidney transplantations without splenectomy, using antigen-specific immunoadsorption and rituximab. *American Journal of Transplantation*, Vol. 5, No.1, (January 2005), pp. 145-148, ISSN 1600-6135

Valli, P.V.; Puga, Y.G.; Fehr, T.; Schulz-Huotari, C.; Kaup, N.; Güngör, T.; Ambühl, P.; Weber, M.; Schanz, U.; Seebach, J.D. & Stussi, G. (2009). Changes of circulating antibody levels induced by ABO antibody adsorption for ABO-incompatible kidney transplantation. *American Journal of Transplantation*, Vol. 9, No. 5, (May 2009), pp. 1072-1080, ISSN 1600-6143

Winters, J.L.; Gloor, J.M.; Pineda, A.A.; Stegall, M.D. & Moore, S.B. (2004). Plasma exchange conditioning for ABO-incompatible renal transplantation. *Journal of Clinical Apheresis*, Vol. 19, No.2, (2004), pp. 79-85, ISSN 0733-2459

Yamamoto F. (2004). Review: ABO blood group system--ABH oligosaccharide antigens, anti-A and anti-B, A and B glycosyltransferases, and ABO genes. *Immunohematology / American Red Cross*, Vol. 20, No. 1, (March 2004), pp. 3-22, ISSN 0894-203X

Yurugi, K.; Kimura, S.; Ashihara, E.; Tsuji, H.; Kawata, A.; Kamitsuji, Y.; Hishida, R.; Takegawa, M.; Egawa, H. & Maekawa, T. (2007). Rapid and accurate measurement of anti-A/B IgG antibody in ABO-unmatched living donor liver transplantation by surface plasmon resonance. *Transfusion Medicine*, Vol. 17, No. 2, (April 2007), pp. 97-106, ISSN 0958-7578

3

Transplantation for the Complex Patient with Hepatitis C and End Stage Renal Disease

Jorge Ortiz, Jason Andre, Kamran Khanmoradi and Victor Araya
Albert Einstein Medical Center, Philadelphia PA
USA

1. Introduction

Hepatitis C (HCV) and End Stage Renal Disease (ESRD) are two major health issues affecting millions worldwide. The diagnosis of HCV in the dialysis patient has significant prognostic indications and specific interventions are necessary in order to evaluate the extent of liver disease and the feasibility of medical treatment or the need for organ replacement therapy. For the transplant candidate, unique issues with respect to immunosuppressive agents and the appropriate use of HCV positive donors may be particularly vexing. Prior reviews have focused on issues classically limited to nephrology or hepatology, this update will address transplantation issues as well.

2. Epidemiology

The Hepatitis C virus (HCV) is a member of the Flaviviridae family. Approximately 150 million people are infected by this single stranded RNA virus, 5 million of whom live in the United States. It is estimated that 85% of patients will develop chronic infection, which is defined as the presence of HCV RNA for six months after presumed onset. Subsequent spontaneous clearing of the virus is rare. Approximately 10-30% will develop cirrhosis. In the renal dialysis population, the incidence of de novo infection is 3-7% per year. The prevalence ranges from 10-20% and may be underestimated due to cases of low viral load.[1,2,3]

Factors associated with virus acquisition in this patient population include the number of blood units transfused (which has decreased with the advent of erythropoietin alpha and blood bank screening), the length of dialysis therapy and the type of renal replacement therapy. Patients on hemodialysis are at higher risk compared to those on peritoneal dialysis.[4] There are at least six genotypes and many subtypes. HCV accounts for 30-50% of liver transplantation procedures performed and is also associated with many extra hepatic manifestations,[5] (Table 1) most importantly diabetes. The mechanisms underlying the diabetogenicity of HCV likely involve insulin resistance, diminished hepatic glucose uptake and the directly injurious effect of the virus on beta cells of the pancreas.[6] In the kidney, HCV is strongly associated with membranoproliferative glomerulonephritis (MPGN), membranous glomerulonephritis, focal segmental glomerulosclerosis, mesangial proliferative glomerulonephritis[7] and albuminuria.[8] Clinically silent immune complex glomerulonephritis was commonly seen in biopsies of patients with end stage HCV liver disease undergoing liver transplantation.[9]

Antiphospholipid syndrome
Aplastic Anemia
Autoimmune hemolytic anemia
Autoimmune thyroiditis
Chronic fatigue syndrome
Behcet's Syndrome
Carotid atherosclerosis
CRST syndrome
Dermatomyositis
Diabetes
Fibromyalgia
Guillain-Barré syndrome
Hypertrophic cardiomyopathy
Hypocholesterolemia
Idiopathic pulmonary fibrosis
Idiopathic thrombocytopenic purpura
IgA deficiency
Lichen planus
MALToma
Mooren corneal ulcers
Multiple myeloma
Non-Hodgkins lymphoma
Neurocognitive impairment
Pancreatitis Polyarteritis nodosa
Polymyositis Porphyria cutanea tarda
Rheumatoid arthritis
Sialadenitis
Sjogren's syndrome
Systemic lupus erythematosis
Uveitis
Waldenstrom's macroglobuminemia

Table 1. Extrahepatic disease manifestations with HCV infection

3. Evaluation for treatment and kidney transplantation

Evaluation of the potential kidney transplant recipient with HCV involves a careful history and physical examination. Patients with encephalopathy, variceal bleeding, ascites and muscle wasting have significant risk of continued deterioration and should be considered for liver (and kidney) transplantation. The presence of hepatocellular carcinoma within the Milan or UCSF criteria[10] should also be considered an indication for combined liver and kidney transplantation.

False positives (and negatives (0.23%)) are not uncommonly seen with the current generation of ELISA blood tests and therefore a confirmatory PCR should be ordered[11]. The mean time from detection of HCV RNA to the appearance of antibody may be as long as six months[12]. Nevertheless, screening with PCR is not recommended. A negative PCR in a previously positive patient should be repeated because frequent variations in the viral load can be seen. The genotype of the virus may determine its susceptibility to interferon treatment. However, early studies in patients with renal replacement therapy failed to demonstrate that HCV genotype is a factor in interferon responsiveness[13]. Additionally, HCV genotype does not seem to influence survival in renal transplant recipients[14].

4. Biopsy

Liver function tests are not sensitive enough to determine whether there is significant inflammation or even cirrhosis[15]. Liver biopsies are therefore indicated in all HCV positive candidates being considered for kidney transplantation and possible treatment. Studies indicate that advanced fibrosis is a common finding despite normal aminotransferase levels[16]. Histologic features of chronic hepatitis will be seen in 100% of ESRD patients with HCV. 60-80% of patients will have significant fibrosis and 10-12% will have cirrhosis[17]. Established cirrhosis was found to be the most important predictor of death after renal transplantation and is considered a relative contraindication to isolated renal transplantation[18]. If the liver biopsy shows cirrhosis mandatory screening for hepatocellular carcinoma must be instituted[19].

Regarding the biopsy technique, obtaining tissue via the transjugular route may be safer than the percutaneous method especially if the patient has ascites, disorders of the coagulation system or undergoes peritoneal dialysis. An additional advantage of the transjugular approach is the determination of portal pressure gradients which may help to diagnose sub clinical portal hypertension. Radiologic imaging or upper endoscopy (another important screening tool) may demonstrate obvious cirrhosis and varices perhaps obviating the need for this particular intervention. In the absence of cirrhosis, biopsies should be performed at five year intervals. Surrogate serum markers for fibrosis and cirrhosis have been investigated but are not yet the standard of care[20].

5. Hepatocellular carcinoma

The incidence of hepatocellular carcinoma (HCC) is increasing in the general population[21] and is higher in patients with ESRD. The prognosis is also worse for patients with ESRD[22]. Screening is crucial as prognosis after the onset of symptoms is dismal while patients with small expeditiously treated lesions reap a significant survival advantage. The yearly risk of HCC in patients with HCV is highest in those with established cirrhosis (about 2-8% per year). HCV infected patients who do not have cirrhosis have a lower risk of developing HCC. Based on current knowledge all patients with HCV and cirrhosis should undergo surveillance. This should entail a radiologic exam (CT scan, MRI or ultrasound) and alpha fetoprotein monitoring. These screens should be performed (in cirrhotics) at 6-12 month intervals. If HCC is found, metastatic workup includes bone scans and chest CT scans. Surgical resection can be safely performed for patients with ESRD and preserved liver function[23]. For patients with decompensated cirrhosis and small solitary HCC or early multifocal disease (up to three lesions, total tumor burden less than 6.5cm) the best option is liver (and kidney) transplantation[24]. Other modalities used to treat HCC include chemoembolization, alcohol infusion, radiofrequency ablation,Y-90, and acetic acid infusion.

Systemic chemotherapy is not associated with improvements in patient survival. Sorafenib (Nexavar) may be associated with survival improvements in untransplantable patients.

6. Anti viral therapy

Antiviral therapy before transplantation with the objective of eradicating the virus is the current standard of care. Secondary benefits may include the prevention of hepatic decompensation and hepatocellular carcinoma. In dialysis patients, the only recommended treatment is Alpha Interferon monotherapy. The average virological response is 40% and is independent of genotype. Interferon therapy interruption, seen in up to 60% of patients, is due to side effects. The most common of which are flu like symptoms, neurologic symptoms and gastrointestinal symptoms. Sustained viral response (SVR) may be durable (22 months average) post transplantation in those patients successfully treated before surgery. Of the sixteen patients studied in one report, HCV viral counts remained negative in all.[25] Immunosuppressive issues remain troublesome in this complex patient population. Others have also indicated that successfully treated dialysis patients may have an improved graft survival and lower incidence of HCV related kidney disease[26] and new onset post transplant diabetes.

The higher rate of SVR after interferon therapy may result from higher levels of interferon in patients with renal failure. The dose of interferon is 3 million units one to three times a week. Pegylated interferons, although commonly used, are not yet recommended. From a pharmacokinetic standpoint dose adjustments would probably be unnecessary in patients with renal impairment[27]. Absorption may vary with a patient on dialysis[28]. One study reported 87.5% viral clearance in 8 patients after 12 weeks of therapy. All of the 6 patients who completed 48 weeks of therapy achieved a biochemical response[28]. In another report, two of six genotype 1 patients completed a 24 week course of Pegylated Interferon and achieved a SVR[30]. The appropriate dose of Pegylated Interferon Alpha-2 is probably 135 micrograms a week, this gives similar serum levels as 180 micrograms per week in patients with preserved renal function. Pegylated Interferon Alpha-2 should probably be dosed between 0.5-1.0 micrograms/kg (as opposed to 1.0-1.5 ug/kg)[31].

Ribavirin is contraindicated, alone and with interferon, because of the hemolytic anemia associated with it. However, some groups have shown that it can be used in combination with interferon at reduced dosages with plasma monitoring and erythropoietin and iron supplementation[32]. These studies did not prove that ribavirin in low doses, in this population, improved response rates. It is very important to note that if hemolysis results in anemia that necessitates blood transfusion, the patient may be rendered untransplantable because of increased immune reactivity. Amantadine has not proven beneficial.

In kidney transplant recipients, interferon treatment is contraindicated because of the increased risk of acute cellular and antibody meditated rejection[33]. An exception is the patient with fibrosing cholestatic hepatitis (FCH). FCH is characterized by cholestasis with only mild to moderate elevation of transaminases and a rapid deterioration in liver function[34]. Some investigators believe that after combined liver and kidney transplantation, the liver protects the kidney from rejection and interferon can therefore safely be administered.

Ribavirin monotherapy may improve serum aminotransferases and proteinuria, but its effect on liver histology is controversial. Chronic hemolysis may prevent its safe use. Some have recommended that ribavirin be dose adjusted for those renal transplant recipients with HCV who have developed significant proteinuria[35].

7. Prognosis

HCV infection in renal failure patients is usually asymptomatic. The virus seems to have a lower impact on the liver histology of dialysis patients than on the histology of the HCV-positive immunocompetent patients with normal renal function[36]. It would appear that histological progression of liver injury after transplantation is minimal in HCV positive kidney recipients. In fact, fibrosis might regress in some patients[37]. Nevertheless, it is a negative prognostic indicator for survival on dialysis and after kidney transplantation. HCV may intensify oxidative stress in patients with uremia, leading to cardiovascular compromise[38]. Diabetes and cardiovascular disease were statistically significantly associated with patient death (while on dialysis) in one study[39]. Those patients with cirrhosis have a 35% higher death rate than noncirrhotic counterparts.[40,41] In another report, HCC was a statistically significantly more common cause of death in HCV positive dialysis patients[42]. Overall survival in these patients is improved after kidney transplantation compared to remaining on dialysis, despite the theoretical risk of accelerating virus replication with immunosuppression[43], but worse than HCV negative counterparts. This might be related to an increased risk of cardiovascular disease, posttransplant diabetes mellitus, sepsis [44,45,46], and rejection[47]. Thrombotic microangiopathy, MPGN and proteinuria are also associated with HCV infection and may result in lower rates of patient and graft survival[48]. The most common cause of proteinuria post transplant is still chronic allograft nephropathy, and a biopsy is crucial for the diagnosis[49]. All cause hospitalizations are significantly higher in HCV positive kidney recipients compared to HCV negative ones. HCV positive kidney transplant recipients are more likely to be African American, male, older, and have a higher rate of alcohol abuse, experience extended time on dialysis, malnutrition (as measured by serum albumin) and prior transplantation. Those patients with concomitant hepatitis B infection do particularly poorly in terms of patient and graft survival[50]. As do patients with HIV co-infection[51].

8. HCV and Tacrolimus

As stated, HCV infection is associated with pre transplant and de novo post transplant diabetes. This is seen more commonly with Tacrolimus compared to Cyclosporine. Nevertheless, the U.S. FK506 multicenter trial demonstrated higher patient survival in those HCV positive patients who received Tacrolimus compared to Cyclosporine. According to a recent query of the UNOS database (Tables 2-3), 1,3,5 year graft survival for HCV positive recipients of HCV negative organs was 89.7%, 76.7% and 61.6% for those patients treated with cyclosporine. 1,3,5 year graft survival with Tacrolimus immunosuppression was 92.2%, 80.6% and 63.3%. If the donor were HCV positive, 1,3,5 year graft survival for HCV positive recipients was 92.7%, 76% and 56.3% for cyclosporine treated recipients and 89.6%, 74.6% and 52.5% for Tacrolimus treated patients. Patient survival at 1,3, and 5 years for HCV negative donor organs was 94.8%, 88.8% and 80.5% with cyclosporine 95.6%, 89.4% and 79.7% with Tacrolimus. If the donor were HCV positive, patient survival at 1,3 and 5 years was 98%, 91.1% and 82% for cyclosporine and 93.9%, 87% and 75.8% for Tacrolimus.[52] The mechanisms behind diminished graft and patient survival with HCV positive donors and Tacrolimus immunosuppression are not entirely clear.

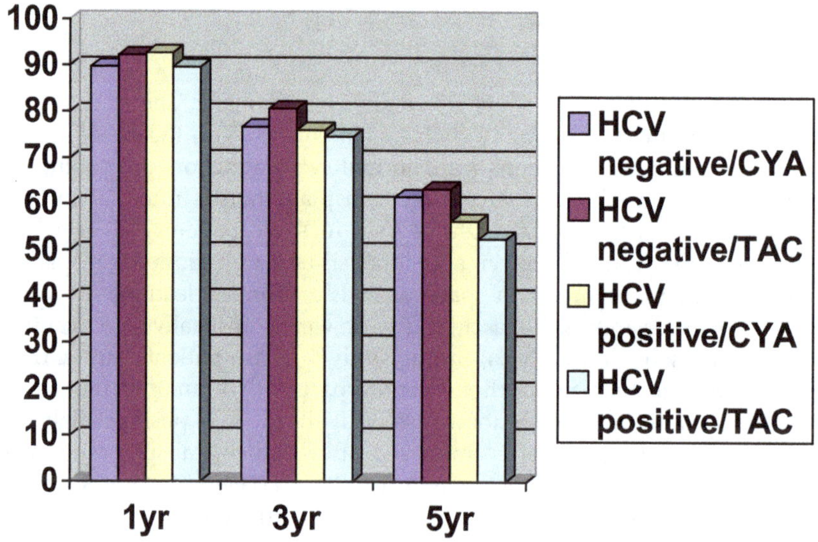

Table 2. Graft Survival by Donor HCV status and Main Maintenance Immunosuppression Agent

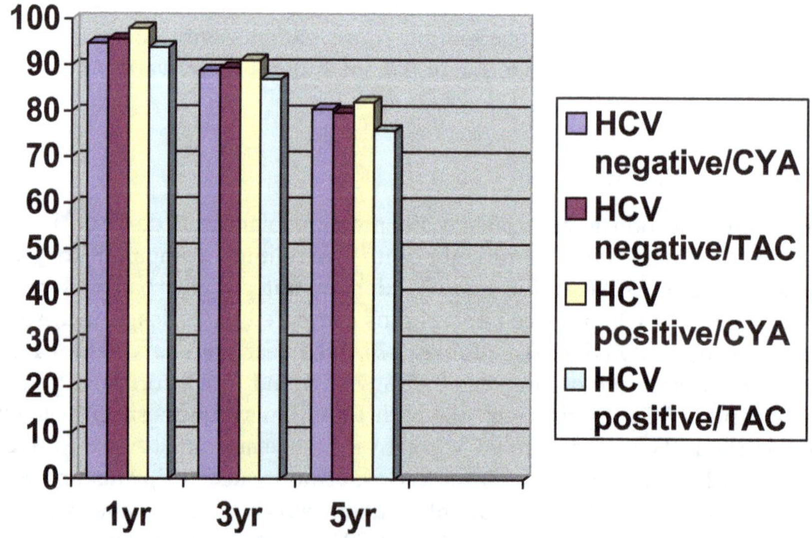

Table 3. Patient Survival By Donor HCV Status and Main Maintenance Immunosuppression Agent

9. Mycophenolate, steroids and induction agents

Another risk factor for diabetes, and a multitude of other complications, is prolonged steroid usage. Early rapid withdrawal has been reported to be safe (at least in the short term) compared with a historic control group[53]. The use of mycophenolate mofetil is associated with improved survival (at least with HCV positive donors) due to fewer infectious deaths[54]. Patients induced with OKT3 or anti-lymphocyte globulin have experienced inferior survivals[54]. The UNOS database was queried for 1,3 and 5 year patient and graft survival for HCV recipients of donor positive and donor negative organs stratified by induction agent (see Table 4). Definitive conclusions pertaining to the best induction agent for the ESRD patient with HCV can not be made until randomized prospective trials are performed.

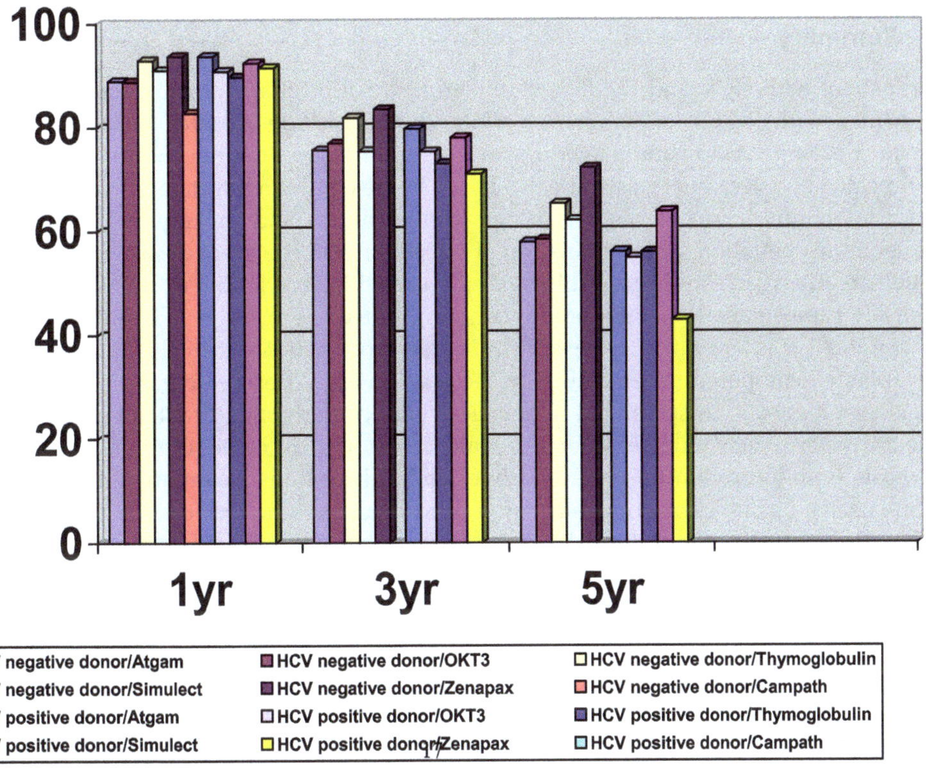

Table 4. Graft Survival by Donor HCV Status and Induction Agent

10. HCV positive donors

The organ donor shortage has compelled centers to transplant kidneys from donors who test positive for HCV. The prevalence and utilization of HCV positive organ donor referrals has increased in the United States. The prevalence of HCV is several fold higher in deceased donors compared to healthy living blood donors. Almost 20% of anti HCV positive donors will be RNA negative[56]. The utilization of HCV positive kidneys for HCV negative recipients is contraindicated[57, 58].

Surprisingly, Bucci et al demonstrated that 34.1% of HCV positive donor kidneys were allocated to HCV negative recipients in the United States in 2000[59]. The use of donor positive kidneys for HCV positive recipients is associated with greater long term mortality compared to virus negative kdneys. Although HCV positive recipients more frequently develop new onset diabetes mellitus (NODM) compared to negative controls, the risk is heightened with HCV positive donors[60]. Nevertheless, in comparison to staying on the waitlist, transplantation with donor virus positive kidneys is associated with increased survival in HCV positive recipients[61]. There is no definitive proof that conversion of genotype after transplantation portends a bad prognosis. Nevertheless, one case reported did implicate a genotypic mismatched kidney transplant in the exacerbation of hepatic dysfunction[62]. Any possible adverse effect of super infection with a different genotype is believed to be outweighed by the beneficial effect of decreased time on dialysis[63].

11. Summary

The patient with HCV and ESRD is very complex. All positive antibody screens should be confirmed with PCR. The standard workup should include a search for clinical signs of hepatic decompensation and a liver biopsy. The biopsy, if it does not show cirrhosis, should be repeated at 5 year intervals. Patients should be treated with interferon if at all possible in order to minimize long term hepatologic complications and to improve outcomes after kidney transplantation. The formulation of interferon and the exact dosing remain a matter of debate. Ribavirin should probably be used only with close follow up and in a setting of a trial. After transplantation, interferon is contraindicated.

Although HCV is a negative prognostic indicator, those patients with HCV are better served transplanted compared to remaining on the waitlist. HCV positive organ donors are also a negative prognostic indicator but nonetheless may confer a significant survival advantage due to the associated decrease in the wait time for a deceased organ. Decompensated cirrhosis is an indication for combined liver and kidney transplantation. At this time well compensated cirrhotics are not considered candidates for single or dual organ transplants, although many centers perform both. Mycophenolate mofetil and steroid freedom have been shown to be safe in this patient population. The results with various calcineurin inhibitors and induction agents have been reviewed. Until randomized perspective trials are performed, the choice of which medication to employ is center specific and experience driven.

12. Conclusion

HCV will remain a major health issue for decades to come. Appropriate communication between disciplines is mandatory in order to ensure excellent patient outcomes. Randomized trials and multi-disciplinary meetings are indicated.

13. References

Hanuka N, Sikueler E, Tovbin D, et al: Hepatitis C virus infection in renal failure patients in the absence of anti-hepatitis C virus antibodies. Journal of Viral hepatitis 2002, 9:141

Lauer GM, Walder BD. Hepatitis C virus infection. N Engl J Med 2001, 345:41

Batty DS Jr, Swanson SJ, Kirk AD, et al. Hepatitis C virus seropositivity at the time of renal transplantation in the United States: associated factors and patient survival. Am J Transplant 2001, 1:179

Pereira BJG. Hepatitis C n organ transplantation: Its significance and influence on transplantation policies. Curr Opin Nephrol Hypertens 1993, 2:912

Agnello V, De Rosa FG. Extrahepatic disease manifestations of HCV infection: some current issues. Journal of Hepatology 2004, 40:341

Masini M, Campani D, Boggi U et al. Hepatitis C virus infection and human pancreatic beta-cell dysfunction. Diabetes care 2005, 28:940

Gopalani A, Ahuja TS. Prevalence of glomerulopathies in autopsies of patients infected with the hepatitis C virus. Am J Med Sci 2001, 322:57

Tsui JI, Vittinghoff E., Shlipak MG, et al., Relationship between Hepatitis C and Chronic Kidney Disease: Results from the Third National Health and Nutrition Examination Survey. J Am Soc Nephrol 2006, 17:1168

McGuire BM, Julian BA, Synon S, et al. Brief Communication: Glomerulonephritis in Patients with Hepatitis C Cirrhosis Undergoing Liver Transplantation. Ann Intern Med 2006, 144:735

Mazzaferro V; Regalia E; Doci R, et al. Liver transplantation for the treatment of small hepatocellular carcinomas in patients with cirrhosis. N Engl J Med 1996, 334(11):693-9

Schneeberger PM, Keur I, Van der Vliet W, et al. Hepatitis C virus infection in dialysis centers in the Netherlands: a national survey by serological and molecular methods. J Clin MIcrobiol 1998, 36:1711

Furusyo N, Hayashi J, Kakuda K, et al. Acute Hepatitis C among Japanese hemodialysis patients: a prospective 9-year study. Am J Gastroenterol 2001, 96:1593

Izopet J, Rostaing L, Moussion F, et al. High rate of hepatitis C virus clearance in hemodialysis patients after interferon-alpha therapy. J Infect Dis 1997; 17:1614

Natov SN, Lau JY, Ruthazaer R, et al. Hepatitis C virus genotype does not affect patient survival among renal transplant candidates. The New England Organ Bank Hepatitis C Study Group. Kidney Int 1999, 56:700

Fabrizi F, Martin P, Dixit V, et al. Acquisition of hepatitis C virus in hemodialysis patients: a prospective study by branched DNA signal amplification assay. Am J Kidney Dis 1998; 31:647

Sterling RK, Sanyal AJ, Luketic VA, et al. Chronic hepatitis C infection in patients with end stage renal disease: characterization of liver histology and viral load in patients awaiting renal transplantation. Am J Gastroenterol 1999, 94:3576

Martin P, Carter D, Fabrizi F, et al. Histopathologic features of hepatitis C in renal transplant candidates. Transplantation 2000, 69:1479

Mathurin P, Mouquet C, Poynard T, et al. Impact of HBV and HCV on kidney transplantation outcome. Hepatology 1999, 29: 257

Llovet JM, Burroughs A, Bruix J. Hepatocellular carcinoma. Lancet 2003; 362:1907-1917 Varaut A, Fontaine H, Serpaggi Je, et al. Diagnostic Accuracy of the Fibrotest in

Hemodialysis and Renal Transplant Patients with Chronic Hepatitis C Virsu. Transplantation 2005, 80:1550

El-Serag HB, Mason AC: Rising incidence of hepatocellular carcinoma in the United States. N Engl J Med 1999; 340:745-750

Hayashi H, Ohtake Y, Kashima T, et al: Hepatocellular carcinoma among hemodialysis patients infected with hepatitis C virus-early evolution and rapid prognosis. Clin Nephrol 1999;51:321-323

Cheng S, Wu C Shu K, Ho W et al. Liver Resection for Hepatocellular Carcinoma in Patients With End-Stage Renal Failure. Journal of Surgical Oncology 2001; 78:241- 247

Bruix J and Sherman M. Management of Hepatocellular Carcinoma. Hepatology, vol 42, No 5, 2005

Kamar N, Toupance O., Buchler M. Evidence that clearance of hepatitis C virus RNA after alpha-interferon therapy in dialysis patients is sustained after renal transplantation. J Am Soc Nephrol 2003, 14:2092

Cruzado J.M., Casanovas-Taltavull T., Torras J. Pretransplant interferonprevents hepatitis C virus-associated glomerulonephritis in renal allografts by HCV - RNA clearance. Am J Transplant 2003, 3:357

Martin P., Mitra S., Farrington K. Pegylated (40kDa)interferon alfa=2a (Pegasys) is unaffected by renal impairment. Hepatology 2000, 32:370

Barril G., Quiroga J.A. Sanz P. Pegylated interferon alfa 2a kinetics during experimental hemodialysis: impact of permeability and pore size of dialyzers. Aliment Pharmacol Ther 2004, 20:37

Sporea I., Sirli R., Golea O., Peg interferon alfa 2a (40kDA) in patients on chronic hemodialysis with chronic C hepatitis: preliminary results. Rom J Gastroenterol 2004, 20:99

Annichiarico A.E., Siciliano M., Pegylated interferon-alpha 2 monotherapy for hemodialysis patients with chronic hepatitis C. Aliment Pharmacol Ther 2004, 20:123

Fried MW, Shiffman ML, Reddy KR, et al. Peginterferon alfa-2a plus ribavirin for chronic hepatitis C virus infection-a pilot study. N Engl J Med 2002, 347:975

Bruchfeld A, Stahle L, Andersson J, et al. Ribavirin treatment in dialysis patients with chronic hepatitis C virus infection-a pilot study. J Viral Hepat 2001, 8:287

Baid S, Tolkoff-Rubin N, Saidman S, et al. Acute Humoral rejection in hepatitis C-infected renal transplant recipients receiving antiviral therapy. Am J Transplant 2003, 3:74

Toth CM, Pascual M, Chung RT, et al. Hepatitis C virus-associated fibrosing cholestatic hepatitis after renal transplantation. Transplantation 1988, 66:1254

Kamar, N, Ribes D, Izopet J, et al. Treatment of hepatitis C Virus Infection (HCV) After renal Transplantation: Implication for HCV-Positive Dialysis Patients Awaiting a Kidney Transplant. Transplantation 2006, 82:853

Alric L, Di-Martino V, Selves J. et al. Long term impact or renal transplantation on liver fibrosis during hepatitis C virus infection. Gastroenterology 2002; 123(5):1494

Kamar N, Rostaing L, Selves J et al. Natural history of hepatitis C virus-related liver fibrosis after renal transplantation. Am J Transplant 2005, 5:1704

Pawlak K, Pawlak D, Mysliwiec M. Hepatitis intensified oxidative stress, MIP-1 beta and RANTES plasma levels in uraemic patients. Cytoine 2004, 28:197

Bloom RD, Sayer G., Kosuntarty F et al. Outcome of Hepatitis C virus Infected Kidney Transplant Candidates Who Remain on the Waiting List. Am J Transplant 2005, 5:139

Fabrizi F, Poordad FF, et al. Hepatitis C Infection and the Patient with End-Stage renal Disease. Hepatology 2002, 36:3

Marcelli D, Stanhard D, Conte F, et al. ESRD patient mortality with adjustment for comorbid conditions in Lobardy (Italy) versus the United States. Kidney Int 1996: 50:1013

Maisonneuve P., Agodoa L., Geller R. Cancer in patients on dialysis for end-stage renal disease: an international collaborative study. Lancet 1999, 354:93

Knoll GA, Tankerserley MR, Lee JY, et al. The impact of renal transplantation on survival in hepatitis C-positive end stage renal patients. Am J Kidney Dis 1997; 29:608

Yunossi Zzm, Braun WE, Protiva DA et al. Chronic viral hepatitis in renal transplant recipients with allografts functioning for more than 20 years. Transplantation 1999, 67:272

Fabrizi F, Martin P, Dixit V, et al. Post-transplant diabetes mellitus and HCV seropositive status after renal transplantation: Meta analysis of clinical studies. Am J Transplant 2005, 5:2433

Pereira BJ, Wright TL, SchmidCH, Levey AS. The impact of pretransplantation hepatitis C infection on the outcome of renal transplantation. Transplantation 1995, 60:799

Sotsky T, Polyak MR, Riggio R et al. Hepatitis C infection confers increased risk of immunologic failure following renal transplantation. Transplantation 1999; 67 Suppl 1):S577

Baid S, Pascual M, Williams WW, et al. Renal thrombotic microangiopathy associated with anticardiolipin antibodies in hepatitis C-positive renal allograft recipients. J Am Soc Nephrol 1999, 10:146

Nampoory MR, Johny KV, Costandi JN, et al. High incidence of proteinuria in hepatitis C virus infected renal transplant recipients is associated with poor patient and graft outcome. Transplant Proc 2001, 33:3639

Breitenfeldt MK, Rasenack J, Berthold H, et al. Impact of hepatitis B and C on graft loss and mortality of patients after kidney transplantation. Clin Transplant 2002, 16:130

Rostaing L, Izopet J, Cisterne JM, et al: Impact of hepatitis C virus duration and hepatitis C virus genotypes on renal transplant patients: Correlation with clinicopathological features. Transplantation 1998, 65:930 www.UNOS.org OPTN data accessed 12/08/06

Akalin E, Murphy B, Sehgal V, et al. Rapid steroid withdrawal in hepatitis C virus-positive kidney transplant recipients Clin Transplant 2004, 18:384

Abbott KC, Bucci JR, Matsumoto CS, et al. Hepatitis C and renal Transplantation in the Era of Modern Immunosuppression. J Am Soc Nephrol 2003, 14:2908

Gentil MA, Rocha JL, Rodriguez-Algarra G et al. Impaired kidney transplant survival in patients with antibodies to hepatitis C virus. Nephrol Dial Transplant 1999, 14:2908

Pereira B, Milford E, Kirkman R, et al. Prevalence of HCV RNA in organ donors positive for HCV antibody and in the recipients of their organs. N Engl J Med 1992, 327:910

http://www.hdcn.com/symp/03asn/09/per/per.htm

Natov SN, Pereira BJ. Transmission of viral hepatitis by kidney transplantation: donor evaluation and transplant policies (Part 2:hepatitis C virus). Transpl Infect Dis 2002, 4:124

Bucci JR, Matsumoto CS, Swanson SJ, et al. Donor hepatitis C seropositivity: clinical correlates and effect on early graft and patient survival in adult cadaveric kidney transplantation. J Am Soc Nephrol 2002, 13:2974

Abbott KC, Lentine KL, Bucci JR, et al. Impact of diabetes and hepatitis after kidney transplantation on patients who are affected by hepatitis C virus. J Am Soc Nephrol 2004, 15:3166

Abbot KC, Lentine KL, Bucci JR, et al. The Impact of Transplantation with Deceased Donor hepatitis C-Positive Kidneys on Survival in Wait-Listed Long Term Dialysis Patients. Am J. Transplant 2004, 4:2032

Schussler T, Staffield-Coit C., Eason J, et al. Severe Hepatitis C Infection in a Renal Transplant Recipient Following Hepatitis C genotype Mismatch Transplant. Am J Transplant 2004, 4:1375

Gane E, Pilmore H. Management of chronic viral hepatitis before and after renal transplantation. Transplantation 2002, 74:427

4

Kidney-Pancreas Transplantation

Farzad Kakaei[1] and Saman Nikeghbalian[2]

[1]Tabriz University of Medical Sciences
[2]Shiraz University of Medical Sciences
Iran

1. Introduction

During the past decade, simultaneous pancreas kidney transplantation has been widely accepted as the most effective way to achieve normoglycemia in patients with type 1 diabetes and end-stage renal disease. This procedure was performed for the first time on a human in 1966 but it was in the 1980s, with advances in surgical technique and introduction of cyclosporine for immunosuppression, that the success rates of SPK became acceptable. According to international pancreas transplant (IPTR) report as of December 31, 2004, 23,043 pancreas transplants were performed worldwide. These included more than 17,000 (17,127) performed in the United States (US) and nearly 6,000 (5,916) from outside the US (non-US). In the US, the majority of the cases, 78% (n=11,898), have been simultaneous pancreas-kidney transplants (SPK); 16% (n=2427) are pancreas after kidney (PAK) transplants; 7% (n=1,008) are pancreas transplants alone (PTA).

Indications for pancreas transplantation include the development of diabetic complications such as ESRD, retinopathy or multiple attacks of hypoglycemic unawareness. Unfortunately, pancreas transplantation has been associated with the highest surgical complication rate of all the routinely performed organ transplant procedures (except for small intestinal or multivisceral transplantation) and the risk of pancreas graft loss from surgical complications (technical failures) is higher than from immunological reasons. The overall incidence of surgical complications in PTx is reported to be around 10% to 38%. This high rate of complications leads US centers to preclude PTA in most centers and now over 95% of pancreas transplantations are performed in patients with renal disease or a previous functioning kidney transplant. One year patient, kidney, and pancreas survival rates for recipients of an SPK transplant are 95%, 91%, and 86%, respectively. Compared to patients with diabetes who receive a kidney alone, the addition of a pancreas improves long-term patient and kidney graft survival. Recipients of a pancreas-after-kidney transplant or a pancreas transplant alone have an average 1-year pancreas graft survival rate of 78-83%.

In this chapter we will thoroughly describe many aspects of this complex transplantation procedure including:

- The history of pancreas transplantation
- Indications for pancreas transplantation
- Surgical aspects of pancreas graft procurement from the deceased donor
- Current surgical techniques for pancreas transplantation
- Immunosuppressive regimens

- Postoperative care of pancreas transplant recipients
- Complications of pancreas transplantation
- Long term results of pancreas transplantation

2. History of pancreas transplantation

Experimental transplantation of the pancreas in animals began as early as 1890 with proved success in the treatment of insulin dependent diabetes mellitus (Burke GW , et al, 2004). Grafting 3 pieces of sheep pancreas into the subcutaneous tissue of a diabetic child by Williams in 1893 was another attempt to treat diabetes but the patient died after 3 days because of severe ketoacidosis (Williams PW, 1903). The first clinical attempt to cure type 1 diabetes by vascular pancreas transplantation was done simultaneously with kidney transplantation, at the University of Minnesota in 1966 three years after first successful kidney transplantation (Kelly WD, et al, 1967), but the procedure was not performed with any frequency until many years later. Only 12 cases were done between 1967 till 1973 at the same center but almost all of them rejected before the first year after the operation. Segmental pancreas transplantation from living donors first introduced in 1979. Besides the rejection and vascular problems, dealing with pancreas exocrine secretion was complicated this type of procedure from the early days. By the mid-70s three different techniques were in use: enteric drainage, urinary drainage (into the ureter or directly into the bladder and duct injection. Ureteral drainage was first introduced by Gleidman et al (Gleidman et al , 1973). Bladder drainage first by direct anastomosis of the pancreatic duct to the bladder by Sollinger et al (Sollinger HW, et al, 1984) and then by duodenocystostomy by Nghiem and Corry (Nghiem DD & Corry RJ, 1987) was the most common method for exocrine drainage during the 1980s and 1990s and was still in use in some centers around the world specially for solitary pancreas transplantation. In the early 80's, a dramatic improvement in outcomes happened due to introduction of cyclosporine for immunosuppression (Squifflet JP, et al, 2008). In 1984, Starzl et al (Starzl et al,1984) reintroduced the technique of enteric drainage as originally described by Lillehei which is now is the routine procedure in most pancreas transplant centers.

In 1992, systemic venous drainage which was done through anastomosis of the portal vein to recipient iliac veins was replaced by direct portal drainage by Rosenlof et al (Rosenlof LK, et al, 1992) and also Shokouh-Amiri et al (Shokouh-Amiri MH, et al, 1992) because of its more physiologic pattern of insulin delivery. Now during the modem era of immunosuppression, the whole pancreas transplantation technique with portal - enteric drainage became the gold standard for simultaneous pancreas and kidney transplantation (SPK), and even for pancreas after kidney (PAK) or pancreas transplantation alone (PTA) and as of December 31, 2004, 23,043 pancreas transplants were reported to the international pancreas transplant registry (IPTR) of whom over 60% were performed in the united states.

3. Indications for pancreas transplantation

Patients with type 1 or insulin dependent type 2 diabetes mellitus are eligible for pancreas transplantation when they have any major complications of their disease, but because of complications of this type of surgery and need for lifetime immunosuppression therapy and frequent interventional surveillance (such as protocol biopsies), both the clinicians and the patients should be aware of those conditions that really might benefit from pancreas transplantation. Most common indications are as follows: diabetic nephropathy, retinopathy, neuropathy, disabling or life threatening hypoglycemic unawareness or incapacitating emotional or clinical problems associated with insulin therapy (White et al, 2009). Some of the rare indications (which are not accepted by all transplant surgeons) are diabetic complications after total pancreatectomy, presence of other autoimmune diseases, insulin allergy or resistance to subcutaneous insulin.

Patients should be considered as potential candidate for pancreas transplantation only when their morbidity or mortality risk of the surgical procedure or long term immunosuppressive treatment are lower than the diabetic complications (Meloche RM, 2007). Unfortunately, most patients with chronic diabetes who develop these complications have major comorbidities such as obesity, cardiovascular, cerebrovascular or peripheral vascular diseases, diabetic gastropathy, and vascular or neuropathic diabetic foot. These patients are most suitable for pancreatic islet cell transplantation which is very simpler and has fewer and more minor complications that the relatively complex surgical procedure of whole pancreas transplantation.

Patients with diabetic nephropathy who need concomitant renal transplantation are the most common eligible patients who benefits from simultaneous kidney pancreas transplantation (SPK). Those who previously underwent kidney transplantation are candidate for pancreas after kidney (PAK) transplantation. According to 2004 annual IPTR report (The University of Minnesota, modified on May 28, 2009, available from www.iptr.umn.edu/annual_reports/2004_annual_report/3_txs_cat/home.html) pancreas transplant alone (PTA) now performed in less than 5% of all pancreas transplant recipients because unlike SPK or PAK recipients they don't otherwise need immunosuppression for their renal allograft and surgical complications of this procedure and higher rejection rate of this type of operation outweigh the potential benefits of glycemic control. PTA is best appropriate for those patients with hypoglycemic unawareness, stable renal function, and minimum proteinuria (White et al, 2009), because calcineurin inhibitor immunosuppressive therapy reduces the glomerular filtration rate at least 20% in the first year after pancreas transplantation (Mazur et al, 2004) PAK transplantation is performed mostly in patients who have an appropriate living donor for kidney graft and also are simultaneously candidate for pancreas transplantation. When coordinate logistics available, these operation using kidney graft from the living donor and pancreas graft from a deceased donor may be performed at the same time and at the same center. In some centers partial segmental pancreas transplantation technique is used for SPK when the living donor is suitable for this complex procedure firstly performed by Merkel in 1973 (Merkel et al, 1973).

The contraindications for pancreas transplantation are the same as other types of transplantations (Tiong & Krishnamurthi, 2011): active infections, coronary angiographic evidence of significant non-correctable or untreatable coronary artery disease, recent myocardial infarction, ejection fraction below 30%, history of recent, incompletely treated malignancy (excluding non-melanoma skin cancer), positive HIV serology, positive hepatitis B surface antigen serology, substance abuse, major ongoing psychiatric illness, recent history of noncompliance, inability to provide informed consent, any systemic illness that would severely limit life expectancy or compromise recovery, significant, irreversible hepatic or pulmonary dysfunction. In major pancreas transplant centers like University of Wisconsin, Minnesota, correctable (by stenting, angioplasty or bypass) coronary artery disease is not considered as a contraindication for pancreas transplantation (Sollinger HW, et al, 2009). Most pancreas transplant programs exclude patients older than 45-50 years of age, because higher age is an independent risk factor for predicting poorer surgical outcome, although the rejection rate is significantly lower in this age group (Gruessner AC & Sutherland DE, 2005).

4. Surgical aspects of pancreas graft procurement from the deceased donor

Not all deceased donors are suitable for pancreas graft procurement. Absolute contraindications for pancreas donation are active infection or malignancy, positive serologic evaluation for hepatitis B surface antigen (HBsAg), hepatitis C virus (HCV), human immunodeficiency virus (HIV), and human T cell lymphotropic virus type 1 (HTLV-1), proved diabetes mellitus, pancreatitis (acute/chronic), severe pancreatic steatosis or edema, previous pancreatic surgery and intra-abdominal sepsis. Donor hyperglycemia is common because of stress condition and use of high dose corticosteroids and not a contraindication for use of the pancreas, although it may contribute as a minor risk factor for long-term graft loss (Gores, et al, 1992). Most surgeons only select younger non-obese donors (age 10-50 years, weight 30-100 kg) who are hemodynamically stable without need to high doses of vasopressors. Also a cardiocerebrovascular cause of brain death and massive volume resuscitation are other risk factors for postoperative complications in the recipients (Troppmann C, 2004). Because of these stringent criteria, according to IPTR report, in the United States only 21% of the deceased donor pancreata were used for transplantation during the year 2004. Because pancreas transplantation is not life saving, procurement of other donor organs are more important. If the surgeon considers that the pancreas is not suitable for transplantation it may be used for research or pancreas islet cell transplantation (Shapiro, et al, 2000).

The procedure starts with a long midline incision from suprasternal notch to symphysis pubis area usually by the liver team. All intrathoracic and abdominal organs are evaluated systematically to rule out any suspicious lesion. First, all usual dissections for controlling supraceliac and infrarenal aorta, arc of thoracic aorta and superior or inferior mesenteric vein should be performed, so in case that patient becomes unstable the surgeon can rapidly proceed with cold perfusion of the organs for their safe retrieval. The right colon is completely mobilized from retroperitoneum and then an extended Kocher maneuver is done. All ligaments of the liver are transected and then arterial anatomy of the liver and pancreas is evaluated by palpating the hepatic artery pulsation in the hepatodudenal portion of lesser omentum. The surgeon should have complete knowledge of hepatic artery abnormalities and possibility of existence of a right accessory or right replaced hepatic artery that originate from superior mesenteric artery. In rare cases the entire hepatic artery are originated from superior mesenteric artery. With novel microsurgical techniques none of these anomalies is considered as a contraindication for concomitant liver, pancreas or small intestinal harvesting from a deceased donor. It's better to perform a dissection of the supraduodenal area to reveal the anatomy of common hepatic artery, gastroduodenal and celiac trunk branches specially the origin of the splenic artery. The other dissections may be performed after cold perfusion. The common bile duct is divided and infrarenal aorta and superior or inferior mesenteric vein are cannulated at the next stage. Supraceliac aorta is clamped 3-5 minutes after systemic heparinization and the heart team also clamps the aortic arc and cold perfusion is started.

The most commonly used solutions for cold perfusion are Belzer University of Wisconsin (UW), histidine - tryptophan - ketoglutarate (HTK) and Celsior solution with no significant difference in the results when cold ischemia time is less than 12 hours, but UW is the standard solution in most centers (Fridell et al, 2010).
The donor blood evacuated through the supradiaphragmatic or in some certain cases (such as history of previous thoracic surgery) infrarenal inferior vena cava (IVC). After removing the heart and lungs, liver, pancreas and small intestine usually are procured en bloc and the remaining dissection may be performed in the bench procedure. The duodenal lumen is irrigated by 500 ml of 20% Betadine, 50 mg/ml amphotericin B and metronidazole solution through the nasogastric tube and distal and proximal part are transected by gastrointestinal (GIA) staplers. The portal vein is divided 1 cm to 2 cm above the pancreas border. The gastroduodenal artery is divided and suture ligated and the splenic artery is divided close to its origin and marked by a nonabsorbable 6-0 suture for future identification. The base of mesentery at the inferior border of pancreas is transected by another GIA stapler and the whole pancreas-duodenum-spleen graft removed.
In back table or bench procedure, all excessive fat tissue and spleen should be removed and the origin of mesentery and all small arterial and venous branches in the inferior border of pancreas is reinforced again for future hemostasis. Duodenum is shortened again and reinforced in both distal and proximal side by non-absorbable sutures. Arterial reconstruction is performed by anastomosis of the donor iliac Y-graft, external and internal iliac branches to the graft superior mesenteric and splenic artery, respectively. We also recommend using a small segment of donor left gastric or inferior mesenteric artery for reperfusion of gastroduodenal artery for better circulation of duodenum and head of pancreas to prevent future frequent duodenal ulcers in the graft.

5. Current surgical techniques for pancreas transplantation

Forty five years after the first SPK, controversy continues regarding the site of both venous effluent and exocrine drainage and also many other aspects in this complex surgical procedure. In most centers, SPK is performed separately by two teams. During kidney transplant procedure, the pancreas team prepares the pancreas graft for transplantation. Usually an intraperitoneal approach is used by a long midline incision and the kidney graft is transplanted by standard technique to left iliac fossa (renal artery to internal or external iliac artery and then renal vein to external iliac vein and at last ureter to the bladder or native ureter as described in other chapters of this book). Use of right side for pancreas transplantation is recommended due to more superficial iliac artery position in this side, which makes arterial anastomosis easier. The next step is arterial or venous reconstruction. Except for a few minor changes in arterial reconstruction technique (such as reperfusion of gastroduodenal artery or changing the site of arterial inflow), there is no significant change in the arterial reconstruction technique during these era. There are at least 2 options for venous drainage: systemic or portal drainage. It's better to reconstruct the venous drainage before arterial anastomoses because a short portal vein of the graft may limit the later maneuvers needs for venous anastomosis. In our center we use the recipient superior mesenteric vein at the base of mesentery below the transverse mesocolon for venous outflow(portal drainage) and right common iliac artery for arterial inflow to the donor iliac Y-graft. Those surgeons that prefer to use systemic venous drainage use the right external or common iliac vein as the venous outflow, perfectly as the same manner that they used external iliac artery and vein for kidney transplantation. After completing the arterial and venous anastomoses, the graft is reperfused and complete hemostasis is done. Usually despite every effort for complete hemostasis during back table preparing of the pancreas graft, there is brisk bleeding around the borders of the graft at the time of reperfusion and crystalloid and blood product replacement should be used to prevent hypotension and subsequent damage to the kidney and pancreas grafts. Graft splenectomy is done at this stage by some surgeons. The next step is anastomosis of the graft duodenum to the recipient jejunum (enteric drainage) or bladder (bladder drainage). When portal drainage is chosen, the pancreas head should be directed cephalad and use of bladder drainage is almost impossible and vice versa. In other words, if the surgeon selects bladder drainage for duct management (as is the case for most PTA surgeries), the pancreas head should be directed caudad and use of portal venous drainage won't be possible. Also if portal drainage is used we need a rather longer donor common iliac artery or even an extension graft for arterial reconstruction of the graft.

Drains are inserted at the end of operation around the kidney and pancreas graft separately to monitor for postoperative bleeding and leakages. We prefer to perform the kidney transplant operation retroperitoneally in the left iliac fossa and at the end use the peritoneum to hide the kidney to be able to monitor the kidney graft complications such a urine leakage and lymphocele s1eparately from the pancreas graft.

It is worthwhile to describe briefly about the evolution of these techniques in the leading center of pancreas transplantation in the world, University of Minnesota (Sutherland DE, 2001). For pancreas graft duct management they used many techniques during this long term period: a cutaneous graft duodenostomy, open duct free intraperitoneal drainage, duct occlusion (simple ligation or polymer-injection), enteric drainage (ED) and urinary drainage (bladder and only 4 cases to the ureter). Except for ED and bladder drainage (BD), the other techniques of duct management were used only in the early years of pancreas transplantation evolution in a small portion of their cases because of their recognized complications and now they (along with most other pancreas centers around the world) lose their early enthusiasm to BD technique because of its chronic complications such as hyperchloremic metabolic acidosis, dehydration, chemical cystitis and urethritis, recurrent hematuria, bladder stones, and recurrent graft pancreatitis, recurrent urinary tract infections, urethral stricture and perineal excoriations (Han DJ & Sutherland DE, 2010). They recommended using BD for duct management because they could monitor the graft function by serial measurement of urinary amylase and they had showed that decrease in urinary amylase always preceded hyperglycemia as a manifestation of rejection in pancreas grafts. For SPK bladder drainage transplants, monitoring of urine amylase was less important to detect rejection because a serum creatinine elevation usually preceded a urine amylase decline when the rejection episode affected both organs. In the past, severe complications would lead to conversion of BD to ED in up to 25% of patients within 10 years (Sollinger HW, et al, 1992). Enteric drainage also has many complications (at least risk of enteric contamination) that may be devastating in case of duodenal necrosis and gastrointestinal leakage.

Several options are available for enteric drainage: side-to-side duodenojejunostomy, or duodenojejunostomy with a Roux-en-Y limb and duodenoduodenostomy (Hummel et al, 2008). The site of duodenojejunostomy (distance from the Treitz ligament) and its length are different between authors. Although duodenoduodenostomy complications are more dangerous but endoscopic biopsy and hemostasis of duodenal ulcers of the transplanted pancreas-duodenum complex will be made feasible by this technique.

Systemic venous drainage is technically less demanding and used with less difficulty and more frequently by those surgeons who are familiar with kidney transplantation technique. In the early days of pancreas transplantation in the University of Minnesota, portal venous drainage was used for the pancreas graft venous effluent only in seven cases. Systemic hyperinsulinemia caused by systemic drainage first was showed by Diem et al (Diem et al, 1990). This concept lead Rosenlof et al (Rosenlof LK, et al, 1992) and Shokouh-Amiri et al (Shokouh-Amiri MH, et al, 1992) to recommend routine use of portal drainage for SPK transplants in 1992 because of its more physiologic pattern of insulinemia, although the carbohydrate metabolism is not different in both groups some authors showed that de-novo hyperinsulinemia predisposes to accelerated atherosclerosis (Fontbonne A, et al, 19991) and increasing the level of low density lipoprotein(LDL) (Hughes TA , et al, 1995) but its relevance to pancreas transplant recipients is not certain.

Some centers now use extra- or retroperitoneal approaches for better accessibility of the pancreas graft for postoperative routine percutaneous biopsies and easier arterial anastomosis and some of them suggest using an en bloc kidney-pancreas transplantation from the same donor. The technique of retroperitoneal pancreas transplantation with portal-enteric drainage was first described by Boggi et al in 2005 (Boggi et al, 2005). This method may be used in patient with severe intraperitoneal adhesions due to multiple previous abdominal surgeries and also for pancreas retransplant. Kahn et al described the same technique by systemic venous drainage (Kahn et al, 2008). They recommend this approach in obese patient with severe iliac artery atherosclerosis because of best exposure of the aorta and inferior vena cava by this method. In the en bloc techniques donor pancreas and left (or right kidney) is harvested en bloc in line with abdominal aorta so that the superior mesenteric, celiac artery and renal artery origins are maintained intact on the aorta and no arterial reconstruction by donor iliac artery would be needed in the back table procedure. Then the aorta could be used as the complex graft inflow conduit. Portal vein and renal vein may be anastomosed separately (Schenker P, et al, 2009) but we recommend to anastomose the graft portal vein to the left renal vein in the bench procedure, and then use the graft renal vein as the venous outflow of the graft. This will reduce the warm ischemia time by reducing the number of vascular dissections and anastomoses.

6. Immunosuppressive regimens

Unlike other solid organ transplantations, pancreas transplantation needs immunosupression for prevention of alloimmune rejection or autoimmune recurrence of diabetes mellitus even in transplant between identical twins (Sutherland DE, et al, 1984). In the early years of pancreas transplantation, only azathioprine and prednisone were used for immunosupression, but such a regimen was not adequate for prevention of rejection in PTA recipients (Sutherland et al, 2001). In the later years Minnesota antilymphocyte globulin added to this regimen for induction and maintenance immunosupression evolved to triple therapy by cyclosporine, azathioprine and prednisone. This change along with better surgical methods and better preservation of the deceased donor pancreas by UW solution resulted in better long term results of pancreas transplantation during the era of late 80's and early 90's. The pancreas rejection rate remained as high as 78% in this era (Stegall MD, et al, 1997). Gradually, cyclosporine and azathioprine were replaced by Tacrolimus

(Prograf™) and Mycophenolate mofetil (MMF, Cellcept™) during the later years and monoclonal anti T cell antibodies such as basiliximab and daclizumab added to induction immunosuppressive regimen of these patients. By use of these new regimens, risk of rejection decreased to less than 8-11% in the modern era of pancreas transplantation (Cantarovich D & Vistoli F, 2009).

The routine immunosupression regimen in most pancreas transplant centers includes a T cell depleting agent such as rabbit antithymocyte globulin (rATG or Thymoglobulin™) with a total dose of 4-12 mg/kg in divided doses, or alemtuzumab (Campath™) or an interleukin-2 receptor antagonist such as basiliximab (Simulect™) or daclizumab (Zenapax™) for induction immunosupression. We add a low dose intravenous methylprednisolone (Solumedrol™) in the day of operation to prevent allergic reactions to these agents. Unfortunately, these induction regimens only reduce the biopsy proven acute rejection (BPAR) episodes, but had no or modest effect on the patient or graft long term survival (Sutherland DE, 2009). Information about use of anti inter leukin-2 receptor antibodies are confounding. For example, Becker *et al.* found no significant differences in patient and graft survival comparing the outcomes of no induction versus daclizumab or basiliximab in 63 SPK transplant recipients receiving tacrolimus, MMF and prednisone. There was, however, a slightly higher rate of deaths due to sepsis in the anti-IL-2R induction group (Becker et al, 2006). Newer data mostly agree with the use of alemtuzumab for induction immunosuppression, without incurring a risk of increased infections or malignancies except for cytomegalovirus. (Sollinger et al, 2011) . A new randomized trial has showed that in the short term follow-up after SPK, alemtuzumab and rATG induction therapies has been similarly safe and effective but alemtuzumab is more cost-effective and has been associated with less BPAR episodes (Farney AC, et al, 2009).

For maintenance immunosupression, perhaps the best current regimen is prednisolone free or rapidly steroid tapering regimens which consist of tacrolimus and MMF combinations. Omitting the steroids from the maintenance regimens results in better wound healing and also prevents from steroid induced insulin resistance. Replacing the MMF with sirolimus has no effect on pancreas rejection rates, but had poorer long term kidney graft survival in the SPK recipients, because sirolimus accentuates the nephrotoxicity of tacrolimus (Gallon LG, et al, 2007). Tacrolimus per se had diabetogenic effects in other solid organ transplant recipients, but such an effect has not been shown in pancreas transplant recipients, may be due to more cautious use of this nephrotoxic drug in SPK recipients or use of healthier donors for pancreas transplantation (Ming CS & Chen ZH, 2007). Because of known nephrotoxicity of calcineurin inhibitors (CNIs) e.g. tacrolimus or cyclosporine, avoidance of these drugs in all pancreas transplant recipients who are potentially at risk of renal damage (SPK or PAK recipients) or future renal failure (PTA recipients) is desirable but all initial attempts with calcineurin inhibitor avoidance or minimization are less promising (Singh RP & Stratta RJ, 2008). Although newer agents such as sirolimus, everolimus, and CTLA-4 Ig are agents known to be either both nonnephrotoxic and nondiabetogenic or less so when compared with CNIs, but their impact on pancreas transplant results are not yet evaluated by randomized trials and their solitary use may be dangerous for the recipients and end up with graft loss (Cantarovich D & Vistoli F, 2009).

7. Postoperative care of pancreas transplant recipients

Perioperative care of pancreas transplant patients has no difference with any other major operation in diabetic patients. Kidney-pancreas recipients should be dilysed briefly for 1-2 hours before the operation to maintain the serum potassium below 5.5 meq/l and also to optimize the platelet function. Complete fluid removal is unnecessary. During the operation all of these patients need routine anesthesiologist monitoring with special attention to hemodynamic stability, tight control of blood sugar (to prevent both hypo- or hyperglycemia) and serum potassium, arterial blood gas and prevention of volume overload by keeping central venous pressure (CVP) around 8-10 mmHg. Ketoacidosis may be occur and should be prevented by intravenous insulin infusion if required. Sterile aseptic techniques are recommended for all venous and arterial line placements.

In kidney-pancreas recipients, usually kidney transplantation is done before the pancreas operation. During the kidney operation the patient is kept mildly volume expanded and before declamping the renal vasculature, the systolic blood pressure should be around 120 mmHg and Mannitol and furosemide should be infused as described in the other chapters of this book. Induction immunosuppressant (methylprednisolone or any types of t-cell receptor or interleukin-2 antibodies) usually started preoperatively and continued throughout the operation. Some surgeons advise to use these agents prior to declamping of vascular anastomoses.

After completion of kidney transplantation, the anesthesiologist should carefully monitor the brisk urine output and maintain it at least around 4 ml/kg/hour with appropriate fluid and electrolyte management throughout the remaining of the operation. Hypovolemia leads to acute tubular necrosis (ATN) of the renal allograft and volume overload will result in bowel and pancreas graft edema and may lead to postoperative abdominal compartment syndrome and graft dysfunction. Anticoagulation is not recommended for general kidney transplant alone recipients unless in the instance of presence of any other indications like mechanical heart valve or history of coagulopathy. But because pancreas is a low blood flow organ, especially when portal drainage is chosen as the preferred method for surgery, before clamping of the inflow veins or arteries, it's better to use systemic heparinization of the patient and we prefer to continue intravenous heparin postoperatively at least for 5 days to maintain the activated partial thromboplastin time (aPTT) around 1.5 times the normal value (between 55 - 85 seconds) to prevent graft vascular thrombosis.

After the operation the patient is transferred to transplant intensive care unit and CVP, vital signs, arterial blood gas, blood pressure, urine output and blood glucose are monitored continuously. Almost all patients are extubated in the operating room and don't need postoperative mechanical ventilation.

Kidney transplant patients usually have large urine outputs (as much as 20 liters/day) that should be replaced according to the patient fluid and electrolyte condition as discussed in the other chapters. Hypotension is usually due to intraabdominal bleeding (even in the absence of drainage from abdominal drains) or gastrointestinal bleeding from duodenal anastomosis and should be treated emergently by reexploration of the patient and fluid management. Hypertension should be avoided and treated appropriately to prevent bleeding and graft malfunction.

Oral immunosuppressive drugs (usually tacrolimus and MMF) are started after the day of operation. Prednisolone replaces intravenous methylprednisolone after 3 days by a dose of 0.5-1 mg/kg/day, but rapidly tapered to near zero during the next 4 weeks-3 months. All patients should receive prophylactic broad spectrum antibiotics for 2-5 days and most centers add antifungal drugs (such as amphotericin B or an azole derivative or caspofungin) and anti cytomegalovirus (CMV) drugs (e.g. gancyclovir) to this regimen. These protocols are different slightly among pancreas transplant centers and its better and mandatory that each physician follow the routines of her/his center to avoid and confusion in the patients and personnel and future evaluations of the center. During the first 24 hours the patient may need small doses of intravenous insulin for maintaining the blood sugar below the 200 mg/dl because of delayed graft function or use of high doses of corticosteroids but after that or in case of any unusual increase in the serum glucose level, prompt assessment of graft vascular status by Duplex ultrasound and appropriate intervention should be done emergently. We routinely monitor the graft vasculature by Duplex ultrasound at least every 12 hours for 5 days after the operation. Many other means are available for continuous monitoring of graft function besides the blood sugar and duplex scanning. Serial measurements of serum amylase and/or lipase, C-peptide, and urine amylase and protocol ultrasonographic or computerized scan (CT) guided biopsies are among them (Han DJ & Sutherland DE, 2010).

Drains should be monitored for unusual leakage or bleeding and removed as soon as possible (usually after 5 days for pancreas drains and 24 after removing the Foley catheter for perirenal drain). Nasogastric tube remains until the return of gastrointestinal function usually for at least 72 hours. A recent study has showed that omission of a nasogastric tube has been associated with earlier return of bowel function, less discomfort, and shorter length of stay (Barth RN, 2008). Ambulation of the patient is desirable in the first 24 hours after the operation to prevent deep vein thrombosis and also other known complications of bedridden patients such as atelectasis or postoperative ileus.

8. Complications of pancreas transplantation

Despite large improvements in immunosuppression and surgical techniques, the history of pancreas transplantation, unlike that of other abdominal organ transplants, has largely been shaped by its associated complications (Troppmann C, 2010). We can discuss about these complications in 3 distinct categories: surgical, infectious, immunologic and other non-immunologic. Infectious complications are not specific for pancreas transplantation and many of their aspects are in common with other solid abdominal organ transplantation and discussion about them is presented in other chapters of this book.

Surgical complications

Surgical complications now decreased to at least 8% in large series reported by experienced pancreas transplant center s around the world and most of them frequently result in graft loss and increase recipient morbidity and mortality significantly and augment transplant cost considerably (Goodman J & Becker YT, 2009). Many of the surgical complications (such as hematuria, duodenocystostomy leakage, reflux pancreatitis, etc) are unique to the bladder drainage as previously discussed. These known complications lead pancreas transplant centers to avoid from bladder drainage and use this technique only for PTA cases. Over 25% of these cases require conversion of BD to ED.

Vascular thrombosis

Vascular thrombosis has remained the most common complication of pancreas transplant procedure with a frequency of 3-10% (Gruessner AC & Sutherland DE, 2009). Other major complications include: intraabdominal bleeding, gastrointestinal bleeding, leakage (from duodenal anastomosis), pancreatitis, pancreatic necrosis, pancreatic fistula, abscess formation and other complications of any other major abdominal surgery such as atelectasis, pneumonia, deep vein thrombosis, wound infection, dehiscence, and cardiovascular problem which is common in diabetic and chronic renal failure patients.

Graft vascular thrombosis has many factors that most of them are technical because of several vascular anastomoses that needs for pancreas transplantation. Rotation during arterial reconstruction at the time of back table preparing, inadvertent intimal damage to the iliac artery Y-graft during harvesting and over inflation of the arteries during flushing are the known causes of arterial thrombosis. Higher donor age, cardiocerebrovascular cause of brain death and massive fluid resuscitation and hemodynamic instability of the donor and use of HTK as the preservation solution, especially when cold ischemia time is over 12 hours, and recipient hypercoagulable states or use of sirolimus are other important factors (Troppmann C, 2010). Venous thrombosis may be secondary to arterial thrombosis, severe pancreas rejection, and severe graft pancreatitis or may be completely technical or due to use of venous extension graft. There is no difference in the rate of graft thrombosis according to the venous drainage (systemic or portal) technique. Also PAK transplantation has been an independent risk factor for graft vascular thrombosis (Troppmann C, et al, 1996). Most centers use systemic heparinization for prevention of vascular thrombosis and continue this treatment for 5-7 days and after that change this regimen to 325 mg/day acetyl salicylic acid (ASA) or warfarin for selected cases (second transplants or confirmed hypercoagulable state), although some authors hadn't agree with this concept in the past (Sollinger HW, 1996). Usually the first sign of graft thrombosis is increasing the blood sugar level that should be promptly assessed by Duplex ultrasound. The patient may complain from abdominal pain and later abdominal tenderness will be revealed. Venous thrombosis will results in dark hematuric urine if bladder drainage had been used. Except for a few case reports most of these cases needs relaparotomy for graft removal, but if diagnosed early interventional radiologists or reanastomosis may be very rarely salvage the graft.

Leakage

Leakage from duodenojejunostomy or duodenoduodenostomy is a devastating complication of pancreas transplantation that may be associated with high morbidity and mortality, if recognized late. Because of spillage of enteric content, the patients develop signs and symptoms of peritonitis such as abdominal pain and tenderness, fever, high leukocytosis, and bilious content in abdominal drains. Sometimes this leakage is minor and the site of leakage contained by the greater omentum. Using broad spectrum antibiotics and Roux-en-Y reconstruction help more to obscuring the symptoms. In this situation, signs and symptoms may be obscure and only developing ileus, low grade fever, tachycardia and tachypnea, mild hyperglycemia, hyperamylasemia, low platelet count, will lead the surgeon to perform additional imaging studies (mostly abdominal CT scan) to diagnose this problem. The patient should be undergone exploration and in most cases the best option is graft pancreatectomy if peritonitis is diffuse or associated by multiple intraabdominal abscesses, or the patient ids unstable. Leakage from bladder drained pancreas may have milder symptoms and treated by combined bladder decompression and percutaneous drainage or conversion to enteric drainage. In cases of severe sepsis or diffuse infection, graft pancreatectomy is inevitable. Obscure leakages may be revealed as late as 2 weeks after the operation by abdominal abscess or pancreatic fistula that may be treated conservatively by percutaneous drainage, but many times the patient will prefer the graft to be removed because of the associated bothering complications such as skin excoriations by pancreas secretions. Also, pancreas fistula may be a complication of focal necrosis (due to

ischemia, rejection or infection) of the pancreas graft which communicate with the pancreatic duct or a complication of graft pancreatitis.
Many factors is contributed to anastomosis leakage, including technical errors, ischemia of the head of pancreas (due to vascular events, previous atherosclerosis of the donor, edematous duodenum at the time of reconstruction), reexploration for another causes, intraabdominal bleeding or diffuse primary peritonitis, severe acute rejections, and CMV infections. Some surgeons suggest that revascularization of the gastroduodenal artery or even the gastroepiploic artery may prevent ischemia of the head of pancreas and the duodenal C-loop (Nghiem DD, 2008 and Muthusamy ASR et al, 2008). We use this technique in every patient that the gastroduodenal artery is relatively large. This may also protect the duodenum from later ulcers and bleeding.

Pancreatitis

There is no uniformly accepted definition for graft pancreatitis, but all of the available definitions include the signs and symptoms of native pancreatitis with rising lipase and amylase, and maintained endocrine function (Troppmann C, 2010). Unfortunately these serum markers associated poorly with graft pancreatitis and may be prolong elevated after pancreas transplantation. Early pancreatitis is the result of poor graft handling, long ischemia time and preservation and reperfusion injury and may be visible during the operation, by graft edema and diffuse or focal fat necrosis around the graft. Prolonged cold ischemia time over 12 hours, use of HTK as the preservation solution and also poor donor quality are other risk factors (Han DJ & Sutherland DE, 2010). In case of bladder drained pancreas, pancreatitis may be the result of urine reflux. Most of these conditions are self limiting and adding the subcutaneous octreotide (0.1-0.2 mg every 8 hours) for 3-5 days after the operation, bowel rest and temporary total parenteral nutrition is the only treatment that needed. In rare cases it is so severe that the only option for treatment will be graft necrosectomy or pancreatectomy. In BD drained cases, the best treatment for resistant cases is conversion to enteric drainage. Rarely the cause of acute pancreatitis in these patients is CMV or other viral infections that if confirmed should be treated by gancyclovir or other antiviral agents.
Graft pancreatitis may be complicated just like the native pancreatitis with infections, pseudocysts, peripancreatic sterile fluid or pancreatic ascites, pancreatic fistula, and arterial or venous thrombosis or bleeding which should be treated accordingly.

Bleeding

Intraabdominal bleeding is relatively common after this operation. In most cases this is a technical error due to poor hemostasis of the pancreatic graft or the so many vascular anastomoses that used. Sometimes it is due to technical errors in the associated kidney transplant procedure. It may be due to heparin overdose that should be diagnosed by measurement of aPTT and if needs treated by protamine sulfate. Severe graft pancreatitis or pseudoaneurysms of the infected vascular anastomoses are another source of late abdominal bleedings in these patients that may be delayed as long as 2 weeks to several months after the operation. Early postoperative hypertension may cause transient bleeding from vascular anastomoses and through the abdominal drains that will be stopped spontaneously when the hypertension controlled appropriately with any need to reexploration.
Gastrointestinal bleeding is unique complication of enteric drainage. The site of bleeding may be duodenojejunostomy, distal jejunojejunostomy of the Roux-en-Y loop,

duodenoduodenostomy (DD) or mucosal ulcers in the graft duodenal C-loop (Nikeghbalian S, 2009) due to ischemia, rejection or CMV infection. One should rule out other sources of bleeding, such as native small bowel CMV infections, stress native gastric or duodenal ulcers by upper GI endoscopy or enteroscopy and also obscure site of bleeding such as neoplasm or angiodyplasia of the colon. If DD had been used for enteric drainage, endoscopy can be used for diagnosis and treatment. In other cases, angiography, red blood cell isotope scan, or enteroscopy may be used for diagnosis, but in most cases at last the best option is to explore the patient (Orsenigo E, et al, 2005).

Lymphocele and chylous ascites

Because of diverse perivascular dissections (around the aorta, IVC, superior mesenteric vein and iliac arteries and veins) in pancreas transplantation surgery, intraabdominal or perigraft sterile collections due to lymphorrehea are common. These collections may be so much that exit through the abdominal drains and when the patient returns on oral diet being frankly chylous. Perigraft collections are one of the causes of graft dysfunction and should be drains percutaneously. Chylous ascites is usually self-limiting and therapy is only supportive (replacing the fluid and electrolytes and use of oral short chain fatty acids and removing the drains to prevent lymphocyte and protein depletion. The best treatment is prevention by meticulous dissections and ligation of all perivascular lymphatics during the dissections.

Immunologic complications

Acute rejection

Rejection of the pancreas graft is as much as 40 % in the past and pancreas transplant recipients receive the highest level of immunosuppressant drugs among other abdominal organ transplantations. One-year rates of rejection have steadily decreased and are currently in the 10–20% range depending on case mix and immunosuppressive regimen (Singh RP &Strata RJ, 2008). The highest rate of graft loss due to immunologic rejection is seen in PTA recipients and the lowest incidence is in SPK patients, probably due to immunologic protective effect of the renal graft or earlier diagnosis of the rejections with better response to therapy. In the era that BD pancreas transplant was a routine the best indicators of pancreas transplant rejection was decreasing urine amylase and lipase which was preceded by hyperglycemia. In other words, BD experience showed that pancreas exocrine function is affected sooner that its endocrine function and when hyperglycemia presents it would be too late to salvage the pancreas from acute rejection. In the SPK patient, increasing the serum creatinine due to rejection usually preceded the hyperglycemia, and then diagnosis of the renal graft rejection actually means the pancreas rejection as well and both can treated simultaneously by the same antirejection treatment except for rare instances. Nowadays, with increasing experience, protocol percutaneous pancreas biopsies are routine procedure in the armamentarium of any major pancreas transplant unit. By these timely scheduled biopsies, every pancreas rejection could be diagnosed before its clinical and paraclinical symptoms present but until now the controversies continued about the candidates and interval of this time of protocol biopsies for the surveillance of pancreas graft rejection (Gaber LW, 2007).

It's shown that HLA mismatch is a major contributor to pancreas rejection and fully HLA matched recipients has the lowest levels of rejections when on the same immunosuppressive protocol (Burke, et al, 2004). Other series showed that combination immunosuppressive therapy including T-cell depleting antibodies for induction, tacrolimus and MMF could improve the outcome significantly, even in poorly HLA matched PTA recipients (Gruber

SA, et al, 2000). However, in the PTA and PAK categories, HLA matching has remained an important outcome factor (Han DJ & Sutherland DE, 2010).
Signs and symptoms of pancreas rejection are obscure. Only 5-20% of patients developed mild fever, abdominal pain or distension or sometimes ileus or diarrhea (Sutherland DE, et al, 2010). The clinicians should be rely on paraclinical markers and after performing the biopsy the best approach is to treat empirically when a combination of paraclinical changes support existence of an acute rejection episode, if the results of the biopsy prepare with delay. The best treatment for confirmed acute rejection episodes is the use of pulse methylprednisolone therapy plus increasing the dose of oral drugs or adding the sirolimus to the previous drugs. Nephrotoxicity and diabetogenic effect of tacrolimus, and effect of corticosteroids on insulin resistance induction should be in mind. In severe cases use of thymoglobulin or other T-cell depleting antibodies may be required. As previously described many immunosuppressive protocol are under investigation now to better prevent these acute rejection episodes which most of them focused on corticosteroid spring and also use of T-cell depleting antibodies for induction.

Chronic rejection

Previously, chronic rejection does not appear to be as large a problem for pancreas-transplant recipients as it does for renal-transplant recipients (Hopt UT & Drognitz O, 2000). As the number of pancreas transplants surviving beyond the first year increases, chronic rejection is becoming increasingly common (Burke, et al, 2004). The rate of pancreas loss to chronic rejection was 8.8% in 914 pancreas transplants followed for 3 years. Chronic rejection was highest in the PAK (11.6%) and PTA (11.3%) and lowest for SPK (3.7%)(Humar A ,et al, 2003). The most important pathologic changes in chronic rejection are replacing the pancreas tissue with fibrous band with distortion of architecture and loss of acini (Gaber LW, 2007). The severity of chronic rejection is not correlated well to the graft loss, but clinically the patients become hyperglycemic, first with response to oral hypoglycemic agents and then low dose insulin injection an at last completely depend on insulin injection for the rest of their lives. There's no definite treatment for this type of rejection, which may be simply a non-immunologic "physiologic wear and tear "of the organ, but some authors try to use sirolimus in these conditions (Matias P, et al 2008).

Non-immunologic complications

One the known complications of every solid organ transplant is primary nonfunction or delayed graft function. Primary non-function is a definition of inclusion. No other cause of graft nonfunction should be found, e.g. graft vascular thrombosis, graft necrosis, or severe acute rejections or pancreatitis. In this condition the graft is viable and non-inflamed with no need for pancreatectomy, but no insulin secretion is found and the patient needs insulin injection as his/she preoperative situation. Some patients transiently need low doses of insulin for their blood glucose hemostasis, but after a maximum of 1 week this requirement decreased to zero. This condition is named "delayed graft function". In both of this condition no frank anatomic or pathologic changes in the graft is found in the postoperative assessment of the patient. Poor donor quality and poor handling of the graft is the only causes that may contribute to these conditions.
Other non surgical and non-immunologic complications also may be seen in these diabetic patients. Many of these are due to preoperative diabetic complications. Delayed gastric emptying (gastroparesis), constipation or diarrhea, dizziness and lightheadedness (all due to autonomic neuropathy), peripheral neuropathy, poor visual acuity (accelerated

retinopathy)and accelerated cataract are among these complications. Many of these diabetic signs and symptoms are multifactorial and side effects of the immunosuppressant drugs and multiple other antifungals and antivirals that used for these patients plus preoperative poor diabetic control accelerates them. Every effort should be used to diagnose the treatable causes and treat them accordingly. For example for diabetic gastroparesis, use of erythromycin or domeperidone has been moderately successful (Zaman f, et al, 2004). Intractable diarrhea may be due to CMV or other microbial or protozoal infections which should be treated. But when no known cause is found, the best treatment is dividing the dose o MMF to 4 times a day and also use of subcutaneous octreotide. Also every transplant team member should be completely remember the common complications of the immunosuppressive drugs and treat them appropriately or change the drugs if possible.

9. Long term results of pancreas transplantation

Long term results of pancreas transplantation improve day by day with better surgical experience and use of more potent immunosuppressive regimen. Pancreas graft 1 year survival rate improves from 75% in 1998 to 85% at the end of 2003 for SPK cases, and from 55 to 77% for PAK and from 45 to 77% in PTA patients (Gruessner AC & Sutherland DE, 2005). This improvement also is seen in PTA patients that traditionally have the worst outcome, as shows in many studies. For example in a report Stratta et al. by 1 year patient and graft survival has increased to 96% and 86%, respectively (Stratta RJ, et al, 2003). In one the largest recently published studies, the 5-year, 10-year, and 20-year patient survival for SPK recipients was 89, 80, and 58%, respectively (Wai PY & Sollinger HW, 2011).
Now, by decreasing the technical failures, the randomized studies to valuate other effective factors can be performed with better accuracy and less confounding bias. Perhaps the best statistics that show the effect of pancreas transplantation is the statistics about comparing the patient survival in kidney transplant alone recipients with SPK patients. Even in older studies, life expectancy of younger recipients (less than 50 years) of SPK is 10 years longer than diabetic patients who only received a kidney graft from deceased donors (23.4 years *vs* 12.9 years) (Tyden G, et al, 1999, Ojo AO,etal, 2001). When both grafts were procured from deceased donors, SPK transplant recipients has better survival rate than kidney transplant alone (KTA) recipients but this difference is not significant when KTA patients received their grafts from living donors. The presence of a functioning pancreas graft improved survival by 20% at 8 years (Reddy KS, 2003).
Patient survival is not statistically different according to the type of exocrine drainage (BD vs. ED), but quality of life is better and overall complications is less when BD is used (Sollinger HW, et al, 2009). Despite the improved survival, the most common type of death in these patients is death with a functioning graft and cardiovascular morbidity remains a major contributor to patient outcome in these patients (Sollinger HW, et al, 2009).
Comparing with KTA recipients, quality of life in those 95% of patient who survive after SPK transplantation is improved significantly, due to cessation of insulin injections, multiple needling for glucose monitoring and better emotional status (Sutherland De, et al, 2001 & Joseph JT, et al, 2003).

Effect on end organ damage

Pancreas transplantation improves glycemic control in long term follow up, manifested by lower hemoglobin A_{1C} level, improved lipid profile and insulin mediated protein kinetics, normal hepatic glucose production and counter-regulatory effects of glucagon to hypoglycemia (White SA, et al, 2009).

Sollinger et al suggests that despite numerous reports of improvement in secondary diabetic complications after SPK, retinopathy and cardiac or vascular complications of diabetes are not reversible and show no improvements after SPK, but severe (peripheral and autonomic) neuropathy is an exception to this rule (Sollinger et al, 2009). Diabetic retinopathy will deteriorate after pancreas transplantation in over 30% of patients if it is in an advanced proliferative phase prior to the operation, but after 3 years the pancreas transplantation results in stabilization of retinopathy progression (Chow VC, et al, 1999). Cataract is a known complication of any organ transplantation and is the results of corticosteroids and calcineurin inhibitors and may become evident after pancreas transplantation as well.

Macrovascular effects of diabetes may not improve after pancreas transplantation, especially because of calcineurin inhibitor (CNI) effect on weight gain, dyslipidemia and hypertension, and many other risk factors that are very common in diabetic patients. Also the peripheral vascular disease in diabetics is often far too advanced to reverse. Because, most centers exclude patient with Macrovascular diabetes complications and no conclusive study exists about effect of pancreas transplantation on natural history of macrovascular disease in these patients (Sutherland De, et al, 2001). Deterioration depends on the ongoing risks. Some centers show the benefits of pancreas transplantation on cerebrovascular system, but again the results are inconclusive. Coronary artery disease, diastolic function, left ventricular geometry and cardiac autonomic function may be improved after SPK comparing with KTA recipients after a few years (White SA et al, 2009).

Normoglycemia also improves the diabetic glumerulopathy (but does not reverse it) and decrease the proteinuria. On the other hand, use of CNIs per results in nephropathy and may decrease the creatinine clearance. SPK recipients may not survive enough to benefit from the effects of normoglycemia on their nephropathy. In diabetic KTA recipients, the diabetic nephropathy is progressively leading to lower kidney graft survival and many studies show that PAK transplantation may improves the kidney graft survival by prevention of accelerated diabetic glumerulopathy in these patients.). Some studies shows that PTA (if done early enough) can preserve renal function, but It takes at least 5 years until a pancreas transplant can reverse the lesions of diabetic nephropathy (Sutherland De, et al, 2001).

10. References

Barth RN, Becker YT, Odorico JS, et al. Nasogastric decompression is not necessary after simultaneous pancreas-kidney transplantation. *Ann Surg*. 2008;247:350 -356.

Becker LE, Nogueira VA, Abensur MP, *et al*. No induction versus anti-IL2R induction therapy in simultaneous kidney pancreas transplantation: A comparative analysis. Transplant Proc 2006; 38:1933–1936

Boggi U, Vistoli F, Signori S, et al: A technique for retroperitoneal pancreas transplantation with portal-enteric drainage. *Transplantation* 79:1137, 2005

Burke GW, Ciancio G, Sollinger HW: Advances in pancreas transplantation. *Transplantation*. 2004 May 15;77(9 Suppl):S62-7. Review.

Cantarovich D, Vistoli F: Minimization protocols in pancreas transplantation. *Transpl Int* 2009; 22: 61–68.

Chow VC, Pai RP, Chapman JR, et al: Diabetic retinopathy after combined kidney-pancreas transplantation. *Clin Transplant*. 1999;13:356-362.

Cohn JA, Englesbe MJ, Ads YM, et al. Financial implications of pancreas transplant complications: a business case for quality improvement. *Am J Transplant* 2007; 7:1656–1660.

Diem P, Abid M, Redmon JB, et al. Systemic venous drainage of pancreas allografts as independent cause of hyperinsulinemia in type I diabetic recipients. Diabetes 1990; 39:534 -540.

Farney AC, Doares W, Rogers J, et al: A randomized trial of alemtuzumab versus antithymocyte globulin induction in renal and pancreas transplantation. *Transplantation*. 2009 Sep 27;88(6):810-9.

Fontbonne A, Charles MA, Thibult N, et al. Hyperinsulinaemia as a predictor of coronary heart disease mortality in a healthy population: the Paris Prospective Study, 15-year follow-up. *Diabetologia* 1991 34: 356–61.

Fridell JA, Mangus RS, Powelson JA: Organ preservation solutions for whole organ pancreas transplantation. *Curr Opin Organ Transplant*. 2011; 16(1):116-122

Gaber LW: Pancreas allograft biopsies in the management of pancreas transplant recipients: histopathology review and clinical correlations. (Arch Pathol Lab Med. 2007;131:1192–1199

Gallon LG, Winoto J, Chhabra D, et al: Long-term renal transplant function in recipient of simultaneous kidney and pancreas transplant maintained with two prednisone- free maintenance immunosuppressive combinations: tacrolimus/ mycophenolate mofetil versus tacrolimus/sirolimus. *Transplantation* 2007; 83: 1324–29.

Gliedman ML, Gold M, Whittaker J, et al: Clinical segmental pancreatic transplantation with ureter-pancreatic duct anastomosis for exocrine drainage. *Surgery*. 1973;74:171–180

Goodman J, Becker YT: Pancreas surgical complications. Curr Opin Organ Transplant. 2009 Feb;14(1):85-9.

Gores PF, Gillingham KJ, Dunn DL, et al: Donor hyperglycemia as a minor risk factor and immunologic variables as major risk factors for pancreas allograft loss in a multivariate analysis of a single institution's experience. *Ann Surg* 1992; 215: 217- 30.

Gruber SA, Katz S, Kaplan B, et al. Initial results of solitary pancreas transplants performed without regard to donor/recipient HLA mismatching. *Transplantation* 2000; 70(2): 388.

Gruessner AC, Sutherland DE. Pancreas transplant outcomes for United States (US) and non-US cases as reported to the United Network for Organ Sharing (UNOS) and the International Pancreas Transplant Registry (IPTR) as of June 2004. *Clin Transplant*. 2005 Aug;19(4):433-55

Han DJ, Sutherland DE: Pancreas transplantation. *Gut Liver*. 2010; 4(4):450-65.

Hopt UT, Drognitz O. Pancreas organ transplantation: short and longterm results in terms of diabetes control. Langenbecks Arch Surg 2000; 385(6): 379.

Hughes TA, Gaber AO, Amiri HS, et al. Kidney-pancreas transplantation. The eff ect of portal versus systemic venous drainage of the pancreas on the lipoprotein composition. *Transplantation* 1995; 60: 1406–1412.

Humar A, Khwaja K, Ramcharan T, et al. Chronic rejection: the next major challenge for pancreas transplant recipients. *Transplantation.* 2003;76:918–923

Hummel R, Langer M, Wolters HH, et al: Exocrine drainage into the duodenum: a novel technique for pancreas transplantation. *Transpl Int* 21:178, 2008

Joseph JT, Baines LS, Morris MC, Jindal RM: Quality of life after kidney and pancreas transplantation: a review. *Am J Kidney Dis.* 2003 Sep; 42(3):431-45

Kahn J, Iberer F, Kniepeiss D, et al: Retroperitoneal pancreas transplantation with systemic-enteric drainage—case report. *Clin Transplant* 22:674, 2008

Kelly WD, Lillehei RC, Merkel FK, Idezuki Y, Goetz FC: Allotransplantation of the pancreas and duodenum along with the kidney in diabetic nephropathy". *Surgery* 1967:61 (6): 827–37

Lillehei RC, Ruiz JO, Aquino C, et al. Transplantation of the pancreas. *Acta Endocrinol (Copenh)* 1976; 83(suppl 205): 303.

Matias P, Araujo MR, Romão JE Jr, Abensur H, Noronha IL.: Conversion to sirolimus in kidney-pancreas and pancreas transplantation. *Transplant Proc.* 2008 Dec;40 (10):3601-5.

Mazur MJ, Rea DJ, Griffi n MD, et al: Decline in native renal function early after bladder-drained pancreas transplantation alone. *Transplantation* 2004; 77: 844–49.

Meloche RM: Transplantation for the treatment of type 1 diabetes. *World J Gastroenterol.* 2007;13(47):6347–6355.

Merkel FK, Ryan WG, Armbruster K, Seim S, Ing TS. Pancreatic transplantation for diabetes mellitus. IMJ Ill Med J 1973;144:477-479 passim.

Ming CS, Chen ZH: Progress in pancreas transplantation and combined pancreas-kidney transplantation. *Hepatobiliary Pancreat Dis Int.* 2007 Feb;6(1):17-23.

Muthusamy ASR, Tzivanakis A, Brockmann JG, et al. Revascularization of the gastroepiploic artery in pancreas transplant. *Transpl Int* 2008; 21:1194- 1195.

Nghiem DD, Corry RJ. Technique of simultaneous renal pancreatoduodenal transplantation with urinary drainage of pancreatic secretion. *Am J Surg* 1987; 153: 405–06.

Nghiem DD. Revascularization of the gastroepiploic artery in pancreas transplant. *Transplant Int* 2008; 21:774–777.

Nikeghbalian S, Bahador A, Salahi H, et al: Non-marginal donor C-loop ulcers as a cause of gastrointestinal bleeding after pancreas transplantation: three case reports. *Transplant Proc.* 2009 Sep;41(7):2930-2.

Ojo AO, Meier-Kriesche HU, Hanson JA, et al: The impact of simultaneous pancreas-kidney transplantation on long-term patient survival. *Transplantation* 2001; 71: 82- 90.

Orsenigo E, Fiorina P, Dell'Antonio G, et al: Gastrointestinal bleeding from enterically drained transplanted pancreas. *Transpl Int.* 2005 Mar;18(3):296-302.

Reddy KS, Stablein D, Taranto S, et al: Long-term survival following simultaneous kidney-pancreas transplantation versus kidney transplantation alone in patients with type 1 diabetes mellitus and renal failure. *Am J Kidney Dis* 2003; 41: 464–70.

Rosenlof LK, Earnhardt RC, Pruett TL, et al. Pancreas transplantation. An initial experience with systemic and portal drainage of pancreatic allografts. *Ann Surg.* 1992;215:586–595.

Schenker P, Flecken M, Vonend O, et al: En bloc retroperitoneal pancreas-kidney transplantation with duodenoduodenostomy using pediatric organs. *Transplant Proc.* 2009 Jul-Aug;41(6):2643-5.

Shapiro AJM, Lakey JRT, Ryan EA, et al : Islet transplantation in seven patients with type I diabetes mellitus using a glucocorticoid-free immunosuppressive regimen. *N Engl J Med* 343:230, 2000

Shokouh-Amiri MH, Gaber AO, Gaber LW, et al. Pancreas transplantation with portal venous drainage and enteric exocrine diversion: a new technique. *Transplant Proc.* 1992;24:776–777.

Singh RP, Stratta RJ: Advances in immunosuppression for pancreas transplantation *Curr Opin Organ Transplant* 13:79–84

Singh RP, Stratta RJ: Advances in immunosuppression for pancreas transplantation. *Curr Opin Organ Transplant.* 2008 Feb;13(1):79-84

Sollinger HW: Pancreatic transplantation and vascular graft thrombosis [editorial]. *J Am Coll Surg* 1996; 182:362.

Sollinger HW, Cook K, Kamps D, Glass NR, Belzer FO: Clinical and experimental experience with pancreaticocystostomy for exocrine pancreatic drainage in pancreas transplantation. *Transplant Proc* 1984; 16: 749–51.

Sollinger HW, Odorico JS, Becker YT, et al: Campath vs. basiliximab after simultaneous pancreas–kidney transplantation. *Am J Transplant* (in press).

Sollinger HW, Sasaki TM, D'Alessandro AM, et al: Indications fo enteric conversion after pancreas transplantation with bladder drainage. *Surgery* 1992; 112: 842–45.

Sollinger HW, Odorico JS, Becker YT, et al: One Thousand Simultaneous Pancreas-Kidney Transplants at a Single Center With 22-Year Follow-Up. *Ann Surg* 2009;250: 618–630

Squifflet JP, Gruessner RW, Sutherland DE: The history of pancreas transplantation: past, present and future. *Acta Chir Belg.* 2008 May-Jun;108(3):367-78.

Starzl TE, Iwatsuki S, Shaw BW, Jr, et al. Pancreaticoduodenal transplantation in humans. *Surg Gynecol Obstet.* 1984;159:265–272.

Stegall MD, Simon M, Wachs ME, Chan L, Nolan C, Kam I. Mycophenolate mofetil decreases rejection in simultaneous pancreas-kidney transplantation when combined with tacrolimus or cyclosporine. *Transplantation* 1997; 64: 1695–700.

Stratta RJ, Lo A, Shokouh-Amiri MH, et al. Improving results in solitary pancreas transplantation with portal-enteric drainage, thymoglobin induction, and tacrolimus/mycophenolate mofetil-based immunosuppression. *Transpl Int* 2003; 16(3): 154.

Sutherland DE, Goetz FC, Najarian JS: Living-related donor segmental pancreatectomy for transplantation. *Transplant Proc.* 1980;12:19–25.

Sutherland DE, Gruessner RW, Dunn DL, et al: Lessons learned from more than 1,000 pancreas transplants at a single institution. *Ann Surg.* 2001 Apr;233(4):463-501. Review.

Sutherland DE, Sibley R, Xu XZ, et al. Twin-to-twin pancreas transplantation: reversal and reenactment of the pathogenesis of type 1 diabetes. *Trans Assoc Am Physicians* 1984; 97: 80–87.

Tiong HY, Krishnamurthi V (2011): Selection and preparation of the pancreas transplant recipient. In: *Kidney and pancreas transplantation, a practical guide.* Srinivas

TR and Shoskesisbn DA, pp. 201-209, Springer science + business media, ISBN: 978-1-60761-641-2, New York

Troppmann C (2004): Surgical complications. In: *Pancreas transplantation.* Gruessner RWG, Sutherland DER, pp. 206–237, Springer, New York.

Troppmann C, Gruessner AC, Benedetti E, et al: Vascular graft thrombosis after pancreatic transplantation: univariate and multivariate operative and nonoperative risk factor analysis. *J Am Coll Surg.* 1996 Apr;182(4):285-316.

Troppmann C: Complications after pancreas transplantation. *Curr Opin Organ Transplant,* 2010;15:112–118

Tyden G, Bolinder J, Solders G, et al:Improved survival in patients with insulin-dependent diabetes mellitus and end-stage diabetic nephropathy 10 years after combined pancreas and kidney transplantation. *Transplantation* 1999; 67: 645–48.

Wai PY, Sollinger HW: Long-term outcomes after simultaneous pancreas-kidney transplant. *Curr Opin Organ Transplant.* 2011; 16(1):128–134.

White SA, Shaw JA, Sutherland DE: Pancreas transplantation. *Lancet.* 2009 May 23; 373(9677):1808-17. Review

Williams PW: Transplantation of Pancreas in Diabetes. *Br Med J* 1903;1:580

Zaman F, Abreo KD, Levine S, Maley W, Zibari GB: Pancreatic Transplantation: Evaluation and Management *J Intensive Care Med* 2004 19: 127

5

Combined Liver and Kidney Transplantation

Cláudia Fagundes and Mónica Guevara*
Liver Unit/Hospital Clinic Barcelona
Spain

1. Introduction

Combined liver and kidney transplant (CLKT) is the procedure of choice for patients with both liver and kidney end-stage-disease. In addition, patients with polycystic liver or kidney disease or with hyperoxaluria, or those with cirrhosis and acute renal failure, including hepatorenal syndrome receiving hemodialysis (HD) for more than two months, may also benefit of CLKT.

The decision to transplant both, the liver and kidney, is more difficult in cases when kidney dysfunction may be temporary. Hepatorenal syndrome is a potentially reversible renal failure caused by advance liver disease. Currently, the treatment of choice of hepatorenal syndrome is liver transplant alone and not a combined liver/kidney transplant.

The model for end-stage liver disease (MELD) replaced the United Network for Organ Sharing status classification for the allocation of liver organs. Due to the heavily weighted serum creatinine value in the calculation of the MELD score, candidates with renal failure have received organs more rapidly. As a result there has been considerable increase in number of combined liver-kidney transplants in the past few years.

The reason to propose both liver and kidney transplant for patients with cirrhosis and renal failure relays on the negative impact that renal failure has on patients submitted to liver transplant alone (LTA). Results of several studies show that renal failure in patients with chronic liver disease is associated with high mortality and morbidity after liver transplant alone. Nevertheless, it's very hard to identify a cut-off point of renal dysfunction that determines those patients who may benefit from combined liver and kidney transplant instead of liver transplant alone.

In this chapter, we will review the main points to be considered when evaluating candidates for combined liver kidney transplant, as well as some concerns that have not been yet clarified.

2.Assessment of renal function and evaluating of CLKT in patients with end stage liver disease

Renal failure in cirrhotic patients is associated with poor prognosis. It is well known that cirrhotic patients with renal failure have decreased survival when compared to patients

* corresponding author. Associate Investigator. IDIBAPS

with normal renal function. This negative effect is also evident when these patients undergo liver transplantation, as shown by reduced graft and patient survival.

Ideally, patients with a high probability of developing end stage renal disease after liver transplantation alone should receive a combination of liver and kidney transplant. However, is still a great challenge to identify these patients who are at higher risk.

The presence and the severity of pretransplant kidney failure are factors independently associated with postoperative sepsis, need for renal replacement therapy and poor graft and patient outcomes.

In addition to the degree of renal dysfunction, duration and cause of renal failure should also be considered when evaluating candidates for liver transplantation alone or combined liver kidney transplantation.

Patients with pretransplant renal dysfunction (defined as pretransplant Scr > 1.5mg/dL) for a period longer than 12 weeks showed higher probability of progression to end-stage renal disease at 3 years post transplant. However in this study the etiology of renal dysfunction was not specified, mainly due to the authors concern of potential bias in classifying renal failure in absence of kidney biopsy.

Renal failure is usually defined by a reduction in glomerular filtration rate (GFR) that can be acute when it occurs in hours to weeks or chronic when it occurs gradually over time.

Currently, serum creatinine remains the most widely used method to assess renal function in cirrhotic patients.

However, patients with liver dysfunction have reduced creatinine production secondary to loss of muscle mass, and therefore, in those patients serum creatinine usually overestimates renal function. As the Cockroft-Gauld and MDRD (Modification of Diet in Renal Disease) formulas are based on serum creatinine concentration, adjusted by race, age, sex and weight, they also overestimate renal function in patients with cirrhosis and should not be used in clinical settings.

In this context, cystatin C has emerged as an option for evaluate renal function since its level is not influenced by muscle mass. Nevertheless, its value has not been well established and is not available as standart test.

More accurate methods, such as determination of inulin clearance or radionuclide markers, represent the gold standard for measuring glomerular filtration rate. Indeed, its use in daily attendance is not feasible, because of its complexity, making repeated measurements that these patients often require difficult. These gold standard methods should be indicated for selected patients when there is a need to accurately assess renal function to decide between performing liver transplantation alone or CKLT. Their routinary use, however, is not mandatory.

Beyond the degree of renal function, the etiology of renal failure should be assessed, as prognosis varies according to the cause of renal failure. In a recent study with a large population of hospitalized patients with cirrhosis, the most common cause of renal failure was due to bacterial infections (46%), followed by hypovolemia (32%), hepatorenal syndrome (13%) and intrinsic nephropathy (9%). Patients with HRS and bacterial infections had lower 3-month survival compare to patients with intrinsic nephropathy. Even though patients with intrinsic nephropathy present better survival among all causes of renal failure in cirrhosis, its chronic form of renal failure has a non-reversible character and are most likely to receive CKLT.

The diagnostic diagram of etiology of renal failure include a complete medical history and physical examination, searching for presence of diabetes and/or hypertension as well as any other evidence of organ damage. Laboratory evaluation should include urinalysis to seek for signs of intrinsic nephropathy, like hematuria, pyuria, cell and granular casts, and 24h urine collection to assess protein excretion.

In addition to urine test, a renal ultrasonography, is useful in evaluating preexisting renal disease. Findings such as alteration of renal echogenicity and reductions in the size of the kidneys indicate the existence of chronic kidney disease.

Finally, a definitive diagnostic may require the realization of a renal biopsy, which may also give prognostic information. In patients with intrinsic nephropathy, marked tubulointerstitial injury is associated with progression to end stage renal disease, even if the primary disease is a glomerulopathy. Among histological findings, the degree of tubular interstitial fibrosis is the most powerful predictor of subsequent progression of renal impairment. There are very limited data on renal biopsies findings in cirrhotic patients. A study evaluated 23 kidney biopsies performed in liver transplant candidates with renal failure of unknown etiology or persisted HRS (> 4 weeks) demonstrated a variety of pathologic findings. These included menbranoproliferative glomerulopathy, IgA nephropathy, diabetes nephropathy and acute tubular necrosis. Of note, 4 patients showed normal histology. In this study CLKT was recommended for 10 of 26 patients with > 40% global glomeruloesclerosis, > 30% of interstitial fibrosis or severe glomerular ischemia/injury. Although these histological criteria have not been evaluated in further studies in patients with cirrhosis, it suggests that renal histopathology changes may alter therapeutic management, including the need for combined liver and kidney transplant.

Therefore according to a recent consensus, a renal biopsy should be performed in patients with an estimated glomerular filtration rate less than 30ml/min with a chronic course .The decision to perform a transjugular or percutaneous renal biopsy should take into account professional experience and patient's clinical conditions, mostly platelet count and coagulation parameters.

Hepatorenal syndrome is a form of kidney failure that is secondary to a severe circulatory disorder in patients with cirrhosis. This particular complication of liver disease can be potentially reversible with the combination of systemic vasoconstrictors and intravenous albumin. Even though the definite treatment of this severe condition remains liver transplantation, the importance of pre-liver transplantation treatment should not be underestimate. Patients with HRS treated with systemic vasoconstrictors and albumin before liver transplantation and pretransplant serum creatinine inferior to 1.5 mg/dL had a three year survival similar to patients transplanted with normal renal function.

Finally, the current criteria to perform CLKT according to the consensus conference is shown in table 1.

1. Evidence of chronic kidney disease and renal biopsy demonstrating more than 30% of glomeruloesclerosis or 30% of interstitial fibrosis.
2. If the biopsy is not possible, the decision is made based on *National Kidney Foundation* criteria for chronic kidney disease, which is an eGFR less than 30ml/min for more than 3 months.
3. Patients with end stage renal disease in renal replacement therapy
4. Patients with hepatorenal syndrome or acute kidney injury with creatinine greater or equal to 2.0 mg/dL and on dialysis for more than 8 weeks.

Table1. Indications for combined liver kidney transplant in patients with end stage liver disease.

3. Evaluation of candidates for CLKT in patients with end stage renal Disease (ESRD)

The benefit of combined liver kidney transplantation is not well established for patients with compensated cirrhosis and ESRD. The decision to perform CLKT or only a liver transplant is matter of debate. In a study of patients with chronic hepatitis C on RRT who underwent kidney transplantation alone, the degree of liver fibrosis correlated with patient and graft survival at 3 years .It is recommended that patients with chronic liver disease and ESRD who are candidates for kidney transplantation should be sought for the presence of significant liver fibrosis and cirrhosis. These patients should be submitted to transjugular liver biopsy with assessment of hepatic venous pressure gradient(HVPG). Patients with cirrhosis and/or clinical significant portal hypertension, determined by an HVPG greater than 10mmHg should be referred to CLKT. The option of kidney transplantation alone should be offered for those patients without these characteristics. Even though most of the data regarding these situations comes from patients with cirrhosis due to hepatitis C, the recommendations are generally applied to all patients irrespective of etiology of cirrhosis.

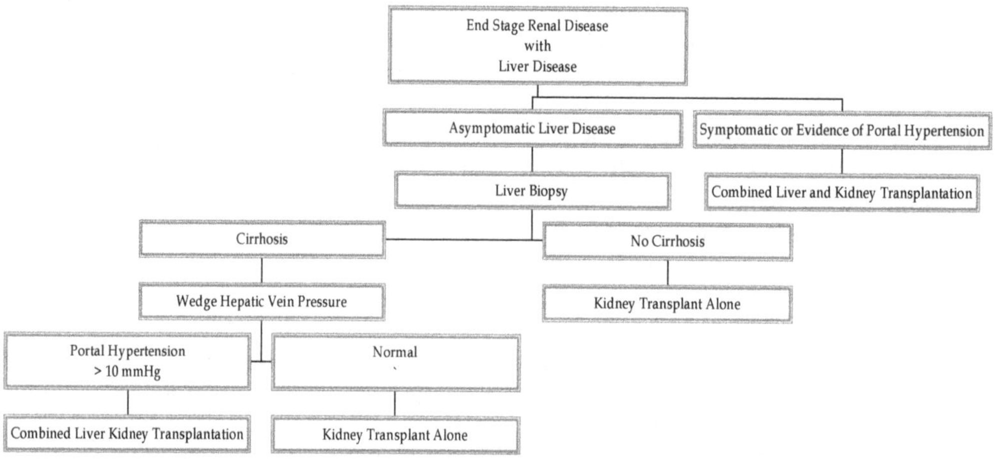

Fig. 1. Diagram for End Stage Renal Disease and Liver Disease (adapted from Consensus Conference on Simultaneous Liver Kidney Transplantation).

4. Outcomes in combined liver and kidney transplantation

Cirrhosis may not be the only indication for CKLT. In a large series of 3520 patients evaluated between 1984-2008, the main indications for combined liver kidney transplantation were: hiperoxaluria type 1 (42.7%), liver cirrhosis and chronic renal failure (23.5%), polycystic liver and kidney disease (15.5%), liver cirrhosis with hepatorenal syndrome (7.1%) and end stage liver disease with renal failure of unknown cause (6%).

Hence, prognosis and outcomes of combined liver kidney transplantation are not well known because most of the data came from series that include patients treated with CLKT not only with end stage liver disease but also patients with inherited diseases without cirrhosis.

In recent years, MELD score has increasingly been used for liver allocation. Due to the presence of serum creatinine in the formula of MELD score, candidates with renal failure are more likely to receive a liver graft. Although pre transplant renal failure is associated with poor outcomes in liver transplantation settings, this modification on organ allocation system was not followed by changes in survival. The 3-year survival of liver transplant recipients remained almost unchanged when compared pre and pos-MELD era (81% vs. 80%, respectively).

A large case-control study compared the outcomes of patients submitted to liver transplant alone with or without renal failure to combined liver kidney transplants (CKLT) between 1987 and 2006. After adjusting for multiple donor (age, race, cause of death) and recipient (MELD, dialysis status at time of transplant) characteristic's, recipients of CLKT had a similar one-year survival compared to liver transplant alone (82 vs. 81.8%). However, the degree of renal failure in both groups was not described. The only subgroup in which CLKT had benefit on survival was in patients on long-term pre transplant hemodialysis (defined as a period equal to or greater than 12 weeks). In this subgroup, CKLT recipients had a higher survival than those submitted to liver transplantation alone (84.5% vs. 70.8%, P=0.008).

Another study demonstrated that patients on hemodialysis prior to transplantation had a significantly higher 1-year survival for CLKT group when compared to LT alone (79.4% vs. 73.7%, p=0.004). This difference, however, was not observed when only patients with renal failure (defined by serum creatinine ≥ 2.5 mg/dL) not on dialysis where analyzed. In this subgroup, 1-year survival was similar for patients who received CLKT or liver transplant alone (81% vs.78.8%, p= n.s.). An important issue to highlight is that patients receiving CLKT, either on hemodialysis or not, had better liver function at the time of transplant compared to those receiving liver transplantation alone. Mean MELD score of patients receiving LTA or CKLT was 36 vs. 31 for recipients on hemodialysis, and 34 vs. 28 for those with renal failure (serum creatinine >2.5 mg/dl) but not on hemodialysis (p<0.01 for both comparisons).

Most studies of survival in combined liver kidney transplantation analyzed a very heterogeneous population respect to the etiology of liver transplantation. Though, a recent study that only included patients with cirrhosis and chronic kidney disease, showed a 1-year survival lower for patients treated with CKLT compared to liver transplant alone group (80 vs. 97%, p=0.014). The probability of survival at 3 years was also lower in the CLKT group, but the difference between both groups did not reach statistical significance (75% and 88%, respectively). The incidence of complications was also higher for CKLT. Patients with CLKT had a higher incidence of bacterial infections and transfusions requirements compared to LTA group. Nevertheless, the comparison group (liver transplant alone) did not present renal failure at the time of transplant (mean serum creatinine value of 0.96±0.27 mg/dL), because all patients with cirrhosis and advanced chronic kidney disease (defined by a glomerular filtration rate below 30ml/min) were considered candidates for CLKT.

Another important point is the potential reversibility of renal failure after liver transplantation. As mentioned previously, patients with HRS should be treated to reverse the renal failure before liver transplantation. Many of these patients, however, do not respond to treatment and eventually undergo CKLT. Only a few single-center series had described outcomes of patients with hepatorenal syndrome submitted to CLKT. One of them compared the results of patients with HRS on hemodialysis who received CLKT (n=22, median time of pretransplant hemodialysis of 41 days) to those with HRS on hemodialysis who received liver transplant alone (n=80, pretransplant hemodialysis time inferior to 30 days). The one-year survival for patients undergoing CLKT or LTA was similar (72% vs. 66%, respectively, p=0.88). Most of the benefit of performing CKLT was observed in patients on hemodialysis for more than 8 weeks pre transplant. This group had higher survival than those receiving CLKT on hemodialysis for a period inferior than 8 weeks (88% vs.66%, respectively). Among patients receiving liver transplantation alone, recovery of renal function was achieved in 90% of patients at one-month, even though most of them required hemodialysis at post transplant period.

The possible benefit of CLKT on LTA in patients with hepatorenal syndrome was also evaluated in a study comparing patients submitted to CLKT to patients with HRS submitted to LTA. Survival at 5 years was similar for CLKT recipients (48.1%) and patients with HRS receiving LTA (67.1%) (p=ns).

Some recent data on patients who received CLKT (n=75) over a 23 year-period show excellent 1-, 3- and 5- year patients survival (81%, 73% and 67%, respectively). However, short-term mortality (< 90 days) was especially high because of sepsis/infection on postoperative period. In addition, there was no difference in patient survival based on whether or not a recipient was on dialysis pre-transplantion. Nevertheless, the need of post transplant renal replacement therapy was significantly associated with poor prognosis (p=0.0012).

Regarding graft survival, it seems that the liver graft has an immune protective effect on kidney graft when both organs came from the same donor. A study comparing renal allograft outcomes of patients who undergone CLKT to kidney after liver transplantation (KALT) demonstrated a higher incidence of chronic rejection in KALT group than CLKT group (4.6 vs. 1.2%, P < 0.001). One and three-year rejection-free renal graft survival of KALT was lower than CLKT group (77% and 67% KALT vs. 85% and 78% CLKT, respectively; P < 0.001). Renal half-life of KALT allograft was shorter than CLKT group (6.6+/-0.9 vs. 11.7+/-1.3 years, P < 0.001). It has been speculated that this effect is secondary to the secretion of soluble HLA antigens by the liver and to phagocytosis of these reactive antibodies by kupffer cells.

Although many theories have been described to explain the possible hepatic protection on renal graft, some recent findings have questioned this statement. A case report of acute humoral rejection in kidney allograft in an ABO compatible CLKT was described. Even treating, the humoral rejection with plasmapheresis, intravenous immunoglobulin and rituximab, the kidney required 3 months to recovery function and finally progressed to chronic allograft nephropathy.

5. Combined liver and kidney transplantation in special conditions

Polycystic kidney diseases (PKD) compass a group of inherited diseases that causes an irreversible decline in kidney function. Autosomal dominant polycystic kidney disease (ADPKD) is associated with cysts in the kidneys and, in many cases, cysts in the liver and pancreas. The autosomal dominant form (ADPKD) is the most common genetic cause of chronic kidney disease .As survival with dialysis or transplant increase, incidence of liver disease will also increase. When cysts are diffused, fenestration/resection procedures are not successful and LKA offers a good survival option. For combined liver and kidney transplantation one- and two-year patient survival rates were similar to combined transplantation for other indications. For patients with acceptable renal function at time of transplantation, solitary liver transplantation has an excellent outcome.

Primary hyperoxaluria (PHO) is a rare metabolic disorder with autosomal recessive inheritance. PHO is induced by one of two enzymatic defects, both of which result in markedly enhanced conversion of glyoxalate to poorly soluble oxalate which is then excreted in the urine. Combined liver-kidney transplantation is probably the treatment of choice for children with type 1 PHO with progressive renal disease. The liver provides the missing enzyme, thereby lowering oxalate production to the normal range. The outcome may be best if transplantation is performed when the GFR falls to 25 mL/min per 1.73 m2 and prior to marked tissue oxalate deposition. Isolated liver transplantation has been proposed for patients with rapidly progressive disease who still have a glomerular filtration rate above 30 mL/min per 1.73 m^2.

6. Conclusion

Since implementation of MELD score as an organ allocation system, a crescent number of cirrhotic patients with renal failure has been submitted to CLKT. Due to increase shortage of organ donors, is of outstanding importance to define which are the patients who benefit most of this procedure.

The decision to perform orthotopic transplant alone or combined kidney-liver transplantation is still challenging, mainly because there is not enough data on factors that can predict renal function recovery. In patients with possible reversible causes of kidney dysfunction, including those with hepatorenal syndrome and acute renal failure, it is difficult to precise the boundaries between functional and irreversible damage. Therefore, in these cases kidney biopsy should be encouraged in order to evaluate interstitial and glomerular injury.

Combined liver kidney transplantation seems to be an adequate treatment in patients with end stage liver disease and chronic kidney disease on renal replacement therapy, as well as for those with inherited disease. The survival advantage in others subsets of patients is not well established and more studies are needed.

7. Acknowledgment

Supported in part by grants from Fondo de Investigación Sanitaria FIS070443 and 080108. Centro de investigaciones en red de enfermedades hepaticas y digestivas. CIBEREHD is supported by the Instituto de Salud Carlos III. Claudia Fagundes is supported by a grant of Fundación Renal Reina Sofía

8. References

Baccaro, ME. (2010). Combined liver-kidney transplantation in patients with cirrhosis and chronic kidney disease. *Nephrology Dialysis Transplantation,* Vol. 25, No. 7, pp. 2356-63, ISSN 0931-0509

Bahirwani, R. (2008). Transplantation: impact of pretransplant renal insufficiency. *Liver Transplantation,* Vol. 14, No. 5, pp. 665-71, ISSN 1527-6473

Barua M. (2009). Family history of renal disease severity predicts the mutated gene in ADPKD. *Journal of American Society of Nephrology*, Vol. 20, No. 8, pp. 1833-8, ISSN 1533-3450

Brinkert, F. (2009). Transplantation procedures in children with primary hyperoxaluria type 1: outcome and longitudinal growth. *Transplantation*, Vol. 87, No. 9, pp. 1415-21, ISSN 1534-0608

Campbell, MS. (2005).Renal Function after Orthotopic Liver Transplantation is Predicted by Duration of Pretransplantation Creatinine elevation. *Liver Transplantation,* Vol. 11, No. 9,pp. 1048-1055, ISSN 1527-6465

Caregaro, L. (1994). Limitations of serum creatinine level and creatinine clearance as filtration markers in cirrhosis. *Archives of Internal Medicine*, Vol. 154, No. 2, pp. 201-205, ISSN 0003-9926

Cochat, P. (1993). Should liver transplantation be performed before advanced renal insufficiency in primary hyperoxaluria type 1?. *Paediatric Nephrology*, Vol. 7, No. 2, pp. 212-8, ISSN 0931-041X.

Davis, CL. (2007).Simultaneous liver-kidney transplantation: evaluation to de decision making. *American Journal of Transplantation*,Vol.7, No. 7,pp. 1702-9, ISSN 1600-6135

D'Amico, G. (1992).Influence of clinical and histological features on actuarial renal survival in adult patients with idiopathic IgA nephropathy, membranous nephropathy, and membranoproliferative glomerulonephritis: survey of the recent literature. *American Journal of Kidney Disease*, Vol.20, No. 4,pp.315-23, ISSN 0272-6386

D'Amico, G. (2006).Natural history and prognostic indicators of survival in cirrhosis: a systematic review of 118 studies. *Journal of Hepatology*, Vol.44, No. 1,pp.217-231,ISSN 0168-8278

De Eason, JD. (2008). Proceedings of consensus conference on simultaneous liver kidney transplantation (SLK). *American Journal of Transplantation*, Vol.8, No. 11,pp. 2243-51,ISSN 1600-6135

Ginès P, Schrier RW. (2009). Renal failure in cirrhosis. *New England Journal of Medicine*, Vol.13, No. 361, pp.1279-1290, ISSN 0028-4793

Gonwa, TA. (1995). Impact of pretransplant renal function on survival after liver transplantation. *Transplantation*,Vol.59, No. 3,pp.361-365, ISSN 0041-1337

Gonwa, TA. (2006).Continued influence of preoperative renal function on outcome of orthotopic liver transplant (OLTX) in the US: where will MELD lead us? *American Journal of Transplantation*, Vol.6, No. 11,pp.2651-2659,ISSN 1600-6135

Jeyarajah, DR. (1997). Hepatorenal syndrome: combined liver kidney transplants versus isolated liver transplant. *Transplantation*, Vol. 64, No. 12, pp. 1760-5, ISSN 1534-0608.

Jeyarajah, DR. (1997).Hepatorenal syndrome : combined liver kidney transplants versus isolated liver transplant. *Transplantation*,Vol.64, No. 12,pp.1760-1765. ISSN 0041-1337

Locke, JE. (2008). Declining outcomes in simultaneous liver-kidney transplantation in the MELD era: ineffective usage of renal allografts. *Transplantation,* Vol. 85, No. 7, pp.935-42, ISSN 1534-0608

Maluf, DG. (2007). Hepatitis C virus infection and kidney transplantation: predictors of patient and graft survival. *Transplantation,* Vol. 83, No. 7, pp. 853-7, ISSN 1534-0608

Martin-Llahí, M. (2010).Prognostic importance of the cause of renal failure in patients with cirrhosis. *Gastroenterology,*Vol.140, No. 2,pp. 488-496, ISSN 0016-5085

McMillan, RW. (1997). Soluble fraction of class I human histocompatibility leukocyte antigens in the serum of liver transplant recipients. *Clinical Transplantation,* Vol. 11, No. 2, pp. 98-103, ISSN 0902-0063

Mehrabi, A. (2009). A single center experience of combined liver kidney transplantation. *Clinical transplantation,* Vol. 23, Suppl. 21, pp. 102-114, ISSN 0902-0063

Millan MT. (2003). One hundred percent patient and kidney allograft survival with simultaneous liver and kidney transplantation in infants with primary hyperoxaluria: a single-center experience. *Transplantation,.* Vol. 76, No. 10, pp. 1458-63, ISSN 1534-0608.

Nair, S. (2002).Pretransplant renal function predicts survival in patients undergoing orthotopic liver transplantation. *Hepatology* ,Vol.35, No. 5,pp.1179-85, Online ISSN 1527-3350

Nath, KA. (1992).Tubulointerstitial changes as a major determinant in the progression of renal damage. *American Journal of Kidney Disease,* Vol.20, No. 1,pp.1-17. ISSN 0272-6386

Pöge, U. (2006).Calculation of glomerular filtration rate based on cystatin C in cirrhotic patients. *Nephrology Dial Transplan,.*Vol.21, No. 3, pp.660-664, ISSN 0931-0509

Reichmann, TW. (2009). Acute humoral rejection in an ABO compatible combined liver-kidney transplant-the kidney is not always protected, Vol. 9, No. 8, pp1957-60, ISSN 1600-6143

Ruiz, R. (2006). Long-term analysis of combined liver and kidney transplantation at a single center. *Archives of Surgery,* Vol. 141, No. 8, pp. 735-41, ISSN 1435-2451

Ruiz, R. (2010). Indications for combined liver and kidney transplantation: propositions after a 23-yr experience. *Clinical Transplantation,* Vol. 24, No. 6, pp. 807-11, ISSN 0902-0063

Schmitt, TM. (2009). Combined liver-kidney and liver transplantation in patients with renal failure outcomes in the MELD era. *Transplantation International,* Vol. 22, No. 9, pp. 876-83, ISSN 1432-2277

Sherman, DS. (2003). Assessing renal function in cirrhotic patients: problems and pitfalls. *American Journal of Kidney Diseases,* Vol. 41, No.2, pp. 269-78, ISSN 0272-6386.

Skulzacek, PA. (2003). Prediction of GFR in liver transplant candidates. *American Journal of Kidney Diseases,* Vol. 42, No. 6, pp. 1169-76, ISSN 0272-6386.

Simpson, N. (2006). Comparison of renal allograft outcomes in combined liver-kidney transplantation versus subsequent kidney transplantation in liver transplant recipients: Analysis of UNOS Database. , Vol. 82, No. 10, pp. 1298-303, ISSN 1534-0608

Ueno,T. (2006). Liver and kidney transplantation for polycystic liver and kidney-renal function and outcome. *Transplantation*, Vol. 82, No. 4, pp. 501-7, ISSN 1534-0608.

6

Clinical Pharmacokinetics of Triple Immunosuppression Scheme in Kidney Transplant (Tacrolimus, Mycophenolate Mofetil and Corticosteroids)

Robles Piedras Ana Luisa and Monroy Funes Manuel Alejandro
Universidad Autónoma del Estado de Hidalgo
México

1. Introduction

Kidney transplantation is now firmly established as the treatment of choice for most patients with End Stage Renal Disease. The short-term outcomes of renal transplantation have dramatically improved over the past several decades; in a large part, this success is due to improvements in immunosuppression and post transplantation medical care. The goal of immunosuppressive strategies in transplantation is to deliver immunosuppression that result in long-term allograft and patient survival, while minimizing the complications of this immunosuppression. Tacrolimus has been one of the cornerstones of immunosuppressive strategies in clinical transplantation. Currently, regimens that are used for induction and maintenance therapy include the concomitant use of Mycophenolate Mofetil and Corticosteroids. The purpose of this chapter is to provide comprehensive and updated information, about the immunosuppressive drugs tacrolimus, mycophenolate mofetil and corticosteroids, which are used as triple immunosuppression scheme to the control of rejection of the transplanted organ.

2. Tacrolimus

Tacrolimus was isolated from Streptomyces tsukubaensis in 1984 and is a potent immunosuppressant widely used to prevent acute rejection after solid-organ transplantation, it has a macrolide lactone structure (C44H69NO12, 803.5 g/mol) comprising a 23-member carbon ring and a hemiketal masked b-diketoamide function(Scott et al., 2003). In 1984, the compound tacrolimus was discovered in a soil sample taken from the foot of Mount Tsukuba in Tokyo that was found to possess potent in vitro immunosuppressive qualities. Initially called FR000506, tacrolimus was subsequently found to suppress interleukin-2 production associated with T-cell activation, thus inhibiting the differentiation and proliferation of cytotoxic T cells (Fung, 2004). Tacrolimus has a greater effect on the T lymphocyte than does an earlier released calcineurin inhibitor, cyclosporine. In a response to antigenic stimulation, in vitro studies on cultured CD4 helper T lymphocytes have demonstrated that tacrolimus is superior to cyclosporine in selectively inhibiting the secretion of various cytokines, including IL-2 and IL-3. This difference may contribute to the greater effect of tacrolimus than cyclosporine on impairing the expression of alloantigen-stimulated T cells in solid organ transplantation (Vicari-Christensen et al., 2009). The calcineurin inhibitor tacrolimus, has a toxicity profile similar to cyclosporine (Winkler & Christians, 1995). Two types of side effects must be differentiated: (1) those caused by (over)immunosuppression and (2) those caused by drug toxicity. Immunosupression itself results in an increased incidence of infectious complications and malignancies, mainly lymphoma, as well as failure of vaccination. The principal adverse effects associated with tacrolimus treatment include nephrotoxicity, neurotoxicity, disturbances in glucose metabolism, gastrointestinal (GI) disturbance and hypertension. Susceptibility to infection and malignancy is also increased. Many of the adverse effects of tacrolimus are dose-related; nephrotoxicity, neurotoxicity, glucose metabolism disturbances, GI disturbances and infections may occur more frequently or be more severe at higher whole-blood tacrolimus concentrations. Importantly, these adverse events can often be managed by dosage reductions. Concomitant drugs such as corticosteroids may also contribute to some adverse effects (Naesens, 2009¸Plosker, 2000). Because of its variable pharmacokinetics and narrow therapeutic index, monitoring drug concentrations is essential to avoid the risks of over- and under-immunosuppression. For routine clinical practice therapeutic drug monitoring of tacrolimus whole blood concentrations is recommended and target ranges have been defined (Jusko, 1995; Plosker & Foster, 2000). Increased tacrolimus toxicity is observed with increased tacrolimus concentrations. The large variability in the pharmacokinetics of this drug, makes it difficult to predict what drug concentration will be achieved with a particular dose or dosage change (Staatz & Tett, 2004; Venkataramanan, 1995). Therapeutic drug monitoring-guided dosing is an important clinical tool to control Tacrolimus exposure and to improve outcome after transplantation. Therapeutic drug monitoring plays an important role in maintaining effective therapeutic levels and avoiding toxic tacrolimus blood concentrations after systemic administration for the treatment of autoimmune diseases (Christians, 2006). Today, tacrolimus has gained worldwide recognition as the cornerstone of immunosuppressant therapy. It is now commercially available in more than 70 countries and has established a significant role in the field of transplantation. According to statistics issued by the Global Observatory on Donation & Transplantation, an average of 69,300 kidney transplants are performed around the world each year, which constitutes nearly 70% of solid organ transplants performed world-wide (WHO, 2008). There are currently over 100,000 transplant recipients being treated with immunosuppressive drugs, and tacrolimus is being prescribed to patients with new liver and kidney transplant recipients around the world. Studies have also shown that other adjunctive agents can be safely prescribed in combination with tacrolimus.

2.1 Mechanism of action

2.1.1 Immunosuppressive activity

Tacrolimus is a macrolide immunosuppressant that acts by a variety of different mechanisms which include inhibition of calcineurin. The drug inhibits T-lymphocyte activation, this may occur through formation of a complex with FK 506-binding proteins (FKBPs). The complex inhibits calcineurin phosphatase. This is believed to inhibit interleukin-2 (IL-2) gene expression in T-helper lymphocytes. Tacrolimus also binds to the steroid receptor–associated heat-shock protein 56. This ultimately results in inhibition of transcription of proinflammatory cytokines such as granulocyte–macrophage colony-stimulating factor (GM-CSF), interleukin-1 (IL-1), interleukin-3 (IL-3), interleukin-4 (IL-4), interleukin-5 (IL-5), interleukin-6 (IL-6), interleukin-8 (IL-8), and tumor necrosis factor alpha (TNF alpha). The mechanism of action of tacrolimus is largely similar to that of cyclosporin, but tacrolimus is 10 to 100 times more potent. The drugs both inhibit calcineurin but do so via formation of complexes with different immunophilins: Tacrolimus binds to FK-506 binding protein, whereas cyclosporin binds to cyclophilin A. The drugs appear to differ in their effects on patterns of TH2 cell cytokine expression and possibly some aspects of humoral immunity. Furthermore, lymphocyte sensitivity to the drugs may differ between patients. Calcineurin is a protein phosphatase known as protein phosphatase 2B. It is responsible for activating the transcription of interleukin 2 (IL-2), which stimulates the growth and differentiation of a T-cell response. Calcineurin dephosphorylates a nuclear factor of activated T cells, and cytoplasmic component transcription factor can then migrate into the nucleus and activate genes involved in IL-2 synthesis. IL-2 is a powerful inflammatory catalyst implicated in allograft rejection. The allograft rejection process begins when an alloantigen is presented to the T-cell receptor and an increase in the cytoplasmic levels of calcium results. This response activates calcineurin by binding regulatory subunits and calmodulin complexes. Calcineurin induces different transcription factors that are important in the IL-2 genes. IL-2 activates helper T lymphocytes and induces the production of other cytokines. In this way, calcineurin governs the process of rejection. The amount of IL-2 produced by the helper T cells is believed to significantly influence the extent of the immune response (Pascual et al., 2002).

2.1.2 Toxicity

Because cyclosporine has been used for a much longer time, most data in this field pertain to cyclosporine. The effects of tacrolimus are considered to be similar (Naesens et al., 2009). Tacrolimus resembles cyclosporine in that it can result in nephrotoxicity and the hemolytic-uremic syndrome, but it is less likely to cause hyperlipidemia, hypertension, and cosmetic problems and more likely to induce post-transplantation diabetes (Halloran, 2002). Because of its similar mechanism of immunosuppressive activity and its similar clinical toxicity spectrum it is generally assumed that the mechanism involved in tacrolimus toxicity are similar to those for cyclosporine (Christians, 2006). Although the use of cyclosporine and tacrolimus has led to major advances in the field of transplantation, with excellent short-term outcome, the chronic nephrotoxicity of these drugs is the Achilles' heel of current immunosuppressive regimens. Chronic calcineurin inhibitor nephrotoxicity is associated with mostly irreversible histologic damage to all compartments of the kidneys, including glomeruli, arterioles, and tubulo-interstitium, but the nonspecificity of most lesions makes the differential diagnosis with other injurious processes cumbersome. The pathophysiologic mechanisms underlying CNI nephrotoxicity are partly elucidated, although the main question whether nephrotoxicity is secondary to the actions on the calcineurin-nuclear factor of activated t cells pathway remains largely unanswered. It becomes clear that local renal factors are more important for susceptibility to CNI nephrotoxicity than systemic exposure to cyclosporine and tacrolimus. These factors include variability in P-glycoprotein and CYP3A4/5 expression or activity, older kidney age, salt depletion, the use of Non-Steroidal anti-inflammatory drugs, and genetic polymorphism (Hesselink, 2010; Naesens, 2009).

Although the exact mechanism is not clear, calcineurin inhibitors are thought to produce nephrotoxicity through their direct action on the kidney. Long-term use of cyclosporine and tacrolimus can also cause hypertension and diabetes, which could contribute to renal failure. Sirolimus, which is not a calcineurin inhibitor but is structurally related to tacrolimus, has also been linked to nephrotoxicity in patients with focal segmental glomerulosclerosis (Bai, 2010). The long term use of cyclosporine produces diminished renal function associated with macrophage infiltration and interstitial fibrosis in the kidney on biopsy. Cyclosporine exposure is also associated with endothelin expression, which is a regulator of inflammation and fibrosis. Hypertension and renal adverse effects are interrelated, so the mechanisms involved in cyclosporine induced hypertension could also influence its adverse effects on the kidney (Bai, 2010). Tacrolimus has been suspected of inducing more BK-related polyomavirus nephropathy than has cyclosporine in patients who have undergone kidney transplantation, especially when used with mycophenolate mofetil, but renal function may be better with tacrolimus (Halloran, 2002; Meier-Kriesche, 2002).

2.2 Clinical pharmacokinetics

Tacrolimus is usually administered orally in capsules containing the equivalent of 0.5 mg, 1 mg or 5 mg in a solid dispersion in hydroxipropylmethylcellulose, and an injection solution is available in 5 mg/mL, swell as an ointment for the topical treatment of skin lesions during autoimmune diseases (Astellas, 2009).

2.2.1 Absorption

After oral administration absorption of tacrolimus from the gastrointestinal tract after oral administration is incomplete and variable. Generally, bioavailability is about 20 to 25%, but can range from 5% to 93%. The relatively low fraction of tacrolimus absorbed most likely reflects incomplete absorption, the extent of absorption of this drug from the gastrointestinal tract is also influenced by the activity of P-glycoprotein (P-gp) in enterocytes. P-gp is a transmembrane transporter that is closely associated with CYP3A4 and secretes tacrolimus and its metabolites (Undre, 2003). In most subjects, absorption is rapid with peak blood concentrations occurring within approximately 0.5–2 hours of administration (Astellas, 2009; Venkataramanan, 1995). However, in some individuals, drug uptake occurs more slowly, yielding an essentially flat absorption profile, an extended lag time or secondary peaks. Poor aqueous solubility of tacrolimus and altered gut motility in transplant recipients may be partially responsible. Tacrolimus is absorbed rapidily in most subjects, an oral dose of 0.15 mg/kg/12 hours at steady state, the peak concentration (Cmax) averages 45 ng/mL, with a corresponding mean time to peak concentration (Tmax) of 1.5 hours. There is a strong correlation between the area under the concentration-time curve (AUC) and the trough concentration of tacrolimus (Cmin) in whole blood, therefore doses are individualized on the basis of target whole blood trough concentrations (Staatz & Tett, 2004; Undre, 1999). In stable liver transplant recipients, the oral bioavailability of tacrolimus is decreased if it is taken after food containing moderate fat content (Bekersky et al., 2001a, 2001b). However in a study in a study in renal transplant recipients where tacrolimus trough levels were evaluated prospectively during fasting ingestion of tacrolimus and 1 week after nonfasting ingestion, the results observed were statistically and clinically not significantly different (van-Duijnhoven et al., 2002). Data from a study in 7 patients with type 1 diabetes mellitus and 10 nondiabetic patients, all with end-stage renal failure, also showed that the rate of absorption was affected when tacrolimus was taken together with a continental breakfast high in fat content, and food had a greater effect on the absorption of tacrolimus in patients with than without diabetes mellitus (Plosker & Foster, 2000; van-Duijnhoven, 1998).To avoid the possible effect of food on tacrolimus bioavailability, the drug should be given at a constant time in relation to meals. Oral tacrolimus should not be taken with grapefruit juice since this vehicle inhibits CYP3A4 and/or P-gp contained in the GI tract and markedly increases bioavailability (Christians, 2006).

2.2.2 Distribution

In plasma, tacrolimus is highly bound to plasma proteins (99%) mainly to serum albumin and α–1-acid glycoprotein, so the pharmacological activity is considered to be a function of the unbound fraction of tacrolimus. Tacrolimus binds strongly to erythrocytes in the systemic circulation, resulting in a whole blood/plasma concentration distribution range of approximately 4-114 times and whole blood is therefore the medium usually used for assessing therapeutic concentrations (Plosker & Foster, 2000; Undre, 2003). Erythrocyte concentrations vary in transplant patients, especially those who have received hematopoietic stem cell or kidney transplants. α-acid glycoprotein concentrations also vary greatly among patients. Lipophilic drugs such as tacrolimus readily cross membranes and are taken up by adipose tissue. Animal studies indicate that tacrolimus is widely distributed into most tissues, including the lungs, spleen, heart, kidney, pancreas, brain, muscle and liver, tacrolimus crosses the placenta and is detected in breast milk (Staatz & Tett, 2004; Venkataramanan et al., 1995). At steady state, tacrolimus is distributed extensively in the body and at steady state the majority of the drug resides outside the blood compartment; that is, in the tissues. The plasma volume of distribution is greater than 1,000 L and in whole blood is approximately 50 L (Undre, 2003).

2.2.3 Metabolism and elimination

Calcineurin inhibitors like tacrolimus and cyclosporine are metabolized by cytochrome P-450 (CYP) isoenzyme systems 3A4 and 3A5 in the gut lumen before they even reach the portal vein. P-glycoprotein prevents drug absorption from the gut by promoting efflux into the lumen of the intestine, it has also has a role in systemic clearance of drugs by promoting efflux into the bile for excretion (Tsuchiya et al., 2004). After drugs are absorbed, they are subject to first-pass metabolism and systemic metabolism by CYP3A4 and CYP3A5 in the liver. When CYP3A5 is expressed, it accounts for 50% of the total hepatic CYP3A content. After administration, tacrolimus, either injected or absorbed into the body, is excreted from the body after receiving extensive metabolism primarily in the liver and to a lesser extent in the intestinal mucosa, by cytochrome P450(CYP)3A4 isoenzymes, with <0.5% of the parent drug appearing unchanged in urine and feces (Venkataramanan et al., 1995). The specific number of metabolites formed is unclear, but appears to be at least eight metabolites of tacrolimus have been identified, with two of these exhibiting some activity (Op den Buijsch, 2007; Plosker & Foster, 2000). Three mono-demethylated metabolites, three di-demethylated metabolites, one mono-hydroxylated metabolite and one metabolite modifed by reactions have been identified. Three metabolites O-demethylated at the 13-, 31- and 15-methoxy group of tacrolimus, respectively, and one monohydroxylated metabolite at the 12-position. The didemethylated metabolites at the 15- and 31, 13- and 31-, and 13- and 15-methoxy groups of tacrolimus and one metabolite produced after O-demethylation at the 31-methoxy group and formation of a fused 10-membered ring structure through the 19- to 22-carbon of the macrolide ring after oxidation of the 19-methyl group, and of the 36- and 37-vinyl group of tacrolimus (Iwasaki, 2007). Compounds such as tacrolimus that display significant presystemic metabolism and have an intrinsic clearance lower than hepatic blood flow should be sensitive to changes in CYP3A expression. The CYP3A subfamily consists of at least four isoforms: CYP3A4, CYP3A5, CYP3A7 and CYP3A43. As these isoforms have overlapping substrate specificity, it is difficult to segregate their relative contributions to the metabolism of tacrolimus (Staatz & Tett, 2004). While it is known that CYP3A4 is predominantly localized to the liver and intestines, CYP3A5, on the contrary, is predominantly localized to the kidney (Joy et al., 2007). The isoform CYP3A4 is generally the most abundantly expressed CYP in the adult liver, accounting for 30–40% of total CYP content, its expression is highly variable, with 10- to 100-fold interindividual differences (Paine et al., 1997). Althoug there is evidence that cytochrome P4503A is mainly responsible for demethylation of tacrolimus, a minor involvement of cytochrome P450 enzymes other than cytochrome P4503A cannot be excluded (Christians, 2006). The reported elimination half-life ($t_{1/2}$) of tacrolimus is variable, with mean values of approximately 12 hours in liver transplant recipients, 19 hours in renal transplant recipients and 35 hours in healthy volunteers (Meier-Kriesche, 2002). Less than 1% of an intravenous dose of tacrolimus is excreted in the urine as unchanged drug, and total urinary elimination (metabolites and unchanged drug) is just over 2%. Faecal elimination accounts for >90% of an administered dose, and animal data indicate that the main excretory pathway of tacrolimus metabolites is biliary (Plosker & Foster 2000; Venkataramanan et al. 1995).

2.3 Pharmacokinetic variability

2.3.1 Oral bioavailability

Tacrolimus is highly lipophilic and insoluble in water, these physicochemical properties of tracrolimus cause a large amount of intrasubject variability in tacrolimus oral absorption. Tacrolimus is metabolized in the intestine and liver by the cytochrome P450 (CYP) 3A4 and 3A5 oxidative enzymes. It is also substrate for the P-gp drug transporter, a product of the multidrug resistance (*MDR1*) gene. Furthermore, CYP3A isoforms and P-gp are under the transcriptional control of the human pregnane X receptor (PXR). Therefore, the interindividual variability of tacrolimus pharmacokinetics might be explained by heterogeneity in CYP3A4, CYP3A5, P-gp or PXR expressions due to genetic polymorphisms (López-Montenegro Soria, et al., 2010). Extrahepatic metabolism by CYP3A4 in the gastrointestinal epithelium is responsible for presystemic elimination of about half of the absorbed dose, whereas first-pass metabolism by CYP3A4 in the liver accounts for an additional 10% of elimination. The extent of absorption of tacrolimus from the gastrointestinal tract is also influenced by the activity of P-glycoprotein (P-gp) in enterocytes. P-gp is a transmembrane transporter that is closely associated with CYP3A4 and secretes tacrolimus and its metabolites back into the lumen of the gut (Undre et al., 199; Undre, 2003). This extensive presystemic metabolism limits the oral bioavailability of tacrolimus to approximately 25%. The activity of the metabolizing enzyme as well as of the P-gp transporter varies considerably between individuals and between races, and this requires the dosage to be individualized to achieve the desired systemic exposure (Felipe, et al., 2002). Nevertheless, the intra-patient variability in systemic exposure is considered to be low. The low intra-patient variability in the bioavailability of tacrolimus is evidenced by the small number of dose changes required to maintain target whole-blood trough concentrations. While the average oral bioavailability of tacrolimus is 25%, there is a large amount of variation in this parameter among patients (4-89%), small intestine metabolism and/or transport processes contribute greatly (Tuteja et al., 2001). Renal transplant patients may have reduced oral bioavailability for tacrolimus. When given with meals, especially with high fat content food, oral bioavailability of tacrolimus decreases (Venkataramanan et al., 1995). To avoid the possible effect of food on tacrolimus bioavailability, the drug should be given at a constant time in relation to meals. Oral tacrolimus should not be taken with grapefruit juice since this vehicle inhibits CYP3A4 and/or P-glycoprotein contained in the gastrointestinal tract and markedly increases bioavailability. The individual pharmacokinetic response of a renal transplant recipient to immunosuppressive drugs is highly variable. Recent studies have shown that specific genetic variations may alter the pharmacokinetics of these drugs (Rosso Felipe et al., 2009). The metabolic enzyme of tacrolimus is the CYP3A subfamily, including the CYP3A4, CYP3A5, CYP3A7, and CYP3A43 isodynamic enzyme. CYP3A4 and CYP3A5 are the main fractions of these isodynamic enzymes. The mutable site of CYP3A5 is multivariate; the wild type of CYP3A5 is defined as *1, while mutation of 6986A_G is defined as *3. As disclosed by many studies, the CYP3A5 genotype has a great effect on FK506 concentrations. The amount of CYP3A5 in the liver is large among patients with the *1 genotype in contrast to the patients with the *3 genotype, which metabolize tacrolimus faster with lower concentrations in patients with the *1 genotype. Patients with the *3/*3 genotype theoretically have high concentration per dosage ratios (Chen et al., 2002; Rosso Felipe et al., 2009; Tuteja et al., 2001). The presence of the CYP3A5*3 genotype is associated with the absence of protein function. López Montenegro et al., demonstrated that Intestinal absorption and metabolism of tacrolimus is significantly affected by the Single Nucleotide Polymorphisms (SNP) in the CYP3A5 and MDR1 genes. Macphee et al., in 2002 in a study with 180 kidney transplant patients, found that a single nucleotide polymorphism in the CYP3AP1 pseudogene (A/G(44)) that previously has been noted to be more common in African Americans and strongly associated with hepatic CYP3A5 activity correlated well with the tacrolimus dose requirement, and found a weaker association for a polymorphism in the MDR-1 gene, which influences intestinal P-glycoprotein expression. They conclude that the CYP3AP1 genotype is a major factor in determining the dose requirement for tacrolimus, and genotyping may be of value in planning patient-specific drug dosing. As substrates for CYP3A enzymes and P-glycoprotein, drugs that inhibit or induce these mechanisms may increase or decrease blood tacrolimus concentrations, respectively (Van Gelder, 2002). In clinical studies, CYP3A/P-glycoprotein inhibitors and inducers primarily affect the oral bioavailability of tacrolimus rather than clearance, indicating a key role of intestinal P-glycoprotein and CYP3A. Drugs that interact with P-gp may change the distribution of tacrolimus in tissue and modify its toxicity and immunosuppressive activity (Christians et al., 2002). Ketoconazole, an azole antifungal agent, is known to be a potent inhibitor of P-gp and CYP3A4 and have even been used to reduce the dose of tacrolimus and thus save money. If possible, drugs interfering at the level of the CYP system should be avoided. If tacrolimus and either of these drugs are used concomitantly, close monitoring of tacrolimus concentrations should be performed (Van Gelder, 2002).

2.3.2 Ethnicity, pharmacogenetic variability

The importance of interethnic differences in the pharmacokinetics of immunosuppressants has been recognized as having a significant impact on the outcome of transplantation.

Between-patient variability in drug absorption may be the major cause of inferior transplant outcome observed in special populations such as African-Americans, children and diabetic patients. For example, the poorer transplant outcome observed among African-Americans has been attributed mainly to differences in absorption of cyclosporine, tacrolimus and mycophenolate mofetil (Hariharan et al., 1993; Schweitzer et al., 1998; Stein et al., 2001). Also, compared with white recipients, black transplant patients may also require higher doses of sirolimus to achieve comparable acute rejection rates, even without displaying significant differences in drug absorption. Whether this effect is the result of pharmacodynamic differences comparing black and white patients is not known (Felipe et al., 2002). In a retrospective analysis Fitzimmons et al. found that the oral bioavailability of tacrolimus in African American healthy volunteers and kidney transplant patients was significantly lower than in non-African Americans (Fitzsimmons, 1998). There was no statistically significant difference in clearance. These results were confirmed in a healthy volunteer study. The absolute oral bioavailability of tacrolimus in African American and Latin American subjects was significantly lower than in Caucasians. The results suggested that the observed ethnic differences in tacrolimus pharmacokinetics were, instead, related to differences in intestinal P-glycoprotein-mediated efflux and CYP3A-mediated metabolism rather than differences in hepatic elimination (Mancinelli et al., 2001). Other ethnic groups such as the Japanese populations are not different from the Caucasian population because their transplant outcomes were comparable under usual tacrolimus dosages (Ochiai et al., 1995). Drugs metabolized by CYP3A4/5 inhibited tacrolimus metabolism, with ketoconazole being the most potent. Ketoconazole, cyclosporine A, diltiazem, erythromycin, and fluconazole were reported as the drugs that elicit clinically relevant drug interactions with tacrolimus (Christians et al., 2002). These results indicate the potential for metabolic interactions between tacrolimus and co-medicated drugs metabolized by CYP3A4/5. Rifampicin decreased the blood levels of tacrolimus in kidney and liver transplant patients. Rifampicin treatment caused a decrease of tacrolimus blood levels in healthy volunteers when compared to pretreatment levels (Hariharan et al., 1993; Stein et al., 2001). Co-administration of rifampicin significantly increased tacrolimus clearance and decreased tacrolimus bioavailavility. A combination of fluconazole and tacrolimus augments tacrolimus blood levels (Mañez et al., 2002). In kidney transplantation, it was also reported that in a combination of fluconazole at 100 mg to tacrolimus, the dosage of tacrolimus could be reduced by forty percent without changing tacrolimus trough levels (Toda et al., 2002). *CYP3A* proteins are involved in the metabolism of more than 50% of the drugs in use, including tacrolimus. Pharmacogenomic studies have shown that SNP in intron 3 of the *CYP3A5* gene correlate with different expression levels, because of the appearance of a cryptic-splice site resulting in either the presence (*1/*1 and SNP *1/*3) or absence (SNP *3/*3) of the protein (Yu et al., 206; Barrera-Pulido et al.,2008). Interindividual CYP3A expression in the liver varies 10- to 100-fold and up to 30-fold in the small intestine, but there is no significant polymorphism of CYP3A4. Only people with at least one CYP3A45*1 allele express significant amounts of CYP3A45*3and CYP3A45*6 cause alternative splicing and protein truncation that results in the absence of CYP3A5 enzyme (Macphee et al., 2002). Greater than 60% of African Americans compared with less than 10% of the Caucasian population possess the CYP3AP1 G_{-44} allele, which is necessary for CYP3A5 expression. In humans expressing CYP3A5, it represents at least 50% of the total hepatic content of CYP3A. Together with CYP3A4 it is the most abundant CYP enzyme in the small intestine. CYP3A5 is probably the most important genetic contributor to interindividual and interracial differences in CYP3A-dependent drug clearance. As discussed above, another important factor affecting the pharmacokinetics of tacrolimus is the expression of MDR1, the gene encoding the active transporter P-glycoprotein. Homozygous individuals for the T-allele for MDR1, C3435T, have significantly lower intestinal and leukocyte P-glycoprotein expression than C homocygotes ((Macphee et al., 2002; Schaeffeler et al., 2001). MDR1 C3435T is significantly more prevalent in the Caucasian than in the African American population. MacPhee (2002) demonstrated that the dose-normalized tacrolimus blood concentration after renal transplantation was associated with a SNP in the CYP3AP1 gene, probably through linkage with an SNP in the CYP3A5 gene. Individuals with at least one CYP3A5*1 allele synthesize CYP3A5 and CYP3A5*3/*3 homozygotes do not (Paine et al., 1997). In another study MacPhee et al. (2005) showed results with direct typing of the CYP3A5 genotype for a group of 180 kidney-only transplant recipients. South Asian and white patients with at least one CYP3A5*1 allele achieved twofold lower dose-normalized tacrolimus blood concentrations compared with CYP3A5*3/*3 homozygotes, confirming their previous findings for the CYP3AP1 SNP. There was a significant delay in achieving target blood concentrations in those with at least one CYP3A5*1 allele. They conclude that the Determination of the CYP3A5*1/*3 genotype could be used to predict the tacrolimus dose requirement and, given incomplete linkage, would be better than determination of the CYP3AP1 genotype. For renal transplant recipients receiving tacrolimus as an immunosuppressant, practitioners can expect *CYP3A5*1* carriers to have a tacrolimus clearance 25-45% greater than that of *CYP3A5*3* homozygotes, with proportional dosing needs to maintain adequate immunosuppression. Since inadequate immunosuppression is linked to graft rejection, evaluation of CYP3A5 polymorphisms may be helpful in determining an appropriate starting dosage, rapidly achieving adequate immunosuppression, and ultimately improving the outcome of renal transplantation (Utecht et al., 2002).

2.3.3 Sex

Gender-related differences in pharmacokinetics have frequently been considered as potentially important determinants for the clinical effectiveness of drug therapy. The human multidrug-resistance gene 1 (MDR1) gene product P-gp has been identified as a major determinant in the pharmacokinetics of numerous drugs. Additional other drug transporters are also assumed to play a major role in absorption, distribution and/or renal and hepatic excretion of therapeutic agents. Gender differences have been noted in the hepatic expression of MDR1, with women displaying only one-third to one-half of the hepatic P-gp level of men. Low P-glycoprotein activity in the liver is suggested to result in increased hepatic CYP3A metabolism for cosubstrates of CYP3A and P-glycoprotein. Low P-gp activity in the gut wall results in shorter gut wall transit time and, hence, decreased gut wall CYP3A metabolism (Lown et al., 1997; Meibohmet al., 2002). The most important pharmacokinetic parameter influenced by sex differences seems to be oral biovailability (Christians, 2006; Harris et al., 2002). Although no difference in dosing by sex was found in the tacrolimus kidney transplant trials and dosing recommendations for male and female patients are the same, sex differences were found when tacrolimus and ketoconazole were coadministered (Fitzsimmons et al., 1998; Tuteja et al., 2001). Female-specific issues such as pregnancy, menopause, oral contraceptive use and menstruation may also have profound effects on drug metabolism. These effects can often be clinically important (Harris et al., 2001).

2.3.4 Age

As already mentioned, tacrolimus is primarily metabolized by cytochrome P450(CYP)3A enzymes in the gut wall and liver. It is also a substrate for P-gp, which counter-transports diffused tacrolimus out of intestinal cells and back into the gut lumen. Age-associated alterations in CYP3A and P-gp expression and/or activity, along with liver mass and body composition changes, would be expected to affect the pharmacokinetics of tacrolimus in the elderly (Staatz & Tett, 2002). Several changes in hepatic function and structure have been noted in the elderly; among them, two of the most important are an absolute (and relative to bodyweight) decrease in the size of the liver, and reduced regional blood flow to this organ (Hämmerlein et al., 2002). It is likely that inter- and intraindividual pharmacokinetic variability associated with tacrolimus increase in elderly populations. In addition to pharmacokinetic differences, donor organ viability, multiple co-morbidity, polypharmacy and immunological changes need to be considered when using tacrolimus in the elderly. Aging is associated with decreased immune responsiveness, a slower body repair process and increased drug adverse effects. Elderly liver and kidney transplant recipients are more likely to develop new-onset diabetes mellitus than younger patients, elderly transplant recipients exhibit higher mortality from infectious and cardiovascular causes than younger patients, but may be less likely to develop acute rejection, also have a higher potential for chronic allograft nephropathy and a single rejection episode can be more devastating (Staatz & Tett, 2002). Pharmacokinetic parameters observed in adults may not be applicable to children, especially to the younger age groups. In general, patients younger than 5 years of age show higher clearance rates regardless of the organ transplanted or the immunosuppressive drug used (del Mar Fernández De Gatta et al., 2002). Only limited information is available on the pharmacokinetics of tacrolimus in pediatric patients, the rate and extent of tacrolimus absorption after oral administration do not seem to be altered in pediatric patients. The volume of distribution of tacrolimus based on blood concentrations in pediatric patients (2.6 L/kg) is approximately twice the adult value. Blood clearance of tacrolimus is also approximately twice as high in pediatric (0.14 L/h/kg) compared with adult (0.06 L/h/kg) patients. Consequently, $t_{1/2}\beta$ does not appear modified in children, but oral doses need to be generally 2-fold higher than corresponding adult doses to reach similar tacrolimus blood concentrations. More pharmacokinetic studies in pediatric patients are, however, needed to rationalize the use of therapeutic drug monitoring for optimization of tacrolimus therapy in this patient population (Wallemacq & Verbeeck 2001).

2.4 Time after initiation of treatment

It is well established that tacrolimus pharmacokinetics changes with the time after transplantation are the results of a reduced clearance or an increase in oral bioavailability (Staatz & Tett, 2004). Possible reasons include stabilization of the patient with reduction of postsurgical stress, hematocrit, ischemia-reperfusion injury and stabilization of transplant organ function, especially if the latter directly affects tacrolimus pharmacokinetics such as the liver. Also, immunosuppressive drugs affect expression and activity of CYP3A enzymes and P-gp (Christians et al., 2002). There is evidence that induction of CYP3A and P-gp by corticosteroids is responsible for the requirement to reduce tacrolimus doses as corticosteroid doses are tapered (Hesselink et al., 2003; Plosker & Foster 2000; Undre 1998). After cessation of concomitant steroid treatment, tacrolimus exposure increase by 25% (del Mar Fernández De Gattaet al., 2002).

2.5 Drug-Drug interactions

Drug interactions occur when the efficacy or toxicity of a medication is changed by coadministration of another drug (Dresser et al., 2000). The clinical relevance of pharmacokinetic drug interactions depends on a number of considerations, of which the therapeutic index of the drug is the most important. Potential sites of pharmacokinetic drug interactions include the gastrointestinal tract, protein- and tissue-binding sites, drug metabolising enzymes, drug transporter systems, biliary excretion and enterohepatic recirculation as well renal excretion (Van Gelder, 2002). There are several factors involved in absorption of a drug after oral administration, all of which can be the target of drug interactions: delivery to the intestine (pH, gastric emptying and food), absorption from the intestinal lumen (dissolution, lipophilicity, stability, active uptake), intestinal metabolism (phase I or II metabolism), active intestinal drug efflux pumps, and subsequent hepatic first pass extraction (Christians et al., 2002). Drug interactions with tacrolimus fall into two basic categories. The first are agents known to cause nephrotoxicity when administered by themselves, the second category of drug interactions involves inhibition or induction of tacrolimus metabolism. Because tacrolimus is metabolized extensively by CYP3A4 isoenzymes and P-glycoprotein, drugs that are either inhibitors or inducers of this system may increase or decrease serum concentrations of tacrolimus. CYP3A4 inhibitors that increase whole blood concentrations of tacrolimus include antifungal agents (fluconazole, voriconazole, ketoconazole, itraconazole, and clotrimazole), calcium channel blockers (diltiazem, nifedipine, nicardipine, and verapamil), macrolide antibiotics (erythromycin, clarithromycin, and troleandomycin), prokinetic drugs (metoclopramide and cisapride), protease inhibitors (indinavir, saquinavir, ritonavir, nelfinavir, amprenavir, and atazanavir), and grapefruit juice. CYP3A4 inducers that are known to decrease tacrolimus concentrations include anticonvulsants (carbamazepine, phenytoin, and phenobarbital); rifamycins (rifampin and rifabutin), and St John's wort (Vicari-Christensen et al., 2009). Potential pharmacokinetic interactions between tacrolimus and mycophenolate mofetil has been evaluated since these drugs are frequently used in combination (Zucker et al., 2002; Undre at al., 2002; Hübner et al., 1999). Results indicate that mycophenolate mofetil does not significantly affect the pharmacokinetics of tacrolimus in renal and hepatic transplant recipients. However, tacrolimus may have an effect on the pharmacokinetics of mycophenolic acid, the active metabolite of mycophenolate mofetil. In renal transplant recipients who were converted from cyclosporin to tacrolimus therapy (while being maintained on the same dosage of mycophenolate mofetil), plasma trough concentrations of mycophenolic acid were significantly increased (approximately doubled) as were AUC values for mycophenolic acid (increased by about one-third) after conversion from cyclosporin to tacrolimus (although there was no mycophenolate mofetil control group in the study) (Plosker & Foster, 2000). Because of the large number of potentially interacting agents, and the critical nature of the drugs involved in the treatment of transplant patients, complete avoidance of drug interactions with tacrolimus is not possible. Thus, most drug interactions with tacrolimus are managed using appropriate tacrolimus dosage modification with tacrolimus concentration monitoring as a guide.

2.6 Adverse reactions

The calcineurin inhibitors tacrolimusa and cyclosporine, are the mainstay of immunosuppressive therapy in solid organ transplantation. These drugs produce severe adverse effects and tended to occur most frequently in the first few months after transplant and decline thereafter, possibly in ther line with reduction in dosages of the immunosuppressants (Bai et al., 2010). There are several principal adverse effects associated with tacrolimus. Nephrotoxic effects can occur in up to 52% of patients and limit the use of the drug. However, nephrotoxic effects may be difficult to distinguish from other causes of renal failure in kidney transplant recipients. Neurotoxic effects may be manifested by tremors (15%-56%), headache (37%-64%), insomnia (32%-64%), and paresthesias (17%-40%). Post-transplant diabetes mellitus is one of the more serious metabolic disorders associated with calcineurin inhibitors treatment (Scott et al., 2003). Cyclosporine appears to be less diabetogenic than tacrolimus, but both agents may impact directly the transcriptional regulation of insulin gene expression in the pancreatic β cells. Based on an analysis of 3365 kidney recipients, the primary risk factors identified for posttransplantation diabetes included older age, female, increased Body Mass Index, and tacrolimus-based therapy.[24] Other studies have also identified tacrolimus as a risk factor for posttransplantation diabetes in addition to older age (> 40 years), Body Mass Index greater than 25 kg/m^2, positive hepatitis C serology, family history of diabetes, metabolic syndrome, African-American or Hispanic race-ethnicity, and higher mean pretransplantation plasma glucose concentration. The risk factors for posttransplantation diabetes are similar to those for type 2 diabetes (Markell, 2004; González-Posada at al., 2004; Kamar et al., 2007). Hypertension (38-89%) is common, as is drug-induced diabetes (24%), exacerbated by the use of corticosteroids. Gastrointestinal disturbances reported are diarrhea (37%-72%), nausea (32-46%), constipation (23-35%), and anorexia (34%). Malignant neoplasms such as lymphoma and lymphoproliferative disease occur rarely (1.5%). Finally, the risk of bacterial, viral and fungal infections is increased (up to 45%), because of the immunosuppressive effect of tacrolimus..

2.7 Therapeutic drug mpnitoring

Therapeutic drug monitoring has been used as an essential tool to individualize immunosuppressive drug therapy in vascularized organ transplant recipients, allowing a more rational use of drugs with narrow therapeutic index such as cyclosporine, tacrolimus, sirolimus, and mycophenolate acid (Rosso Felipe et al., 2009). Tacrolimus whole-blood through concentrations have been found to correlate well with the area under the concentration-time curve measurements in liver, kidney and bone marrow transplant recipients (r= 0.91-0.99). Thus, through concentrations are a good index of overall drug exposure, and are currently used for routine monitoring as part of patient care posttransplantation (Jusko, 1995; Staatz et al., 2001). This approach offers the opportunity to reduce the pharmacokinetic variability by implementing drug dose adjustments based on plasma/blood concentrations. Drug levels are obtained as predose (12 hours after previous dose) trough concentrations in whole blood (Cattaneo et al., 2009). These trough levels correlate reasonably well with area under the curve, with total area under the curve being an accurate measure of drug exposure (Kapturczak et al., 2004). Therapeutic ranges of tacrolimus after kidney transplantation are reported as a range for various times after transplant: 0-1 month, 15-20 μg/L; 1-3 months, 10-15 μg/L; and more than 3 months, 5-12 μg/L (Scott et al., 2003). Pharmacokinetic therapeutic drug monitoring can only be of clinical relevance when the pharmacodynamics response is correlated to drug exposure. In a retrospective analysis based on adult renal transplant recipients during the first month after transplantation, tacrolimus through blood concentrations measured, were correlated with rejection episodes. The median through blood concentration in patients with rejections (5.6±1.6 ng/mL) were significantly lower than in patients without rejection (9.2±3.5 ng/mL). A rejection rate of 55% was found for patients with median tacrolimus through blood concentrations between 0 and 10 ng/mL, whereas no rejection was observed in patients with median tacrolimus through blood concentrations between 10 and 15 ng/mL (Staatz at al., 2001). Tacrolimus blood concentrations are monitored 3 to 7 days a week for the first 2 weeks, at least three times for the following 2 weeks, and whenever the patient comes for an outpatient visit thereafter (Jusko & Kobayashi, 1993). On the basis of the terminal half-life of tacrolimus, it was suggested to start monitoring tacrolimus blood concentrations 2 to 3 days after initiation of tacrolimus treatment after the drug has reached steady state. However it is important to reach effective drug concentrations early after transplantation to decrease the risk of acute rejection and to avoid excessive early calcineurin inhibitors concentrations that may be severely damaging after reperfusion of the transplanted organ (Shaw et al., 2002). The frequency of therapeutic drug monitoring of tacrolimus should be increased in the case of suspected adverse events or rejection, when liver function is deteriorating, after dose adjustments of the immunosuppressants, change of route of administration, or change of drug formulations, when drugs that are known to interact with CYP3A or P-gP are added or discontinued, or when their doses are changed, in case of severe illness that may affect drug absorption or elimination such as severe immune reactions and sepsis, or if noncompliance is suspected (Christians at al., 2006). Recent advances in molecular biology and genetic information made available through the Human Genome Project has had a great influence in the biomedical and pharmaceutical area. It is well established that large numbers of patients demonstrate great differences in drug bioavailability. Nowadays the advent of the genomic era has brought several new fields of study, including pharmacogenomics, which seek to link drug treatment with the individual's genetic makeup. Pharmacogenomics holds many promises for improved treatment of a large variety of medical conditions, including immunosuppression for organ transplantation (Cattaneo et al., 2004; Danesi et al., 2000). In recent years, extensive studies on pharmacogenetics of immunosuppressive drugs have been focused on the contribution of drug metabolizing enzyme cytochrome P450 (CYP) 3A (CYP3A4 and CYP3A5) and the drug transporter P-gp to the individual administration of cyclosporine and tacrolimus, for they are thought to be the main determinant of the pharmacokinetics of currently used immunosuppressive drugs (Macphee et al., 2002). Those involved in therapeutic drug monitoring are now realizing the potential role of pharmacogenomics in influencing individual patient's exposure to immunosuppressive agents and concomitant therapy. As rapid techniques for assessing genetic polymorphisms become available, they are likely to play a significant part in planning the initial doses of immunosuppressive drugs and tailor maintenance therapy (Cattaneo et al., 2004).

3. Mycophenolate

The search for inhibitors of the *novo* purine synthesis led to the ancient compound mycophenolic acid discovered in 1896. MPA was known to be immunosupresive, to inhibit lymphocyte DNA synthesis, and to inhibit guanine nucleotide synthesis in tumor cells. It was found to block the *novo* purine biosynthesis by inhibit the key enzyme in this pathway, inosine monophosphate dehydrogenase (IMDPH). The principle of the Mycophenolate mofetil arose from de observation that defects in the *novo* purine biosynthesis create immunodeficiency without affecting other tissues. Mycophenolate mofetil (MPM) is the 2-

morpholinoethyl ester of mycophenolic acid (MPA), an immunosuppressive agent IMPDH inhibitor. The chemical name for MMF is 2-morpholinoethyl (E)-6-(1,3-25 dihydro-4-hydroxy-6-methoxy-7-methyl-3-oxo-5-isobenzofuranyl)-4-methyl-4-6 hexenoate. It has an empirical formula of $C_{23}H_{31}NO_7$, a molecular weight of 433.50 (Christians et al., 2006), is a potent, selective, noncompetitive, reversible inhibitor of IMPDH, an essential enzyme in *de novo* synthesis of purines (i.e. guanosine), MPA has potent cytostatic effects on lymphocytes. Inhibits proliferative responses of T and B-cells to both mitogenic and allospecific stimulation and suppresses antibody formation by B-cells. By preventing glycosylation of lymphocyte and monocyte glycoproteins involved in intracellular adhesion to endothelial cells, MPA may inhibit recruitment of leukocytes to sites of inflammation and graft rejection (Pillans et al., 2001; Kiberd, et al., 2004; van Gelder et al., 1999).

3.1 Mechanism of action

The salvage pathway of purine synthesis in lymphocytes is less active than the de novo synthesis of purines. Inosine monophosphate is converted to guanosine monophosphate by inosine monophosphate dehydrogenase. During T-cell activation, the activity of both types I and II inosine monophosphate dehydrogenase enzymes increases by tenfold. Mycophenolate mofetil is converted in the liver by ester hydrolysis to mycophenolic acid, which in turn non-competitively and reversibly inhibits types I and II inosine monophosphate dehydrogenase activity during DNA synthesis in the S phase of the cell cycle. In the salvage pathway, guanine is converted to guanine monophosphate by the enzyme hypoxanthine-guanine phosphoribosyltransferase. MPM is commonly used in transplanted patients; it is a non-competitive reversible inhibitor of 5'-mono phosphate inosine dehydrogenase, which controls the synthesis of guanosine triphosphate; its mechanism of action is by depletion of intracellular levels of guanosine triphosphate (GTP) and deoxyguanosine triphosphate (dGTP), which leads to suppression of DNA synthesis in T and B lymphocytes stimulated with antigens or mitogens. It does not inhibit early events of lymphocytes activation including cytokine production. It also inhibits antibody formation and production of adhesion molecules on the cellular surface. It has been used to prolong transplant survival in animal and human models in 5/6 nephrectomy to reduce cellular infiltration within the tubule and interstitium with decreased renal damage been observed in the remnant kidney (Bullingham, 1996a, 1996b).

3.2 Clinical pharmacokinetics

3.2.1 Onset & plasma concentrations

Peak mycophenolic acid levels occur approximately one hour post dose, with a secondary peak occurring 6 to 8 hours later, due to enterohepatic recirculation of MPA glucuronide (MPAG) and its hydrolysis back to mycophenolic acid in the gastrointestinal tract. The apparent elimination half-life of mycophenolic acid after a single oral dose of MMF is approximately 18 hours. The AUC is found to increase following renal transplantation, stabilising after about a month of therapy. Food reduces the Cmax but has no effect on the AUC. Single dose studies in chronic renal impairment (creatinine clearance < $25 mL/min/1.73m^2$) showed that the AUC for mycophenolic acid was 28-75% higher than in individuals with no or milder renal impairment (Christians et al., 2006). A secondary plasma MPA peak is often seen 6 to 12 h after oral administration of MMF, suggesting enterohepatic circulation of the drug. Because of this secondary rise in plasma MPA concentration, the apparent mean terminal half-life of MPA is 17.9 h in healthy subjects. MPA is converted in the liver to the pharmacologically inactive MPAG, which is excreted by the kidney. Plasma MPA is extensively bound to albumin, and a mean protein binding of 97% has been reported in normal plasma (Bullingham, 1996a, 1996b). Renal transplant patients who received oral mycophenolate mofetil 1.5 g twice daily achieved maximal plasma concentrations of 13.5 µg/mL early postransplant (less than 40 days) and 24.1 µg/mL late posttransplant (at least 3 months). The maximum plasma concentrations were achieved at 1.21 hours and 0.9 hours, respectively. Following kidney transplantation, 10 patients who received oral mycophenolate mofetil 1 g twice daily achieved mean maximum plasma concentrations of mycophenolic acid of 11.1 µg/mL, 11.9 µg/mL, and 14.9 µg/mL on days 2, 5, and 28, respectively. The maximum concentration was achieved at 2.18 hours, 1.9 hours, and 1.63 hours (Johnson et al., 1999). Renal transplant patients (n=12) who received oral mycophenolic acid 720 mg twice daily achieved maximal plasma concentrations of 15 µg/mL, 26.2 µg/mL, and 24.1 µg/mL at 2 weeks, 3 months, and 6 months posttransplant, respectively. The maximum plasma concentrations were achieved at 1.8 hours, 2 hours, and 2 hours (Sollinger et al., 1992).

3.2.2 Absorption

MPM is well absorbed orally with a mean bioavailability of 94%. After oral administration, it is rapidly and essentially completely absorbed, and then essentially completely converted to MPA, the active immunosuppressant species. In renal transplant recipients, very low serum levels of mycophenolic acid were achieved after oral mycophenolate mofetil therapy in the early posttransplantation period; serum levels increased significantly after 20 days of treatment, suggesting potentially impaired absorption or altered metabolism of the ester in uremic patients. Following oral and IV administration, MPM undergoes rapid and complete metabolism to MPA, the active metabolite; however, Mycophenolate sodium (MPA 720 mg) and MPM 1 g result in bioequivalent MPA exposure. Food decreases peak plasma concentrations of MPA by 33-40%; no effect on the MPA AUC (Bullingham, et al., 1998).

3.2.3 Distribution

MPA plasma protein binding is ≥ 97-98%, mainly in albumin. Severe renal impairment has been shown to decrease the binding of mycophenolic acid to albumin, thereby elevating the concentration of mycophenolic acid free fraction in serum. In addition, increased levels of the mycophenolic acid glucuronide metabolite in these patients may compete with free mycophenolic acid for binding with albumin. In patients with renal impairment or delayed graft function, protein binding may be decreased (Meier-Kriesche et al., 2000). MPM hydrochloride protein binding is 97%, in albumin principally. MPA half-life is about 8 - 17.9 hours. MPM volume of distribution is approximately 4 L/Kg. The mean volume of distribution for mycophenolic acid was 54 L at steady state and 112 L at elimination phase (Bullingham, et al., 1998).

3.2.4 Metabolism and excretion route

MPM undergoes complete metabolism to MPA; metabolism occurs presystemically following oral administration. MPA is metabolized by glucuronyl transferase to the phenolic glucuronide of MPA. The phenolic glucuronide is converted to MPA via enterohepatic recirculation. MPM is rapidly hydrolysed extensively in the liver to MPA; this metabolite is conjugated to form the pharmacologically inactive mycophenolic acid glucuronide. Approximately 87% of the oral dose is excreted as MPAG in the urine. MPM is excreted in urine (93%) as the phenolic glucuronide of MPA (87%) and in feces (6%). MPS is excreted principally in urine as phenolic glucuronide of MPA (> 60%) and as unchanged MPA (3%). The mean renal clearance of MPA glucuronide was 15.5 mL/min following the administration of delayed release mycophenolic acid to stable renal transplant patients (Christians et al., 2006). Deconjugation of the glucuronide to mycophenolic acid may occur in humans via the action of intestinal or intestinal microflora beta-glucuronidase, with subsequent reabsorption of mycophenolic acid (Mourad et al., 2002; Platzet al., 2002). *In vivo*, mycophenolic acid glucuronide is converted to mycophenolic acid via enterohepatic recirculation. MPM total body clearance is 140 to 193 mL/min. The plasma clearance of MPA is 193 mL/min following oral administration of mycophenolate mofetil. The mean clearance of mycophenolic acid was 140 mL/min following oral administration of the delayed release mycophenolic acid tablet to stable renal transplant patients. The plasma clearance of MPA is 177 (+/- 31) mL/min following IV administration of MPM (Bullingham, et al., 1998; Meier-Kriesche et al., 2000).

3.3 Pharmacokinetic variability

The pharmacokinetics of MMF is complex; some patients achieve a peak in 1 to 2 h and a second peak at 5 to 6 h due to enterohepatic circulation. In some patients, the second peak (Cmax) is as much as 50% of the total peak concentration. A maximum concentration of >10 µg/mL is associated with side effects. There is little correlation with area under the concentration curve (AUC) and dose. The AUC in the first 12 h does correlate with propensity to reject if it is <30 µg.h/mL or toxicity if it is >60 µg.h/mL. The desired exposure is 35 to 60 µg.h/mL (Shaw et al., 2000). Mycophenolic acid AUC is increased by renal dysfunction, which may be clinically relevant early after transplantation or during rejection episodes. Plasma concentrations of MPA glucuronide higher in nontransplant subjects with severe renal impairment than in those with mild impairment or normal renal function. At the same time, plasma concentrations of MPA glucuronide higher in transplant patient with delayed renal graft function than in patients not experiencing delayed graft function. Dialysis does not remove MPA. Plasma concentrations of free (unbound) MPA and total MPA glucuronide have increased in nontransplant individuals with severe chronic renal impairment (GFR < 25mL/minute per 1.73 m^2). Plasma MPA concentrations in patients with delayed graft function similar to values in patients not experiencing delayed graft function. In hereditary deficiency of hypoxanthine-guanine phosphoribosyl-transferase (HGPRT), such as Lesch-Nyhan and Kelley-Seegmiller syndrome, the use of MPM (a inosine monophosphate dehydrogenase inhibitor) is not recommended (Ahsan et al., 1999).

3.3.1 Effect of food consumption, ethnicity and sex

Food delayed MPM absorption, the extent of absorption was not affected by food; however, the maximum concentration of the active metabolite was reduced by 40%. Administration of MPA delayed release tablet with a high fat meal did not affect the extent of absorption of mycophenolic acid, but the maximal plasma concentration was reduced by 33%, and there was a 5 hours delay in the time to reach maximal concentration (Bullingham et al. 1998). A pharmacokinetic study showed that the rate but not the extent of absorption of mycophenolate is affected by food, indicating that mycophenolate may be administered with food (Christians et al., 2010).

Ethnicity and sex do not significantly affect the primary pharmacokinetic parameters of MPA. A study examine MPA pharmacokinetics in 13 African American and 20 Caucasian renal transplant recipients during the first 4 to 90 posttransplant days and found No significant differences in either MPA AUC or free MPA AUC values (Shaw et al., 2000). Another investigation compared MPA pharmacokinetics in 39 African American and 43 Caucasian renal allograft recipients with stable graft function, There were no significant differences in MPA AUC, Cmax and tmax values between the two groups (Pescovitz et al., 2003). MPA pharmacokinetic parameters did not differ significantly in the males versus females in this study. No differences between diabetic and nondiabetic stable renal transplant recipients were found in this study. Limited studies comparing pharmacokinetics parameters between African-American and white renal transplant patients have shown few differences, suggesting that the differences in rejection rates between these two populations are not explained by pharmacokinetic differences alone but are more likely related to differences in innate immunologic response (Ahsan et al., 1999).

3.3.2 Relationship between adult and pediatric patients

There was a considerable inter- and intraindividual variability of pharmacokinetic parameters in both patient groups. Some of this variability appears to be related to the function of the kidney transplant, because in patients with primary transplant dysfunction a bower maximal MPA concentration and a longer time to maximum concentration were observed. This may be due to slower absorption of MMF, most likely as a result of uremic dysmotility of the gastrointestinal tract (Halloran et al., 1997). Because for MMF there is a relationship between the immunosuppressive efficacy in renal transplant recipients and the MPA-AUC, this fact predict that MMF in a dose of 600 mg/m^2 twice a day displays a comparable effectiveness in pediatric transplant recipients, as observed previously in adult patients. This hypothesis is currently being investigated in a large multicenter study. A dose of 600 mg MMF/m2 BSA in children between the ages of 6 and 15 year yielded comparable AUC for MPA and free MPA at 3 weeks after renal transplantation as adults who received 1 g of MMF, the recommended twice daily oral dose in adults (Bullingham, 1996a). Hence, the body surface area (BSA) -adjusted dosing of MMF appears to be appropriate in pediatric renal transplant recipients. MPM pharmacokinetic parameters, including AUC, in children 1 to 18 years of age receiving MPM 600 mg/m^2 (in oral suspension) twice daily following renal transplantation similar to values in adult renal transplant recipients receiving 1 g twice daily. MPS peak plasma concentrations and AUC of MPA in stable pediatric renal transplant patients 5 to 16 years of age receiving a single dose of MPS (MPA 450 mg/m^2) increased (33 and 18% respectively) relative to adults receiving the same dose based on body surface area. Clinical importance is not determined yet (Halloran et al., 1997).

3.4 Effect of time after transplantation on MPA Pharmacokinetics

The dose-interval MPA AUC in renal transplant recipients increases as a function of time. The dose-normalized mean MPA AUC in renal transplant patients is at least 30 to 50% lower in the first few weeks after transplantation than in the later period (1-6 months after transplantation). It has been demonstrated that most of this phenomenon is accounted for in the novo renal transplant patients with impaired renal function. The reason for lower MPA AUC in this patients in the early posttransplant compared with the time when graft function has stabilized (about 1 month after transplant surgery) is most likely the decreased plasma protein binding of MPA leading to an increase clearance of drug by the liver (Shaw et al., 1998). This theory is supported by observations of elevated free MPA fraction values in the early posttransplantation period in patients with impaired renal function that return to normal values by 1 month posttransplantation. A possible additional factor that could contribute to the higher oral clearance of MPA early after transplantation is corticosteroid therapy, which is significantly higher in that period but then is tapered to low dose levels or completely withdrawn. In pediatric patients, as in adult subjects, the median AUC values increase as a function of time after transplantation (from approximately 35 mg.h/L at weeks to approximately 65 mg.h/L at 3 months after transplantation). The intraindividual variability of AUC was high in the immediate posttransplant period, but decline in the stable phase, whereas the wide interindividual variability remained significant (Oellerich et al., 2000).

3.5 Pharmacokinetic Interactions with mycophenolate mofetil

Since mycophenolate mofetil is solely metabolized by glucuronidation, direct pharmacokinetic interactions with drugs metabolised by cytochrome P450 oxidation are not generally expected. Pharmacokinetic interaction with other drugs metabolised by glucuronidation is a theoretical possibility, although a clinically significant interaction is very unlikely. Potential general mechanisms for interactions with mycophenolate mofetil involve either entrohepatic cycling, or renal tubular competition between MPAG and other drugs undergoing transport mediated renal excretion. As regards the former, competitive interaction could occur between MPAG and other drugs at the biliary transporter, although no example has been reported. Once MPAG is excreted into the gut, cholestyramine and other bile acid sequestrants can clearly reduce the plasma mycophenolic acid AUC and hence clinical effectiveness. Deglucuronidation of MPAG in the colon is mediated by the gut flora, and in particular by the Gram-negative anaerobes which contain most of the glucuronidase activity. Antibiotics with activity against such organisms may reduce entrohepatic cycling and hence the mycophenolic acid AUC. With a renal tubular interaction, plasma mycophenolic acid is not affected. No major clinical sequelae appear to follow from raised plasma MPAG concentrations. The clinical significance of any tubular interaction will thus depend on the magnitude and consequence of raised plasma concentrations of the other interacting drug. Being a competitive interaction, high plasma MPAG concentrations are likely to increase the magnitude of the interaction. Renal impairment may thus be the clinical situation where such interactions need special consideration (Bullingham et al. 1998).

3.6 Clinical efficacy

The relationship between MPA pharmacokinetics and clinical outcomes has been reported in at least 1o investigations. The association between MPA AUC and the risk for acute rejection was first noted in a retrospective analysis of pharmacokinetic data obtained during the first 3 weeks after transplantation, in a dose-escalation study of MMF in 41 adult kidney transplant patients (Jeong & Kaplan, 2007; Takahashi et al., 1995). In mid-1990s, three large clinical trials were conducted in kidney transplant recipients to prove clinical efficacy of MMF. These were the largest prospective, randomized, double blind trials ever performed in transplantation, using the incidences of acute rejection as a primary end point. The results demonstrated the superior efficacy of MMF (1.0 or 1.5 g twice daily), combined with cyclosporine and steroids, in reducing the rate of acute rejection during 6 months after kidney transplantation as compared with azathioprine or placebo treatment (Jeong & Kaplan, 2007). Also, they established the safety of MMF in adult renal transplant patients; overall incidence of adverse effects was comparable between groups. The prominent adverse effects of MMF included nausea, vomiting, diarrhea, and hematologic effects, with a high dosage (3 g/d) being associated with increased risk for the adverse effects. Subsequent long-term (1- and 3-years) follow-up studies reported the similar efficacy and safety of MMF. Other maintenance immunosuppressants that have been evaluated in combination with MMF include tacrolimus. A randomized, clinical trial in renal transplant patients who were treated with tacrolimus-based triple regimens (tacrolimus/MMF/steroid) demonstrated a significant reduction in the incidence of rejection compared with the double regimen group when MMF was given at a dosage of 1g twice a day for 1 year after transplantation. However, in the first 6 months of this trial, MMF was discontinued in half of the patients because of gastrointestinal complications or hematologic adverse effects, indicating the need for lower MMF dosages. It was understood later to be because tacrolimus does not inhibit biliary excretion of MPAG, whereas cyclosporine disrupts enterohepatic cycling and intestinal reabsorption of MPA by inhibiting biliary transporters. Subsequent monitoring of MPA levels in renal transplant patients revealed that MPA plasma levels were lower in the cyclosporine-based regimen compared with the tacrolimus combination. In conclusion, MMF is effective in preventing acute rejection and improving graft and patient survival in combination with cyclosporine and tacrolimus. Tacrolimus-based treatment requires a lower dosage of MMF compared with a cyclosporine-based regimen to maintain the similar MPA plasma levels. (Pawinski et al., 2006).

3.7 Therapeutic drug monitoring

The incorporation of MMF into immunosuppressive regimens has been associated with decreased rates of acute rejection and decreased chronic allograft loss. When the drug was introduced into clinical practice, routine therapeutic drug monitoring was not recommended and empiric dosing became the norm of many centers. However, a deeper appreciation for the highly variable pharmacokinetic behavior of MPA and the relationship between concentration of the drug and risk for acute rejection, combined with an increased emphasis on the need for further improvements in clinical outcomes, treatment of patients with greater risk for graft loss than ever before, and the use of strategies for lowering or eliminating concomitant agents such as corticosteroids or CNI, have led to increasing interest in the role of MPA therapeutic drug monitoring in optimizing immunosuppression. Recent reviews have suggested provisional target therapeutic ranges for MPA AUC and trough concentrations when using MMF in combination with either cyclosporine or tacrolimus. When combined with cyclosporine, the recommended target ranges are 1 to 3.5 mg/L and 30 to 60 mg/h per L for trough concentrations and AUC, respectively. For the combination with tacrolimus, the target ranges of 1.9 to 4.0 mg/L and 30 to 60 mg/h per L for trough and AUC measurements, respectively, have been suggested (Van Gelder et al., 2006). Two ongoing concentration-control *versus* fixed dosage trials in renal transplant patients will hopefully provide the basis for rigorous assessment of these target ranges in the setting of contemporary practice. A proposed schedule for objective assessment of MPA exposure is presented in Table 4. We hope that the ongoing trials will provide more definitive data on which to base the selection of sample type, test schedule, and the cost-benefit analysis of MPA therapeutic monitoring (Shaw et al., 2007).

4. Corticosteroids

4.1 Mechanism of action

Glucocorticoids exert their effects by binding to a glucocorticoid receptor (GR) localized in the cytoplasm of target cells. There is a single class of GR that binds glucocorticoids, with no evidence for subtypes of differing affinity in different tissues. Recently a splice variant of GR, termed GR-b, has been identified that does not bind glucocorticoids but binds to DNA and may therefore potentially interfere with the action of glucocorticoids (Bamberger et al., 1995).

4.2 Pharmacokinetics

The pharmacokinetic characteristics of the various glucocorticoids depend on their physicochemical properties. Glucocorticoids are lipophilic and are usually administered as prodrugs when given intravenously (Mager & Jusko, 2002).

4.2.1 Absorption and distribution

Glucocorticoids are well absorbed after oral administration and have a bioavailability of 60–100%. They have moderate protein binding and a moderate apparent volume of distribution (Derendorf et al., 1991; Varis et al., 2000). Over 90% of circulating plasma corticosteroids attached to two types of proteins: (1) a non-specific albumin, and (2) a high affinity transcortin, an α-2-globulin important in regulating corticosteroid flowing freely, as allows greater freedom in tissues with an inflammatory response. Transcortin has a high affinity and a low capacity for hydrocortisone and prednisolone, whereas albumin has a low affinity but high capacity. This leads to an increase in the free glucocorticoid fraction once transcortin is saturated at concentrations of about 400 μg/L. Such concentrations are achieved after administration of hydrocortisone or prednisolone doses >20mg (Czock et al., 2005). Protein binding is biologically relevant, because only free drug can reach the biophase (i.e. the site of action) and interact with the receptor. Therefore, pharmacodynamic considerations have to include protein binding. Clinically, decreased protein binding due to low plasma albumin concentrations correlated with glucocorticoid adverse effects in prednisone therapy (Lewis et al., 1971). Generally, however, alterations in protein binding do not have much impact on drug action (Benet et al., 2002; Czock et al., 2005).

4.2.2 Metabolism and excretion

The renal excretion of unchanged glucocorticoids is only 1–20% (Garg & Jusko, 1994). Glucocorticoid metabolism is a two-step process. Firstly, oxygen or hydrogen atoms are added then secondly, conjugation takes place (glucuronidation or sulphation). Subsequently the kidney excretes the resulting hydrophilic inactive metabolites. Intracellular metabolism by 11β-hydroxysteroid dehydrogenase (11β-HSD) controls the availability of glucocorticoids for binding to the glucocorticoid and mineralocorticoid receptors. Type 1 dehydrogenase (11β-HSD1) is widely distributed in glucocorticoid target tissues and has its highest activity in the liver. 11β-HSD1 acts mainly as a reductase, converting the inactive cortisone to the active cortisol (Czock et al., 2005). Type 2 dehydrogenase (11β-HSD2) is found in mineralocorticoid target tissues (kidney, colon, salivary glands, placenta). 11β-HSD2 has a high affinity for endogenous cortisol and by oxidation, converting cortisol to cortisone, it protects the mineralocorticoid receptor from occupation by cortisol. The activity of 11β-HSD2 varies depending on the type of glucocorticoid, which explains to some extent the different mineralocorticoid activities of different glucocorticoids (Diederichet al., 2002).

4.2.3 Prednisolone and prednisone

The pharmacokinetics of prednisolone and prednisone are complicated by dose-dependency due to nonlinear protein binding (Wald et al., 1992). Protein binding of prednisolone decreases nonlinearly from 95% to 60–70%, while the concentration increases from 200 60–70%, while the concentration increases from 200 μg/L to 800 μg/L when protein binding of prednisolone reaches the stationary state (Rose et al., 1981). In consequence, a dose-dependent increase in the volume of distribution (Vd) and drug clearance (CL) is observed at doses over 20mg (Frey et al., 1990; Rohatagi et al., 1997). However, the elimination half-life remains constant and the dose dependencies of Vd and CL disappear when free prednisolone concentrations are measured (Möllmann et al., 1989; Rohatagi 1997). Prednisolone clearance decreases again only at very high doses, which can be explained by saturation of elimination mechanisms. The affinity of prednisone for transcortin is 10-fold lower than that of prednisolone (Czock et al., 2005).

4.2.4 Methylprednisolone

Methylprednisolone (6α-methylprednisolone) has no affinity for transcortin and binds only to albumin (Czock et al., 2005). Accordingly, methylprednisolone pharmacokinetics are linear, with no dose-dependency. The disposition of methylprednisolone is biexponential (Möllmann et al., 1989). A two-compartment model is appropriate for intravenous administration of very high doses. A one compartment model can be used with lower intravenous doses and oral administration (Booker et al., 2002; Lewis et al. 1971).

4.3 Interactions between glucocorticoids and tacrolimus

Corticosteroids are an essential component of most immunosuppressive regimens currently used in renal transplantation because of their efficacy in reducing acute rejection and improving graft survival. The precise mechanism of action of glucocorticoids is not fully understood, although it is apparent that it is multifaceted, involving both direct and indirect mechanisms and affecting proximal and distal events of T cell activation (Almawi et al., 1999). Long-term administration of corticosteroids also is known to be associated with numerous adverse effects that lead to increased patient morbidity and mortality after renal transplantation. The adverse effects of corticosteroids, including new-onset diabetes, hyperlipidemia, hypertension, growth retardation, accelerated bone loss, weight gain, avascular necrosis, cataracts, cosmetic changes, depression, psychotic behavior, and others, have been well documented Hricik et al., 1993; Grotz et al., 1998; Kobashigawa & Kasiske, 1997; Schulak & Hricik, 1994). There also is evidence that they may interfere with the tolerogenic pathways of organ acceptance (Qian et al., 1997; Wang et al., 2001). In addition to affecting the morbidity and the quality of life of renal transplant recipients, corticosteroids increase the long-term cost of their medical. Because glucocorticoids are inducers of the CYP34A4 enzyme involved in tacrolimus metabolism, theoretically glucocorticoid use would be expected to necessitate increased tacrolimus dosing. Indeed, studies in adults have documented increased tacrolimus levels upon steroid withdrawal, but similar data on pediatric patients are not available. In recent years, tacrolimus has been used both steroid based and steroid-free immunosuppressive protocols (van Duijnhoven et al., 2003; Anglicheau et al., 2003). Steroid avoidance or rapid elimination of steroids may have an advantage over steroid withdrawal. Steroid avoidance protocols may avoid the long-term risks of steroid use and the increased risk for rejection when the steroids are withdrawn. Birkeland and Khwaja reported excellent long term graft survival and function (3 and 4 year, respectively) with very low rejection rates. In other studies, a slight increase in acute rejection episodes, especially in the early posttransplantation period, was observed; these were easily reversible, and their impact on long-term graft survival is unclear at this time (Borrows et al., 2004; Cole et al., 2001; Grewal et al., 1998; ter Meulen et al., 2004). Steroids, once thought to be a mandatory component of immunosuppression to preserve graft survival, are gradually being eliminated from current protocols. It has long been recognized that despite the efficacy of maintenance corticosteroids that these medications are far from benign (Jaber et al., 2007). Consequently, corticosteroid-free immunosuppression has become a desirable goal for many in the transplant community. A potential problem of eliminating corticosteroids from an immunosuppressive regimen, however, is an increased risk for acute rejection (Vanrenterghem et al., 2000).

5. References

Ahsan, N., Hricik, D., & Matas, A., Rose, S., Tomlanovich, S., & Wilkinson, A., Ewell, M., McIntosh, M., & Stablein, D., Hodge E. Prednisone withdrawal in kidney transplant recipients on cyclosporine and mycophenolate mofetil--a prospective randomized study. Steroid Withdrawal Study Group. *Transplantation*, Vol. 68, No. 12, (December 1999), pp. 1865-1874, ISSN 1534-0608

Almawi, W.Y., Melemedjian, O.K., & Rieder, M.J. An alternate mechanism of glucocorticoid anti-proliferative effect: Promotion of a Th2 cytokine-secreting profile. *Clinical Transplantation*, Vol. 13, No. 5, (October 1999), pp. 365-374, ISSN 0902-0063

Anglicheau, D., Flamant, M., & Schlageter, M.H., Martinez, F., Cassinat, B., & Beaune, P., Legendre, C., & Thervet, E. Pharmacokinetic interaction between corticosteroids and tacrolimus after renal transplantation. *Nephrology Dialysis Transplantation*, Vol. 18, No. 11, (November 2003), pp. 2409-14, ISSN 1460-6235

Bai, J.P., Lesko, L.J., & Burckart, G.J. Understanding the genetic basis for adverse drug effects: the calcineurin inhibitors. *Pharmacotherapy*, Vol. 30, No. 2, (February 2010), pp. 195-209, ISSN 0277-0008

Bamberger, C.M., Bamberger, A.M., & de Castro, M., Chrousos, G.P. Glucocorticoid receptor beta, a potential endogenous inhibitor of glucocorticoid action in humans. *Journal of Clinical Investigation*, Vol. 95, No. 6, (Jun 1995), pp. 2435-2441, ISSN 0021-9738

Barrera-Pulido, L., Aguilera-García, I., & Docobo-Pérez, F., Alamo-Martínez, J.M., & Pareja-Ciuró, F., Nuñez-Roldán, A., & Gómez-Bravo, M.A., Bernardos-Rodríguez, A. Clinical relevance and prevalence of polymorphisms in CYP3A5 and MDR1 genes that encode tacrolimus biotransformation enzymes in liver transplant recipients. *Transplantation Proceedings*, Vol. 40, No. 9, (November 2008), pp. 2949-2951, ISSN 0041-1345

Bekersky, I., Dressler, D., & Mekki, Q. Effect of time of meal consumption on bioavailability of a single oral 5 mg tacrolimus dose. *Journal of Clinical Pharmacology*, Vol. 41, No. 3, (March 2001), pp. 289-297, ISSN 1552-4604

Bekersky, I., Dressler, D., & Mekki, Q.A. Effect of low- and high-fat meals on tacrolimus absorption following 5 mg single oral doses to healthy human subjects. *Journal of Clinical Pharmacology*, Vol. 41, No. 2, (February 2001), pp. 176-182, ISSN 1552-4604

Benet, L.Z. & Hoener B.A. Changes in plasma protein binding have little clinical relevance. *Clinical Pharmacology and Therapeutics*, Vol. 71, No. 3, (March 2002), pp. 115-121, ISSN 0009-9236

Birkeland, S.A. Steroid-free immunosuppression in renal transplantation: A long-term follow-up of 100 consecutive patients. *Transplantation*, Vol.71 , No. 8, (April 2007), pp. 1089-90, ISSN 1534-0608

Booker, B.M., Magee, M.H., & Blum, R.A., Lates, C.D., Jusko, W.J. Pharmacokinetic and pharmacodynamic interactions between diltiazem and methyl prednisolone in healthy volunteers. *Clinical Pharmacology and Therapeutics*, Vol. , No. , (October 2002), pp. 370-382, ISSN 0009-9236

Borrows, R., Loucaidou, M., & Van Tromp, J., Cairns, T., Griffith, M., & Hakim, N., McLean, A., Palmer, A., & Papalois, V., Taube, D. Steroid sparing with tacrolimus and mycophenolate mofetil in renal transplantation. *American Journal of Transplantation*, Vol. 4, No. 11, (November 2004), pp. 1845-51, ISSN 1600-6143

Bullingham, R., Monroe, S., & Nicholls, A., Hale, M. Pharmacokinetics and bioavailability of mycophenolate mofetil in healthy subjects after single-dose oral and intravenous administration. *Journal of Clinical Pharmacology*, Vol. 36, No. 4, (April 1996b), pp. 315-324, ISSN 1552-4604

Bullingham, R., Nicholls, A., & Hale, M. Pharmacokinetics of mycophenolate mofetil (RS 61443): A short review. *Transplantation Proceedings*, Vol. 28, No. 2, (April 1996a), pp. 925-929, ISSN 0041-1345

Bullingham, R.E., Nicholls, A.J., Kamm, .BR. Clinical pharmacokinetics of mycophenolate mofetil. Clinical Pharmacokinetics, Vol. 34, No. 6, (1998), pp. 429-455, ISSN 0312-5963

Cattaneo, D., Perico, N., & Remuzzi, G. From pharmacokinetics to pharmacogenomics: a new approach to tailor immunosuppressive therapy. *American Journal of Transplantation*, Vol. 4, No. 3, (March 2004), pp. 299-310, ISSN 1600-6143

Chen, J.S., Li, L.S., & Cheng, D.R., Ji, S.M., & Sun, Q.Q., Cheng, Z., & Wen, J.Q., Sha, G.Z., & Liu ZH. . Effect of CYP3A5 genotype on renal allograft recipients treated with tacrolimus. *Transplantation Proceedings*, Vol. 41, No. 5, (June 2002), pp. 1557–6, ISSN 0041-1345

Christians, U., Jacobsen, W., & Benet, L.Z., Lampen, A. Mechanisms of clinically relevant drug interactions associated with tacrolimus. *Clinical Pharmacokinetics*, Vol. 41, No. 11, (2002), pp. 813-51, ISSN 0312-5963

Christians, U., Klawitter, J., & Clavijo, C.F. *Kidney International, Supplement*, No.115, (March 2010), pp. S1-S7, ISSN 0085-2538

Christians, U., Pokaiyavannichkul, T., & Chan, L. (2006). Tacrolimus, In: *Applied Pharmacokinetics and Pharmacodynamics, Principles of Therapeutic Drug Monitoroing*, M.E. Burton, L.M. Shaw, J.J. Schentag, W.E. Evans, (Ed.), pp. 529-562, Lippincott, Williams and Wilkins, ISSN 0-7817-4431-8, Philadelphia, United States of America

Cole, E., Landsberg, D., & Russell, D., Zaltzman, J., & Kiberd, B., Caravaggio, C., and Vasquez, A.R., Halloran, P. A pilot study of steroid-free immunosuppression in the prevention of acute rejection in renal allograft recipients. *Transplantation*, Vol. 72, No. 5, (September 2001), pp. 845-50, ISSN 1534-0608

Czock, D., Keller, F., & Rasche, F.M., Häussler, U. Pharmacokinetics and pharmacodynamics of systemically administered glucocorticoids. *Clinical Pharmacokinetics*, Vol. 44, No. 1, (2005), pp. 61-98, ISSN 0312-5963

Danesi, R., Mosca, M., & Boggi, U., Del Tacca, M. Genetics of drug response to immunosuppressive treatment and prospects for personalized therapy. *Molecular Medicine Today*, Vol. 6, No. 12, (December 2000), pp. 475-482. [Abstract] ISSN 1357-4310

del Mar Fernández De Gatta, M., Santos-Buelga, D., & Domínguez-Gil, A.,García, M.J. Immunosuppressive therapy for paediatric transplant patients: pharmacokinetic considerations. *Clinical Pharmacokinetics*, Vol. 41, No. 2 (2002), pp. 115-135, ISSN 0312-5963

Derendorf, H., Möllmann, H., & Barth, J., Möllmann, C., & Tunn, S., Krieg, M. Pharmacokinetics and oral bioavailability of hydrocortisone. *Journal of Clinical Pharmacology*, Vol. 31, No. 5, (May 1991), pp. 473-476, ISSN 1552-4604

Diederich, .S, Eigendorff, E., & Burkhardt, P., Quinkler, M., & Bumke-Vogt, C., Rochel, M., & Seidelmann, D., Esperling, P., & Oelkers, W., Bähr, V. 11 β-hydroxysteroid dehydrogenase types 1 and 2: an important pharmacokinetic determinant for the activity of synthetic mineralo- and glucocorticoids. *The Journal of Clinical Endocrinology and Metabolism*, Vol. 87, No. 12, (December 2002), pp. 5695- 5701, ISSN 1945-7197

Dresser, G.K., Spence, J.D., & Bailey, D.G. Pharmacokinetic-pharmacodynamic consequences and clinical relevance of cytochrome P450 3A4 inhibition. *Clinical Pharmacokinetics*, Vol. 38, No. 1, (2000), pp. 41-57, ISSN 0312-5963

Felipe, C.R., Silva, H.T., & Machado, P.G., García, R., & da Silva Moreira, S.R., Pestana, J.O. The impact of ethnic miscegenation on tacrolimus clinical pharmacokinetics and therapeutic drug monitoring. *Clinical Transplantation*, Vol. 16, No. 4, (August 2002), pp. 262–272, ISSN 0902-0063

Fitzsimmons, W.E., Bekersky, I., & Dressler, D., Raye, K., & Hodosh, E., Mekki, Q. Demographic considerations in tacrolimus pharmacokinetics. *Transplantation Proceedings*, Vol. 30, No. 4, (June 1998), pp. 1359-1364, ISSN 0041-1345

Frey, B.M. & Frey, F.J. Clinical pharmacokinetics of prednisone and prednisolone. *Clinical Pharmacokinetics*, Vol. 19, No. 2, (1990), pp. 26-46, ISSN 0312-5963

Fung, J.J. Tacrolimus and transplantation: A decade in review. *Transplantation*, Vol. 77, No. 9, (May 2004), pp. S41-S43, ISSN 1534-0608

Garg, V. & Jusko, W.J. Bioavailability and reversible metabolism of prednisone and prednisolone in man. *Biopharmaceutics and Drug Disposition*, Vol. 15, No. 2, (March 1994), pp. 163-172, ISSN 0142-2782

González-Posada, J.M., Hernández, D., & Bayés Genís, B., García Perez, J., & Rivero Sanchez M. Impact of diabetes mellitus on kidney transplant recipients in Spain. *Nephrology Dialysis Transplantation*, Vol. 19, No. S3, (June 2004), pp. iii57–61, ISSN 1460-6235

Grewal, H.P., Thistlethwaite, J.R. Jr., & Loss, GE. Corticosteroid cessation 1 week following renal transplantation using tacrolimus/mycophenolate mofetil based immunosuppression. *Transplantation Proceedings*, Vol. 30, No. 4, (June 1998), pp. 1378-1379, ISSN 0041-1345

Grotz, W.H., Rump, L.C., & Niessen, A., Schmidt-Gayk, H., & Reichelt, A., Kirste, G., & Olschewski, M., Schollmeyer, P.J. Treatment of osteopenia and osteoporosis after kidney transplantation. *Transplantation*, Vol. 66, No. 8, (October 1998), pp. 1004-1008, ISSN 1534-0608

Halloran, P., Mathew, T., & Tomlanovich, S., Groth, C., Hooftman, L., & Barker, C. Mycophenolate mofetil in renal allograft recipients: a pooled efficacy analysis of three randomized, double-blind, clinical studies in prevention of rejection. *Transplantation*, Vol. 63, No. 1, (January 1997), pp. 39-47, ISSN 1534-0608

Halloran, P.F. Immunosuppressive Drugs for Kidney Transplantation. *New England Journal of Medicine*, Vol. 351, No. 26, (December 2002), pp. 2715-2729, ISSN 0028-4793

Hämmerlein, A., Derendorf, H., & Lowenthal, D.T. Pharmacokinetic and pharmacodynamic changes in the elderly. Clinical implications. *Clinical Pharmacokinetics*, Vol. 35, No. 1, (2002), pp. 49-64, ISSN 0312-5963

Hariharan, S., Schroeder, T.J., & First, M.R. Effect of race on renal transplant outcome. *Clinical Transplantation*, Vol. 7, No. 3, (June 1993), pp. 235, ISSN 0902-0063

Harris, R.Z., Benet, L.Z., & Schwartz, J,B. Gender effects in pharmacokinetics and pharmacodynamics. *Drugs*, Vol. 50, No. 2, (2002), pp. 222-239, ISSN 0012-6667

Hebert, M.F., Fisher, R.M., & Marsh, C.L., Dressler, D., & Bekersky, I. Effects of rifampin on tacrolimus pharmacokinetics in healthy volunteers. *Journal of Clinical Pharmacology*, Vol. 39, No. 1, (February 1999), pp. 91-96, ISSN 1552-4604

Hesselink, D.A., Bouamar, R., & van Gelder, T. The pharmacogenetics of calcineurin inhibitor-related nephrotoxicity. *Therapeutic Drug Monitoring*, Vol. 32, No. 4, (August 2010), pp. 387-393, ISSN 0163-4356

Hesselink, D.A., Ngyuen, H., & Wabbijn, M., Gregoor, P.J., Steyerberg, E.W., & van Riemsdijk, I.C., Weimar, W., & van Gelder T. Tacrolimus dose requirement in renal transplant recipients is significantly higher when used in combination with corticosteroids. *British Journal of Clinical Pharmacology*, Vol. 56, No. 3, (September 2003), pp. 327-30, ISSN 1552-4604

Hricik, D.E., O'Toole, M.A., & Schulak, J.A., Herson, J. Steroid-free immunosuppression in cyclosporine treated renal transplant recipients: a meta-analysis. *Journal of the American Society of Nephrology*, Vol. 4, No. 6, (December 1993), pp. 1300-1005, ISSN 1046-6673

Hübner, G.I., Eismann, R., & Sziegoleit, W. Drug interaction between Mycophenolate mofetil and tacrolimus detectable within therapeutic mycophenolic acid monitoring in renal transplant recipients. *Therapeutic Drug Monitoring*, Vol. 21, No. 5, (October 199), pp. 536-539, ISSN 0163-4356

Iwasaki, K. Metabolism of Tacrolimus (FK506) and Recent Topics in Clinical Pharmacokinetics. *Drug Metabolism and Pharmacokinetics*, Vol. 22, No. 5, (October 2007), pp. 328-335, ISSN 1347-4367

Jaber, J.J., Feustel, P.J., & Elbahloul, O., Conti, A.D., & Gallichio, M.H., Conti, D.J. Early steroid withdrawal therapy in renal transplant recipients: a steroid-free sirolimus and CellCept-based calcineurin inhibitor-minimization protocol. *Clinical Transplantation*, Vol. 21, No. 1, (January-February 2007), pp. 101-109, ISSN 0902-0063

Jeong, H. & Kaplan, B. Therapeutic monitoring of mycophenolate mofetil. *Clinical Journal of the American Society of Nephrology*, Vol. 2, No. 1, (January 2007), pp. 184-191, ISSN 1555-9041

Johnson, A.G., Rigby, R.J., & Taylor, P.J., Jones, C.E., Allen, J., & Franzen, K., Falk, M,C., & Nicol, D. The kinetics of mycophenolic acid and its glucuronide metabolite in adult kidney transplant recipients. *Clinical Pharmacology and Therapeutics*, Vol. 66, No. , (November 1999), pp. 492-500, ISSN 0009-9236

Joy, M.S., Hogan, S.L., & Thompson, B.D., William, F., & Finn, W.F., Nickeleit, V. Cytochrome P450 3A5 expression in the kidneys of patients with calcineurin inhibitor nephrotoxicity. *Nephrology Dialysis Transplantation*, Vol. 22, No. 7, (July 2007), pp. 1963–1968, ISSN 1460-6235

Jusko, W.J. Analysis of tacrolimus (FK 506) in relation to therapeutic drug monitoring. *Therapeutic Drug Monitoring*, Vol. 17, No. 6, (December 1995), pp. 596-601, ISSN 0163-4356

Jusko, W.J. & Kobayashi, M. Therapeutic monitoring of tacrolimus (FK 506). *Therapeutic Drug Monitoring*, Vol. 15, No. 4, (August 1993), pp. 349, ISSN

Jusko, W.J., Thomson, A.W., & Fung, J., McMaster, P., & Wong, S.H., Zylber-Katz E. Consensus document: therapeutic monitoring of tacrolimus (FK506). *Therapeutic Drug Monitoring*, Vol. 17, No. 6, (December 1995), pp. 606-614, ISSN 0163-4356

Kamar, N., Mariat, C., & Delahousse, M., Dantal, J., Al Najjar, A., & Cassuto, E., Lefrançois, N., Cointault, O., & Touchard, G., Villemain, F., & Di Giambattista, F., Benhamou, P.Y. Diabetes mellitus after kidney transplantation: a French multicentre observational study. *Nephrology Dialysis Transplantation*, Vol. 22, No. 7, (July 2007), pp. 1986-1993, ISSN 1460-6235

Kaplan, B., Meier-Kriesche, H.U., & Friedman, G., Mulgaonkar, S., Gruber, S., & Korecka, M., Brayman, K.L., Shaw, L.M. Pharmacokinetics of mycophenolic acid in renal transplant patients whit delayed graft function. *Journal of Clinical Pharmacology*. 1998;39(7):715-20

Kapturczak, M.H., Meier-Kriesche, H.U., & Kaplan, B. Pharmacology of calcineurin antagonists. *Transplantation Proceedings*, Vol. 36, No. 2S, (March 2004), pp. 25S-32S, ISSN 0041-1345

Khwaja, K., Asolati, M., & Harmon, J., Melancon, J.K., & Dunn, T., Gillingham, K., & Kandaswamy, R., Humar, A., & Gruessner, R., Payne, W., & Najarian, J., Dunn, D., & Sutherland, D., Matas AJ. Outcome at 3 years with a prednisone-free maintenance regimen: A single-center experience with 349 kidney transplant recipients. *American Journal of Transplantation*, Vol. 4, No. 6, (June 2004), pp. 980-987, ISSN 1600-6143

Kiberd, B.A., Lawen, J., & Fraser, A.D., Keough-Ryan, T., & Belitsky, P. Early adequate mycophenolic acid exposure is associated with less rejection in kidney transplantation. *American Journal of Transplantation*, Vol. 4, No. 7, (July 2004), pp. 1079–1083, ISSN 1600-6143

Kobashigawa, J.A. & Kasiske, B.L. Hyperlipidemia in solid organ transplantation. *Transplantation*, Vol. 63, No. 3, (February 1997), pp. 331-338, ISSN 1534-0608

Lewis, G.P., Jusko, W.J., & Graves, L., ND Burke, C.W. Prednisone side-effects and serum-protein levels: a collaborative study. *The Lancet*, Vol. 2, No. 7728, (October 1971), pp. 778-780, ISSN 0140-6736

López-Montenegro Soria, M.A., Kanter Berga, J., & Beltrán Catalán, S., Milara Payá, J., & Pallardó Mateu, LM., Jiménez Torres, N.V. Genetic Polymorphisms and Individualized Tacrolimus Dosing. *Transplantation Proceedings*, Vol. 42, No. 8, (October 2010), pp. 3031-3033, ISSN 0041-1345

Lown, K.S., Mayo, R.R., & Leichtman, A.B., Hsiao, H.L., & Turgeon, D.K., Schmiedlin-Ren, & P., Brown, M.B., Guo, W., & Rossi, S.J., Benet, L.Z., & Watkins, P.B. Role of intestinal P-glycoprotein (MDR1) in interpatient variation in the oral bioavailability of cyclosporine. *Clinical Pharmacology and Therapeutics*. Vol. 62, No.3 , (September 1997), pp. 248-260, ISSN 0009-9236

Macphee, I.A., Fredericks, S., & Mohamed, M., Moreton, M., & Carter, N.D., Johnston, A., & Goldberg, L., Holt, D.W. Tacrolimus pharmacogenetics: the CYP3A5*1 allele predicts low dose-normalized tacrolimus blood concentrations in whites and South Asians. *Transplantation*, Vol. 79 , No. 4, (February 2002), pp. 499-502, ISSN 1534-0608

Macphee, I.A., Fredericks, S., & Tai, T., Syrris, P., & Carter, N.D., Johnston, A., & Goldberg, L., Holt, D.W. Tacrolimus pharmacogenetics: polymorphisms associated with expression of cytochrome p4503A5 and P-glycoprotein correlate with dose requirement. *Transplantation*, Vol. 74, No. 11, (December 2002), pp. 1486-1489, ISSN 1534-0608

Mager, D.E. & Jusko W.J. Quantitative structure-pharmacokinetic/pharmacodynamic relationships of corticosteroids in man. *Journal of Pharmaceutical Sciences*, Vol. 91, No. 11, (November 2002), pp. 2441-2451, ISSN 0022-3549

Mancinelli, L.M., Frassetto, L., & Floren, L.C., Dressler, D., & Carrier, S., Bekersky, I., & Benet, L.Z., Christians, U. The pharmacokinetics and metabolic disposition of tacrolimus: a comparison across ethnic groups. *Clinical Pharmacology and Therapeutics*, Vol. 69, No. 1, (January 2001), pp. 24-31, ISSN 0009-9236

Mañez, R., Martin, M., & Raman, D., Silverman, D., & Jain, A., Warty, V., & Gonzalez-Pinto, I., Kusne, S., & Starzl, T.E. Fluconazole therapy in transplant recipients receiving FK506. *Transplantation*. Vol. 57, No. 10, (May 2002), pp.1521-1523 , ISSN 1534-0608

Markell M. New-onset diabetes mellitus in transplant patients: pathogenesis, complications, and management. *American Journal of Kidney Disease*, Vol. 43, No. 6, (June 2004), pp. 953-965, ISSN 0272-6386

Meibohm, B., Beierle, I., & Derendorf, H. How important are gender differences in pharmacokinetics? *Clinical Pharmacokinetics*, Vol. 41, No. 5, (2002), pp. 329-342, ISSN 0312-5963

Meier-Kriesche, H.U. & Kaplan, B. Cyclosporine microemulsion and tacrolimus are associated with decreased chronic allograft failure and improved long-term graft survival as compared with Sandimmune. *American Journal of Transplantation*, Vol. 2, No. 1, (January 2002), pp. 100-104, ISSN 1600-6143

Meier-Kriesche, H.U., Shaw, L.M., & Korecka, M., Kaplan, B. Pharmacokinetics of mycophenolic acid in renal insufficiency. *Therapeutic Drug Monitoring*, Vol. 22, No. 1, (February 2000), pp. 27-30, ISSN 0163-4356

Möllmann, H., Rohdewald, P., & Barth, J., Verho, M., Derendorf H. Pharmacokinetics and dose linearity testing of methylprednisolone phosphate. *Biopharmaceutics and Drug Disposition*, Vol. 10, No. 5, (September-October 1989), pp. 453-64, ISSN 0142-2872

Mourad, M., Wallemacq, P., & König, J., de Frahan, E.H., & Eddour, D.C., De Meye,r M., & Malaise, J., Squifflet, J.P. Therapeutic monitoring of mycophenolate mofetil in organ transplant recipients. Is it necessary? *Clinical Pharmacokinetics*, Vol. 41, No. 3, (2002), pp. 319-327, ISSN 0312-5963

Naesens, M., Kuypers, D.R., & Sarwal, M. Calcineurin Inhibitor Nephrotoxicity. Clinical *Journal of the American Society of Nephrology*, Vol. 4, No. 2, (February 2009), pp. 481–508, 1555-9041

Ochiai, T., Fukao, K., & Takahashi, K., Endo, T., & Oshima, S., Uchida, K., & Yokoyama, I., Ishibashi, M., & Takahara, S., Iwasaki, Y. Phase III study of FK 506 in kidney transplantation. *Transplantation Proceedings*, Vol. 27, No. 1, (February 1995), pp. 829-833, ISSN 0041-1345

Oellerich, M., Shipkova, M., & Schütz E., Wieland, E., Weber, L., & Tönshoff, B., Armstrong, V.W. Pharmacokinetic and metabolic investigations of mycophenolic acid in pediatric patients after renal transplantation: implications for therapeutic drug monitoring. *Therapeutic Drug Monitoring*, Vol. 22 No. 1, (February 2000), pp. 20-26, ISSN 0163-4356

Op den Buijsch, R.A., Christiaans, M.H., & Stolk, L.M., de Vries J.E., & Cheung, C.Y., Undre, N.A., & van Hooff, J.P., van Dieijen-Visser, & M.P., Bekers, O. Tacrolimus pharmacokinetics: infuence of adenosine triphosphate-binding cassette B1 (ABCB1) and cytochrome (CYP) 3A polymorphisms. *Fundamental & Clinical Pharmacology*, Vol. 21, No. 4, (August 2007), pp. 427-35, ISSN 0767-3891

Paine, M.F., Khalighi, M., & Fisher, J.M., Shen, D.D., & Kunze, K.L., Marsh, C.L., & Perkins, J.D., Thummel, KE. Characterization of interintestinal and intraintestinal variations in human CYP3A dependant metabolism. *The Journal of Pharmacology and Experimental Therapeutic*, Vol. 283, No. 3, (December 1997), pp. 1552-1562, ISSN 0022-3565

Pascual, M., Theruvath, T., & Kawai, T., Tolkoff-Rubin, N., & Cosimi, A.B. Strategies to improve long-term outcomes after renal transplantation. *New England Journal of Medicine*, Vol. 346, No. 8, (February 2002), pp. 580-590, ISSN 0028-4793

Pawinski, T., Durlik, M., & Szlaska, I., Urbanowicz, A., & Majchrnak, J., Gralak, B. Comparison of mycophenolic acid pharmacokinetic parameters in kidney transplant patients within the first 3 months post-transplant. *Journal of Clinical Pharmacy and Therapeutics*, Vol. 31, No. 1, (February 2006), pp.27-34, ISSN 0009-9236

Pescovitz, M.D., Guasch, A., & Gaston, R., Rajagopalan, P., & Tomlanovich, S., Weinstein, S., & Bumgardner, G.L., Melton, L., & Ducray, P,S., Banken, L., & Hall, J., Boutouyrie, B.X. Equivalent pharmacokinetics of mycophenolate mofetil in African-American and Caucasian male and female stable renal allograft recipients. *American Journal of Transplantation*, Vol. 3, No. 12, (December 2003), pp.1581-1586, ISSN 16006143

Pillans, P.I., Rigby, R.J., & Kubler, P., Willis, C., & Salm, P., Tett, S.E., & Taylor, P.J. A retrospective analysis of mycophenolic acid and ciclosporin concentrations with acute rejection in renal transplant recipients. *Clinical Biochemistry*, Vol. 34, No. 1, (February 2001), pp. 77-81, ISSN 0009-9120

Platz, K.P., Eckhoff, D.E., & Hullett, D.A., Sollinger, H.W. RS-61443 studies: review and proposal. *Transplantation Proceedings*, Vol. 23, No. 2S2, (April 2002), pp. 33-35, ISSN 0041-1345

Plosker, G.L., & Foster, R.H. Tacrolimus: a further update of its pharmacology and therapeutic use in the management of organ transplantation. *Drugs*, Vol. 59, No. 2, (2000), pp. 323-89, ISSN 0012-6667

Prograf Product Monograph Astellas Pharma Canada, Inc. Revision 2009.

Qian, S., Lu, L., & Fu, F., Li, Y., & Li, W., Starzl, T.E., & Fung, J.J., Thomson, A.W. Apoptosis within spontaneously accepted mouse liver allografts: evidence for deletion of cytotoxic T cells and implications for tolerance induction. *Journal of Immunology*, Vol. 158, No. 10, (May 1997), pp. 4654-4661, ISSN 1550- 6606

Rohatagi, S., Barth, J., & Möllmann, H., Hochhaus, G., & Soldner, A., Möllmann, C., & Derendorf H. Pharmacokinetics of methylprednisolone and prednisolone after single and multiple oral administration. *Journal of Clinical Pharmacology*, Vol. 37, No. 10, (October 1997), pp. 916-925, ISSN 1552-4604

Rose, J.Q., Yurchak, A.M., & Jusko, W.J. Dose dependent pharmaco kinetics of prednisone and prednisolone in man. *Journal of Pharmacokinetics and Biopharmaceutics*, Vol. 20, No. 6, (August 1981), pp. 389-417, ISSN 0090-466X

Rosso Felipe, C., de Sandes, T.V., & Sampaio, E.L., Park, S.I., & Silva, H.T. Jr., Medina, and Pestana, .JO. Clinical impact of polymorphisms of transport proteins and enzymes involved in the metabolism of immunosuppressive drugs. *Transplantation Proceedings*, Vol. 41, No. 5, (June 2009), pp. 1441-1455, ISSN 0041-1345

Salvadori, M., Holzer, H., & de Mattos, A., Sollinger, H., & Arns, W., Oppenheimer, F., & Maca, J., Hall, M. Enteric-coated mycophenolate sodium is therapeutically equivalent to mycophenolate mofetil in de novo renal transplant patients. *American Journal of Transplantation*, Vol. 4, No. 2, (February 2004), pp. 231-236, ISSN 1600-6143

Schaeffeler, E., Eichelbaum, M., & Brinkmann, U. Frequency of C3435T polymorphism of MDR1 gene in African people. *The Lancet*, Vol. 358, No. 9279, (August 2001), pp. 383-384, ISSN 0140-6736

Schulak, J.A., & Hricik DE. Steroid withdrawal after renal transplantation. *Clinical Transplantation*, Vol. 8, No. 2 Pt 2, (April 1994), pp. 211-216, ISSN 0902-0063

Schweitzer, E.J., Yoon, S., & Fink, J., Wiland, A., & Anderson, L., Kuo, P.C., & Lim, J.W., Johnson, L.B., & Farney, A.C., Weir, M.R., & Bartlett, S.T. Mycophenolate mofetil reduces the risk of acute rejection less in African-American than in Caucasian kidney recipients. *Transplantation*, Vol. 65, No. 2, (January 1998), pp. 242-248, ISSN 1534-0608

Scott, L.J., McKeage, K., & Keam, S.J., Plosker, G.L. Tacrolimus: a further update of its use in the management of organ transplantation. *Drugs*, Vol. 63, No. 12, (2003), pp. 1247-97, ISSN 0012-6667

Shaw, L.M., Figurski, M., & Milone, M.C., Trofe, J., & Bloom, R.D. Therapeutic drug monitoring of mycophenolic acid. *Clinical Journal of the American Society of Nephrology*, No. 2, Vol. 5, (September 2007), pp. 1062-1072, ISSN 1555-9041

Shaw, L.M., Holt, D.W., & Keown, P., Venkataramanan, R., & Yatscoff, R.W. Current opinions on therapeutic drug monitoring of immunosuppressive drugs. *Clinical Therapeutics*, Vol. 21, No. 10, (October 2002), pp. 1632-1652, ISSN 0149-2918

Shaw, L.M., Holt, D.W., & Oellerich, M., Meiser, B., & van Gelder, T., Shaw, L.M., & Holt DW, Oellerich M. Current issues in therapeutic drug monitoring of mycophenolic acid: report of a roundtable discussion. *Therapeutic Drug Monitoring*, No. 23, Vol. 4, (August 2001), pp. 305-315, ISSN 0163-4356

Shaw, L.M., Korecka, M., & Aradhye, S., Grossman, R., & Bayer, L., Innes, C., & Cucciara, A., Barker, C., & Naji, A., Nicholls, A., & Brayman, K. Mycophenolic acid area under the curve values in African American and Caucasian renal transplant patients are comparable. *Journal of Clinical Pharmacology*, Vol. 40, No. 6, (June 2000), pp. 624-633, ISSN 1552-4604

Shaw, L.M., Mick, R., & Nowak, I., Korecka, M., & Brayman, K.L. Pharmacokinetics of mycophenolic acid in renal transplant patients with delayed graft function. *Journal of Clinical Pharmacology*, Vol. 38, No. 3, (March 1998), pp. 268-275, ISSN 1552-4604

Sollinger,. H.W., Belzer, F.O., & Deierhoi, M.H., Diethelm, A.G., & Gonwa, T.A., Kauffman, R.S., & Klintmalm, G.B., McDiarmid, S.V., & Roberts, J., Rosenthal, J.T. RS-61443 (mycophenolate mofetil). A multicenter study for refractory kidney transplant rejection. *Annals of Surgery*, Vol. 216, No. 4, (October 1992), pp. 513-518, ISSN 1528-1140

Staatz, C., Taylor, P., & Tett, S. Low tacrolimus concentrations and increased risk of early acute rejection in adult renal transplantation. *Nephrology Dialysis Transplantation*, Vol. 16, No. 9, (September 2001), pp. 1905-1909, ISSN 1460-6235

Staatz, C.E., & Tett, S.E. Clinical pharmacokinetics and pharmacodynamics of tacrolimus in solid organ transplantation. *Clinical Pharmacokinetics*, Vol. 43, No. 10, (2004), pp. 623-53, ISSN 0312-5963

Staatz, C.E., & Tett, S.E. Pharmacokinetic Considerations Relating to Tacrolimus Dosing in the Elderly. *Drugs Aging*, Vol. 22, No. 7, (2002), pp. 541-557, ISSN 1170-229X

Stein, C.M., Sadeque, A.J., & Murray, J.J., Wandel, C., & Kim, R.B., Wood, A.J. Cyclosporine pharmacokinetics and pharmacodynamics in African American and white subjects. *Clinical Pharmacology and Therapeutics*, Vol. 69, No. 5, (May 2001), pp. 317-323, ISSN 0009-9236

Takahashi, K., Ochiai, T., & Uchida, K., Yasumura, T., & Ishibashi, M., Suzuki, S., & Otsubo, O., Isono, K., & Takagi, H., Oka, T. Pilot study of mycophenolate mofetil (RS-61443) in the prevention of acute rejection following renal transplantation in Japanese patients. *Transplantation Proceedings*, No. 27, Vol. 1, (February 1995), pp. 1421-1424, ISSN 0041-1345

ter Meulen, C.G., van Riemsdijk, I., & Hené, R.J., Christiaans, M.H., & Borm, G.F., van Gelder, T., & Hilbrands, L.B., Weimar, W., & Hoitsma, A.J. Steroid-withdrawal at 3 days after renal transplantation with anti-IL-2 receptor alpha therapy: A prospective,randomized, multicenter study. *American Journal of Transplantation*, Vol. 4, No. 5, (May 2004), pp. 803-10, ISSN 1600-6143

Toda, F., Tanabe, K., & Ito, S., Shinmura, H., Tokumoto, T., & Ishida, H., Toma, H. Tacrolimus trough level adjustment after administration of fluconazole to kidney recipients. *Transplantation Proceedings*, Vol. 34, No. 5, (August 2002), pp. 1733-1735, ISSN 0041-1345

Tsuchiya, N., Satoh, S., & Tada, H., Li, Z., & Ohyama, C., Sato, K., & Suzuki, T., Habuchi, T., & Kato, T. Influence of CYP3A5 and MDR1 (ABCB1) polymorphisms on the pharmacokinetics of tacrolimus in renal transplant recipients. *Transplantation*, Vol. 78, No. 4, (October 2004), pp. 1182-1187, ISSN 1434-0608

Tuteja, S., Alloway, R., & Johnson, J., Gaber, O. The effect of gut metabolism on tacrolimus bioavailability in renal transplant recipients. *Transplantation*, Vol. 71, No. 9, (April 2001), pp. 1303–1307, ISSN 1534-0608

Undre, N.A., & Schäfer, A. Factors affecting the pharmacokinetics of tacrolimus in the first year after renal transplantation. *Transplantation Proceedings*, Vol. 30, No. 4, (June 1998), pp. 1261-1263, ISSN 0041-1345

Undre, N.A. Pharmacokinetics of tacrolimus-based combination therapies. Nephrology Dialysis Transplantation, Vol. 18, No. S1, (May 2003), pp. i12-i15, ISSN 1460-6235

Undre, N.A., Stevenson, P., & Schäfer, A. Pharmacokinetics of Tacrolimus: Clinically Relevant Aspects. *Transplantation Proceedings*, Vol. 31, No. S7A, (November 1999), pp. 21S–24S, ISSN 0041-1345

Undre, N.A., van Hooff, J., & Christiaans, M., Vanrenterghem, Y., & Donck, J., Heeman, U., & Kohnle, M., Zanker, B., & Land, W., Morales, J.M., & Andrés, A., Schäfer, A., & Stevenson, P. Pharmacokinetics of FK 506 and mycophenolic acid after the administration of a FK 506-based regimen in combination with mycophenolate mofetil in kidney transplantation. *Transplantation Proceedings*, Vol. 30, No. 4, (June 2002), pp. 1299-1302, ISSN 0041-1345

Utecht, K.N., Hiles, J.J., & Kolesar, J. Effects of Genetic Polymorphisms on the Pharmacokinetics of Calcineurin Inhibitors. *American Journal of Health-System Pharmacy*, Vol. 63, No. 23, (December 2002), pp. 2340-2348, ISSN 1079-2082

van Duijnhoven, E.M., Boots, J.M., & Christiaans, M.H., Stolk, L.M., & Undre, N.A., van Hooff, J.P. Increase in tacrolimus trough levels after steroid withdrawal. *Transplant International*, Vol. 16, No. 10, (October 2003), pp. 721-725, ISSN 0934-0874

Van Gelder T. Drug interactions with tacrolimus. *Drug Safety*, Vol. 25, No. 10, (2002), pp. 707-12, ISSN 0114-5916

van Gelder, T., Hilbrands, L.B., & Vanrenterghem, Y., Weimar, W., & de Fijter, J.W., Squifflet, J.P., & Hené, R.J., Verpooten, G.A., & Navarro, M.T., Hale, M.D., Nicholls, A.J. A randomized double-blind, multicenter plasma concentration controlled study of the safety and efficacy of oral mycophenolate mofetil for the prevention of acute rejection after kidney transplantation. *Transplantation*, Vol. 68, No. 2, (July 1999), pp. 261-266, ISSN 1534-0608

Van Gelder, T., Le Meur, Y., & Shaw, L.M., Oellerich, M., & DeNofrio, D., Holt, C., & Kaplan, B., Kuypers, D., & Meiser, B., Toenshoff, B., & Mamelok, R.D. Therapeutic drug monitoring of mycophenolate mofetil in transplantation. *Therapeutic Drug Monitoring*, Vol. 28 No. 2, (April 2006), pp. 145-154, ISSN 0163-4356

van-Duijnhoven, E.M, Christiaans, M., & Undre, N., Stevenson, P., &van Hooff, J. The effect of breakfast on the oral bioavailability of tacrolimus in diabetic and nondiabetic patients before transplantation. *Transplantation Proceedings*, Vol. 30, No. 4, (June 1998), pp. 1268-1270, ISSN 0041-1345

van-Duijnhoven, E.M., Christiaans, M.H., & Boots, J.M., van Hooff, J.P. Evidence That Fasting Does Not Significantly Affect Trough Levels of Tacrolimus in Stable Renal Transplant Recipients. *Transplantation Proceedings*, Vol. 34, No. 5, (August 2002), pp. 1723-1725, ISSN 0041-1345

Vanrenterghem, Y., Lebranchu, Y., & Hené, R., Oppenheimer, F., & Ekberg, H. Double-blind comparison of two corticosteroid regimens plus mycophenolate mofetil and cyclosporine for prevention of acute renal allograft rejection. *Transplantation*, Vol. 70, No. 9, (November 2000), pp. 1352-1359, ISSN 1534-0608

Varis, T., Kivistö, K.T., & Backman, J.T., Neuvonen, P.J. The cytochrome P450 3A4 inhibitor itraconazole markedly increases the plasma concentrations of dexamethasone and enhances its adrenal-suppressant effect. *Clinical Pharmacology and Therapeutics*, Vol. 68, No. 5, (November 2000), pp. 487-494, ISSN 0009-9236

Venkataramanan, R., Swaminathan, A., & Prasad, T., Prasad, T., & Jain, A., Zuckerman, S. Clinical pharmacokinetics of tacrolimus. *Clinical Pharmacokinetics*, Vol. 29, No. 6, (December 1995), pp. 404-430, ISSN 0312-5963

Vicari-Christensen, M., Repper, S., & Basile, S., Young, D. Tacrolimus: review of pharmacokinetics, pharmacodynamics, and pharmacogenetics to facilitate practitioners understanding and offer strategies for educating patients and promoting adherence. *Progress in Transplantation*, Vol. 19, No. 3, (September 2009), pp. 277-842, ISSN 1526-9248

Wald, J.A., Law, R.M., & Ludwig, E.A., Sloan, R.R., & Middleton, E. Jr., Jusko, W.J. Evaluation of dose-related pharmacokinetics and pharmacodynamics of prednisolone in man. *Journal of Pharmacokinetics and Biopharmaceutics*, Vol. 20, No. 6, (December 1992), pp. 567-589, ISSN 0090-466X

Wallemacq, P.E., & Verbeeck, R.K. Comparative Clinical Pharmacokinetics of Tacrolimus in Paediatric and Adult Patients. *Clinical Pharmacokinetics*, Vol. 40, No. 4, (2001), pp. 283-295, ISSN 0312-5963

Wang, C., Sun, J., & Sheil, A.G., McCaughan, G.W., & Bishop, G.A. A short course of methylprednisolone immunosuppression inhibits both rejection and spontaneous acceptance of rat liver allografts. *Transplantation*, Vol. 72, No. 1, (July 2001), pp. 44-51, ISSN 1534-0608

Winkler, M., & Christians, U. A risk-benefit assessment of tacrolimus in transplantation. *Drug Safety*, No. 12 Vol. 5, (May 1995), pp. 348-57, ISSN 0114-5916

World Health Organization (WHO). Global Activity in Organ Transplantation. Estimates 2008.

Yu, S., Wu, L., & Jin, J., Yan, S., & Jiang, G., Xie, H., & Zheng, S. Influence of CYP3A5 gene polymorphisms of donor rather than recipient to tacrolimus individual dose requirement in liver transplantation. *Transplantation*, Vol. 81, No. 1, (January 2006), pp. 46-51, ISSN 1534-0608

Zucker, K., Rosen, A., & Tsaroucha, A., de Faria, L., & Roth, D., Ciancio, G., & Esquenazi, V., Burke, G., & Tzakis, A., Miller, J. Augmentation of mycophenolate mofetil pharmacokinetics in renal transplant patients receiving Prograf and CellCept in combination therapy. *Transplantation Proceedings*, Vol. 29, No. 1, (February-March 2002), pp.334-336, ISSN 0041-1345

7

Desensitization and Induction Immunosuppressive Therapy in Highly HLA-Sensitized Patients Receiving Cadaveric Renal Allograft

Juana Margarita Rufino Hernández[1], José Manuel González-Posada Delgado[1] and Domingo Hernández Marrero[2]

[1]*Nephrology Section. Hospital Universitario de Canarias, Tenerife*
[2]*Nephrology Section. Hospital Universitario Carlos Haya, Málaga*
Spain

1. Introduction

Approximately 15-20% of patients on the waiting list for cadaveric renal transplant are highly HLA-sensitized. It is well known that the presence of alloantibodies against human class I (A, B, C) and class II (DR, DQ) HLA antigens in transplant recipients waiting for a renal transplant has a significant increase in acute and chronic rejection rates and a poor graft outcome. There are interesting options for minimizing these immunological problems such as national paired kidney exchange program or acceptable mismatch program similar to the one developed by Eurotransplant program. However, despite these efforts, these patients can wait up to 5 years for a kidney graft and just get it finally only 30% of them. It is therefore vital to develop strategies to reduce waiting time and decrease the risk of transplant rejection, through the elimination or reduction of circulating lymphocytotoxic antibodies.

There have been several retrospective and prospective studies that have used immunoabsorption or plasmapheresis together with immunosuppressants and intravenous immune globulins with highly variable success rates that, while not providing a high level of evidence, constitutes a promising therapeutic alternative for these patients.

In addition, the use of rituximab in living donor transplantation ABO incompatible, hypersensitive patients with positive crossmatch, acute rejection resistant to standard treatments and pretransplant desensitization are running with very interesting results. Moreover, newer approaches for treating acute humoral rejection such as the proteosome inhibitor (bortezomib) or eculizumab (an anticomplement monoclonal antibody), are emerging as successful therapeutic options (Gloor J& Stegall, 2010).

Long-term follow- up of these patients and the application on a wider scale of these treatments, will provide the definitive answers about their real efficacy (Nocera, 2009). Nevertheless, acute antibody-mediated rejection (AMR), occurring in 20-50% of patients, and subclinical AMR even in the absence of allograft dysfunction, may decrease allograft survival by chronic histological abnormalities.

The aim of this chapter is to review the current data about approach therapy in highly HLA-sensitized patients receiving deceased renal allograft.

2. Definition of highly HLA-sensitized patients

Patients with PRA (panel reactive antibodies) permanently > 75%, plus HLA-polyspecific reactivity by complement dependent cytotoxicity (CDC) or flow cytometry and multiple previous positive crossmatch, should be considered highly HLA-sensitized patients. HLA antibodies, are present in hyperimmunized patients as a result of pregnancies, blood transfusions and previous failed grafts, and make up an important barrier to renal transplantation.

There are different assays that can be used to determine the PRA, but it is necessary to ensure efficiency and reliability of these tests, so that that each laboratory must continuously monitor its processes and results (Ercilla MG, 2010). Monitoring is guaranteed by the accreditation of processes as well as quality control of results, evaluated by external organisations of experts on histocompatibility (for example, the accreditation programme of the European Federation for Immunogenetics and the American Society for Histocompatibility and Immunogenetics).

2.1 The complement dependent cytotoxicity (CDC) assay

A complement-mediated cytotoxicity reaction occurs when an IgM or IgG reacts against an antigen present on the cell surface of specific tissues. After this reaction, the complement system activation leads to cell membrane damage and, secondarily, cell lysis. In addition, the cells covered by the antibody (opsonized) are susceptible to be ingested by the monocyte-macrophage system, as it reduces the ionic charge of the cell surface directly through immune adherence or by binding to C3.

The complement dependent cytotoxicity (CDC) assay estimates PRA by adding potential recipient serum to microtiter plates that contain a pool of lymphocytes with defined HLA antigens. Rabbit complement is added and the plates are viewed after addition of a vital stain. The PRA can then be determined based upon the number of cytotoxic reactions that are observed. The classic assay CDC crossmatch has a high positive predictive value for graft loss in the first 48 hours if positive, which therefore contraindicates transplantation. Alloantibody testing should be performed every three months in all candidate patients for renal transplantation and 15 days after each sensitising event (transfusion, graft loss and pregnancy). This sequential study helps to reveal antibodies that may have been identified in the past but that may not have been detected at the time of transplantation. If the crossmatch is positive by CDC, the process is repeated with the addition of Dithiothreitol (DTT). This step reduces the disulfide bonds present when the antibody is IgM.

A test that is CDC positive/DTT negative (presence of an IgM antibody only) should not preclude transplantation: in this case, the determination of solid-phase anti-HLA alloantibody screening (by immunoabsorption ELISA or flow cytometry, Luminex) is negative in serum that was CDC-PRA positive. By comparison, the presence of a CDC positive/DTT positive test is an indication of IgG anti-donor antibody and is a contraindication to transplantation without the use of a desensitization procedure, especially if a donor specific antibody has been defined. (Klein, 2010; Ercilla MG, 2010)

2.2 The enzyme-linked immunoabsorption (ELISA)

This assay uses microtest trays containing known HLA antigens to which potential recipient serum is added. This test is faster than the CDC assay and the HLA antigens used for screening can be adjusted as necessary to reflect the presumed potential donor pool. As in the cytotoxicity technique, the mix of antigens should be representative of the general population. In case of anti-HLA antibodies, a colorimetric reaction enzyme occurs. This reaction is quantified by spectrophotometer.

By ELISA assay, we detect all anti-HLA antibodies, including complement fixing and non-fixers. Once it has detected the presence of anti-HLA antibodies (class I or II), specificity against which these antibodies are directed can also be determined by a high definition ELISA plates or unique antigens with the same methodology. Solid-phase anti-HLA alloantibody screening is useful when autoantibodies are suspected and there is a need to rule out them in a patient with positive CDC-PRA. This indicates presence or absence of type IgG anti-HLA antibodies against anti-HLA-I and anti-HLA-II and, in some kits, anti-MICA. By using purified HLA antigens, non-anti-HLA antibodies are not identified. If anti-HLA antibodies are not revealed by cytotoxicity but are detected by solid phase, it is highly recommended that more sensitive crossmatch techniques should be used, such as flow cytometry or virtual crossmatch (VCM) in order to better define the risk for these patients. (Klein, 2010; Ercilla MG, 2010).

2.3 Flow cytometry. Single-antigen bead flow cytometry (SAB-FC)

Flow cytometry measures the fluorescence after patient serum has been added to a defined set of HLA antigen flow beads. A positive test is determined by the mean channel shift in intensity, that is, mean intensity of fluorescence (MFI). This assay allows to identify specific HLA antigens to which the patients are sensitized and constitutes what we know as "virtual lymphocyte crosssmatch (VCM)." VCM is indicated in patients who are candidates for retransplantation, women who have previously been multiple pregnant and those with positive results in the solid-phase screening but negative for CDC as well as also is recommended for all living-donor transplants.

In the event that the only positive result is that of the positive VCM, this will indicate a 55% probability of an antibody-mediated rejection episode in the first year versus a 5% probability in the case of a negative VCM and the graft survival at one year is slightly lower. However, a positive VCM, by itself, does not imply that a transplant is necessarily contraindicated, but a careful monitoring and immunosuppression aimed to controlling alloantibody production are needed for a thorough treatment.

A positive B-cell negative T-cell crossmatch usually occurs in presence of anti-HLA-II antibodies, presence of low-titre anti-HLA-I antibodies detectable only in B lymphocytes and presence of specific B lymphocytes autoantibodies. In these cases, the decision for transplantation must be individualised. In others words, T cell negative/B cell positive reactions may be secondary to either class I or class II antibodies, while a T cell positive/B cell negative reaction most likely results from a non-HLA antibody, as class I antigen is expressed on both T and B cells. For living donor recipients, perform a monocyte crossmatch should be useful as may help to detect anti-endothelial antibodies.

Clearly identifying the reactivity of antibodies with the donor (DSAs) is logistically difficult because it requires donor cells which may be stored frozen in liquid nitrogen, or determined of the living donor who has to be present for each determination. Therefore, is in these cases, when the crossmatch cannot be performed due to lack of donor cells, where this assay plays an important role as it allows identify specific HLA antigens to which the patient is sensitized (virtual lymphocyte crosssmatch).

Singh N et al showed the impact that produces pre-Tx DSAs detected by SAB-FC on early clinical outcomes. They tested pre-Tx sera from all consecutive deceased-donor kidney transplants performed between January 2005 and July 2006 (n=237), 66% had a high-immunologic risk. MFI more than or equal to 100 for class I and more than or equal to 200 for class II were the lowest DSA thresholds associated with inferior antibody-mediated rejection-free graft survival (Singh N et al., as cited in Ercilla MG, 2010). The presence of class I-anti-HLA antibodies post-transplant precedes, even by years, the development of glomerulopathy. In addition, the presence of anti-class II antibodies is strongly associated with chronic rejection in living-donor kidney recipients, but it appears that the worst prognosis is associated with the simultaneous detection of anti-HLA-I and anti-HLA-II antibodies.

There is evidence that it is possible to reduce pre-existing circulating alloantibodies in some patients to levels where the antibodies are unable to trigger hyperacute rejections. This does not imply that there are no B lymphocytes with the capacity to restart alloantibody production, but the short-term survival of grafts transplanted in some centres under these conditions is acceptable. (Klein, 2010; Ercilla MG, 2010).

Compared with the cell-based method, the fluorometric bead system is not as susceptible to drug interference, such as antithymocyte globulin, intravenously administered immunoglobulin (IVIG), and rituximab. IVIG may interfere with the bead assay for a few days after administration. Nonetheless, these new techniques allow for greater identification of HLA antibody specificities and a more accurate interpretation of cross-match results. Patients with high DSA and donor-specific cross matches SFI units are considered at high risk for AMR and warranted more frequent antibody-level monitoring posttransplantation, may need desensitization treatments, or plan biopsies, in order to reduce DSA levels or detect early AMR respectively; sometimes, increase in DSA imply retreatment as can result in reduction in DSA, levels to $\leq 10^5$ SFI units is usually associated with a low risk of AMR.

3. Immunosuppressive therapy in high immunologic risk patients receiving cadaveric renal allograft

3.1 Immunosuppressive agents

3.1.1 Anti-lymphocyte antibodies

Thymoglobulin is a polyclonal immunosuppressive agent that is generated in rabbits, containing antibodies to a wide variety of human T-cell surface antigens, including the major histocompatibility complex (MHC) antigens. These antibodies have the ability to block a number of adhesion molecules, cytokines, chemokines, among others. Anti-lymphocyte antibodies have long been an integral part of induction regimens and, nowdays, continue to be used in the management of patients at risk of early rejection. They are used in combination with steroids, mycophenolate and calcineurin inhibitors or, less frequently, proliferation signal inhibitors and are treatment of choice for acute graft rejection grade II and III of Banff or unresponsive to steroid boluses. Among the available polyclonal globulin, thymoglobulin, has shown a great efficacy and typically requires between 7 and 10 doses.

The reaction of these globulins with some lymphocyte antigens can trigger activation of these cells to release cytokines, which may present with chills, fever and systemic symptoms, mainly with the first dose. Steroids, antihistamines and antipyretics intravenous infusion may prevent these early reactions; polyclonal antibodies will be made through a central venous catheter in at least 6 hours.

Side effects in the medium and long term are related to its immunosuppressive effect. Polyclonal antibodies can increase the risk of infection (herpes simplex virus, varicella-zoster virus, cytomegalovirus or Epstein-Barr virus) and patients may benefit from prophylactic antiviral strategies. Other opportunistic infections may be due to pneumocystis jiroveci and aspergillus, but are related to immunosuppression accumulated by the patient rather than the administration of polyclonal antibodies. Treatment with antilymphocyte globulin and a serum test for Epstein-Barr virus receptor are associated with the risk of lymphoproliferative disorders in renal transplant population. (Gaber ,AO et al., 2010; Oppenheimer, F et al., 2010) .

Currently almost 70% of renal transplant patients in the United States receive antibody induction, either antithymocyte globulin (Thymoglobulin) or inhibitors of IL-2. Brennan, D et al. (Brennan, C et al., 2006) compared the efficacy and safety of randomized use of basiliximab versus thymoglobulin in patients at high risk of rejection (retransplantation, PRA greater than 20% black, one or more HLA incompatibilities) or delayed graft function who received a cadaveric renal transplantation. After 12 months of follow-up, incidence of biopsy proven acute rejection was 15.6% for Thymoglobulin, and 25.2% for basiliximab ($p = 0.02$) and the antibody-treated acute rejection was lower in patients with thymoglobulin (1.4% vs 8.0%, $p = 0{,}005$). The overall rate of adverse events was 99.3% to 98.5%, was similar between boths induction treatment. The overall incidence of infection was 85.8% to 75.2% with thymoglobulin and basiliximab ($p = 0.03$). This difference appears to be attributable to a higher frequency of urinary tract infection and no CMV viral infections. CMV infection was lower with Thymoglobulin (7.8% vs 17.5%, $p = 0.02$), probably due that a prophylactic antibiotics were used less in patients with thymoglobulin (18.9% vs 30.9%, $p = 0.03$).

3.1.2 Alemtuzumab

Alemtuzumab is a humanized IgG1 kappa monoclonal antibody, genetically engineered, specific for a surface glycoprotein of lymphocytes, 21-28 kD (CD52) present on T and B lymphocytes, natural killer cells and to a lesser extent on monocytes and macrophages. It is indicated for the treatment of patients with chronic lymphocytic leukemia who have been treated with alkylating agents and who have not achieved a complete or partial response. Alemtuzumab causes lysis of lymphocytes by binding to CD52, the antibody mediates lysis of lymphocytes by complement fixation and cell-mediated cytotoxicity, antibody-dependent. The antigen has been detected in a small percentage (<5%) of granulocytes, but not detected in erythrocytes or platelets. Alemtuzumab does not appear to damage the hematopoietic stem cells or progenitor cells. Side effects include first-dose reactions, less severe than those due to OKT3, as well as anemia, leukopenia and pancytopenia. Further long-term controlled studies are needed to establish the potential benefit in terms of efficacy and safety after kidney transplantation.

3.1.3 OKT3

OKT3 is a murine monoclonal antibody against the T3 antigen of human lymphocytes which acts as an immunosuppressant by blocking a molecule (CD3) located in the membrane of human T cells. This molecule appears to be associated with the structure of antigen recognition of T cells. It is indicated to treat acute rejection reaction in renal transplant patients. It must be only used in intravenous form and the dose of other immunosuppressive agents used concomitantly with OKT3 should be decreased to minimal levels and restarted about three days before the end of treatment with OKT3. It produces a rapid and concomitant decrease in the number of circulating T cells (CD3, CD4 and CD8) after the administration. After discontinuation of treatment, CD3 cells reappear rapidly and reach pretreatment levels within a week. OKT3 should not be used in patients with hypersensitivity to this or any other product of murine origin and in patients with fluid overload or with a history of seizures or a predisposition to allergies. After the first dose of OKT3 patients may experience fever, chills, malaise, encephalopathy, aseptic meningitis, dysnea and with minor frequency, fatal severe pulmonary edema. The most common infections were cytomegalovirus (19%) and herpes simplex (27%). To summarize, OKT3 was the first monoclonal antibody against CD3 used but adverse effect profile makes little used today.

3.1.4 Intravenous immunoglobulin (IVIG)

Intravenous immunoglobulin (IVIG) products: are derived from pooled human plasma and have been used for the treatment of primary immunodeficiency disorders, autoimmune and inflammatory disorders and recently in the treatment of sensitized patients. Mechanism of action: neutralization of circulating antibodies through idiotype-idiotype interactions to inhibit the binding of Ac antiHLA to their target cells in a dose-dependent form; inhibition of secretion of cytokines and other soluble mediators; stimulation of cytokine receptor antagonists; interaction with antigen-presenting cells by blocking T cell activation through the Fc receptor; inhibition of binding of the fractions of complement to target cells because they have a high affinity for activated complement components C3b and C4b resulting in decreased formation of the potent anaphylatoxin C5a and the C5b-C9 membrane attack complex, inhibition of proliferation of T and B cells and "down regulation" of the synthesis of antibodies and others.

Plasmapheresis, in combination with intravenous immunoglobulin, produces durable, donor-specific antibody suppression as effect of plasmapheresis is short-lived, and a rebound occurs usually when plasmapheresis is discontinued and half-life of IVIg is about 3 weeks; therefore, in most protocols its administration is repeated every 4 weeks. In adition, IVIG are useful in the treatment and prevention of posttransplant infectious complications including cytomegalovirus, parvovirus B19 and polyoma BK virus. Adverse effects are minor: headaches, fever, fatigue, myalgia, hypotension, sweating, dizziness, chills, chest tightness, wheezing. They all probably are secondary to increased levels of inflammatory cytokines and vasoactive substances and with high velocity perfusion. Anaphylactic reaction and shock can occur in patients with total or partial deficiency of IgA. In these cases, epinephrine, and diazepam for muscle spasms are indicated. Another adverse effect is renal dysfunction, because of the content of sucrose or sorbitol which can cause osmotic nephrosis in the proximal tubule. This can be avoided by reducing the osmolarity of immunoglobulin products containing sucrose, using restorative with sterile water instead of saline and lowers the concentration of Igs and sucrose to <9%. Other life-threatening side effects are thrombotic events. Very slow infusion using IVIG at a concentration of 5%, with low or no sodium content and low osmolarity, and using molecular weight heparin reduces the incidence.

3.1.5 Rituximab

It is a chimeric antibody mouse / human directed against the CD20 antigen on B lymphocytes (expressed in mature B lymphocytes and prelinfocito B). Directly inhibits B cell proliferation, induces apoptosis and reduces the production of antibodies. It has been used for the treatment of non-Hodgkin's lymphoma B cells, rheumatoid arthritis, autoimmune diseases such lupus, idiopatic thrombopenic purpure, cryoglobulinemia and organ transplantation. It produces rapid reduction of B cells with subsequent recovery at 12 months. Recent clinical data suggest that the beneficial effects of rituximab may be due to depriving T cells of antigen-presenting cell activity provided by antigen-specific B cells, thus altering effect or functions and inducing a regulatory profile. These data suggest that the beneficial effects of rituximab on autoimmune disease are more likely related to modification of dysfunctional cellular immunity rather than simply a reduction in antibody. A single dose of 375 mg/m2 in renal transplantation produces depletion of CD19 and CD20 cells for long periods in peripheral blood and tissue level.

Rituximab can be administered in a peripheral vein and, although rare, can cause anaphylactic reactions, which suggests his administration under close monitoring. The use of rituximab, which is directed against the CD20 antigen, would seem to be a logical strategy, since reduction or elimination of B cells that express CD20 and make anti-HLA antibodies, should have a beneficial effect. However, there are problems with this concept. First, anti-CD20 activity has no effect on plasma cells, which are the primary source of acute antibody production and second, rituximab has no immediate effect on circulating antibody levels. These problems might limit the benefit of rituximab if were used as the sole treatment, however, it appears that the use of rituximab in combination with other treatments, e.g., plasmapheresis which eliminates circulating antibodies, and intravenous immune globulin, that acts neutralizing circulating antibodies through idiotype-idiotype interactions to inhibit the binding of Ac antiHLA, or both, might constitute an improved approach for the management of allosensitization.

There are concerns regarding the use of rituximab, because it has been reported to induce reactivation of polyomavirus JC virus, resulting in progressive multifocal leukoencephalopathy. Optimal treatment of AMR probably requires a combination of rituximab with PP and low-dose IVIG or with high-dose IVIG (1-2 gm/kg) due to the inability of rituximab to deplete CD20-negative plasma cells that continue to produce DSA and mediate graft injury.

3.1.6 Calcineurin-inhibitors

Cyclosporine A binds to an intracellular receptor (cyclophilin) and form an active complex that binds and inhibits the phosphatase activity of calcineurin. Calcineurin participates in the transcriptional control of ribonucleic acid for the synthesis of cytokines (IL-2, IFN-γ, IL-4 and TNF-α). Thus, inhibits the proliferation of T cells preventing clonal expansion of helper and cytotoxic T cells; suppressor T cells are not affected.

Tacrolimus is a macrolide that forms a complex intracytoplasmic with a specific immunophilin (FKBP) capable of blocking the phosphatase activity of calcineurin, and thereby inhibit transcription of different genes (IL-2 and others). It inhibits the activation and proliferation of T cells and the synthesis of cytotoxic T lymphocytes. It also slows the growth and differentiation of B cells by interfering with the expression of IL-4 receptor and IL-5 synthesis. Unlike cyclosporin, tacrolimus does not interact with the receptor of transforming growth factor beta (TGF-β) type 2, which would provide more efficacy in preventing chronic graft rejection. Tacrolimus is used to prevent acute graft rejection and for treatment of corticosteroids-resistant acute rejection. It is administered in combination with steroids and derivatives of mycophenolic acid and mTOR inhibitors.

Adverse effects with greater clinical significance are nephrotoxicity, similar to that produced by cyclosporine A, carbohydrate intolerance and diabetes mellitus, neurological disorders: tremor, headache, dizziness, and severe neurological (seizures, encephalopathy, etc.) and also increased susceptibility to development of infections and malignancies. (Oppenheimer, F et al., 2010).

3.1.7 Derivatives of mycophenolic acid, mycophenolate mofetil or enteric-coated mycophenolic acid

Mycophenolate is an ethyl ester of mycophenolic acid that selectively inhibits de novo synthesis of purines, the proliferation of T and B lymphocytes, the expression of adhesion molecules and proliferation of smooth muscle cells of the vascular wall. The enteric-coated mycophenolic acid sodium salt is designed to try to improve gastrointestinal tolerance. The efficacy and safety of both drugs are similar. Its main indication is the prevention of acute graft rejection and may play an important role in preventing chronic rejection. Commonly used with cyclosporine A or tacrolimus to prevent acute graft rejection and have also been proposed for the treatment of corticosteroid-resistant acute rejection or refractory to treatment. May appear blood disorders (anemia, leukopenia and thrombocytopenia), which are not severe. Viral infections, especially citomegalolvirus are more frequent than when used in place of mTOR inhibitors. (Oppenheimer, F et al., 2010)

3.1.8 mTOR inhibitors, sirolimus and everolimus

Anti-mTOR drugs, sirolimus and everolimus are potent immunosuppressants with antiproliferative and anti-migratory capacity that act by blocking the intracellular signalling that regulates the growth and proliferation of T2 cells. mTOR inhibitors are macrolide acting in a late stage cell proliferation by inhibiting cytokine-specific signals. To act it requires form a complex with an immunophilin, but unlike the tacrolimus, do not inhibit calcineurin. Everolimus is a derivative of sirolimus with a shorter elimination half-life and greater oral bioavailability.

In primary immunosuppression, associated with cyclosporine A, have a synergistic immunosuppressive effect, and the incidence of acute rejection varies between 10 and 20%. While competing for the same tacrolimus cyclophilin, the association of mTOR inhibitor-tacrolimus is, at least, as effective as tacrolimus, mycophenolic acid association. Its main advantage is a reduction in the appearance of de novo tumours and the absence of nephrotoxicity, although significant proteinuria has been reported, especially after late use in grafts with impaired function. In cases of nephrotoxicity may be useful in association with mycophenolate, after discontinuation of calcineurin. An additional advantage is the lower rate of cytomegalovirus infection. Its side effects are: hypercholesterolemia, hypertriglyceridemia and thrombocytopenia, which are related to the administered dose. These side effects may offset their benefits in the longer term in highly renal transplant considering that are patients with high immunological risk whose should remain on full-dose triple therapy.

3.1.9 Proteosome inhibitor (bortezomib)

Bortezomib, a proteasome inhibitor approved for the treatment of multiple myeloma, induces plasma cell apoptosis. Its role in desensitization protocols and treatment of humoral rejection may offer promise results in transplant recipients. The pharmacokinetics of bortezomib can be characterized by rapid and wide distribution, a prolonged elimination half life, and hepatic cytochrome P-450 (CYP) isoenzyme metabolism. Side effects more frequent are a low-grade gastrointestinal side effect, mild to moderate anemia, neutropenia, and thrombocytopenia, and primarily mild cases of peripheral neuropathy. Despite the mild decrease in PRA levels, bortezomib therapy led to more than 50% decrease in the levels of anti-HLA antibodies triggering C4d deposition on single antigen Luminex beads as measured in MFI with single-antigen bead flow cytometry.

Results in desensitization of patients with this agent before transplantation are less consistent. Wahrmann et al. could not observe a significant decrease of circulating HLA antibodies in two highly sensitized dialysis patients who were treated with two cycles of bortezomib, indicating that this agent is not able to eliminate long-lived plasma cells. Furthermore, in vitro studies indicate that contact with alloantigen enhances the susceptibility of plasma cells to proteasome inhibition-mediated apoptosis, which might also serve as an explanation for the observed differences in the effectivity of bortezomib in the pre- and posttransplant phases.

In the study by Walsh et al., two patients undergoing acute AMR with high DSA and positive C4d staining on biopsy two weeks after kidney transplantation were treated with a multiday regimen consisting of plasmapheresis, methylprednisolone and bortezomib along with a single dose of rituximab. By nearly 14 days after treatment, DSA levels had dropped significantly as well as repeat biopsy showed faint peritubular capillary C4d labeling and decreased glomerular C4d deposition.

Trivedi et al. (Trivedi et al., 2009, 2010) reported thirteen living donor renal transplant patients treated with bortezomib one to two cycles and plasmapheresis to remove HLA antibodies posttransplant. All patients treated with bortezomib/plasmapheresis resulted in a primary DSA reduction of more than 50% measured by means of single antigen bead on Luminex. In 10 of 13 patients, complete DSA removal, below than 1000 mean fluorescent intensity occurred. At 1 year posttreatment, antibody intensity remains significantly depressed in the group as a whole, despite tetanus toxoid and measles IgG levels remained unchanged and above the level of protection. These data suggest that proteasome inhibitors plus plasmapheresis results in prolonged reduction of HLA antibodies while leaving protective immunity intact. Some patients had reappearance of anti-HLA antibodies despite initial effective reduction, and the authors suggested that certain patients may need more than one cycle of treatment to decrease DSA levels.

3.1.10 Eculizumab (anti-C5, anticomplement monoclonal antibody)

The monoclonal antibody eculizumab, which binds to complement factor C5 and prevents formation of the membrane attack complex C5b-9, is currently in clinical use for the treatment of paroxysmal nocturnal hemoglobinuria and being tested for the treatment of atypical hemolytic uremic syndrome. Its use combined with plasmapheresis or IVIg decrease C5b-C9 complex deposition in the kidney. It is very important to be immunized against meningitis (Neisseria meningitidis) to all patients two weeks before the administration of eculizumab as due to its mechanism of action, the use of this drug increases the patient's sensitivity to meningococcal infection.

Eculizumab selectively inhibits the human complement protein C5, preventing its division into C5a and C5b, thus annulling the formation of C5b-9 terminal complement, which is behind the formation of transmembrane channels that cause cell lysis. The adverse reactions most frequently reported are headache, nasopharyngitis, nausea, pyrexia, myalgia, fatigue and herpes simplex, observed in at least 5 of every 100 patients. The most serious side effect was meningococcal septicemia.

Complement activation plays a critical role in mediating AMR after kidney transplantation. As eculizumab has the ability to inhibit C5b-C9 MAC and C5a generation, it should act as a strong accommodation promoter and prevent AMR. Fortunately, recent data presented by Stegall et al. (Stegall et al.,2010, as cited in Jordan, S, 2010) supports this contention. These investigators treated ten patients who underwent desensitization with plasmapheresis + IVIG with eculizumab after transplantation. After nearly 12 months of follow-up for all patients, none developed AMR. Several protocol biopsies showed C4d deposits but no evidence of AMR. This finding is suggestive of incomplete complement activation, which is permissive for accommodation. This author says, that a combination of high-dose IVIG with eculizumab maybe act to modify elements of cellular immunity, humoral immunity, and complement effectors. Confirmation of these ideas awaits clinical trials.

3.1.11 Receptor antagonists interleukin-2 (I1-2R): Basiliximab

This anti-CD25 monoclonal antibody, one chimeric (basiliximab) are widely used in renal transplantation patients with low-moderate immunological risk during the induction phase. Usually, induction therapy with basiliximab is used in combination with calcineurin-inhibitors, derivatives of mycophenolic acid and prednisone This antibody is directed against a chain of IL-2 receptor, whose expression on the cell surface requires activation of the T cell. Basiliximab is used in two doses of 20 mg each, for intravenous injection at time of transplantation and on the fourth day after transplantation, respectively. The first dose should be administered before reperfusion of the organ. Hypersensitivity reactions, including anaphylaxis, have been reported in isolation with the use of these antibodies, which, moreover, are considered safe and an adverse event profile similar to those reported with placebo.

3.1.12 Therapeutic apheresis

Plasmapheresis is a plasma exchange procedure to removal from blood plasma molecules with specific antigen recognition like antibodies or autoantibodies, molecules that alter the physical properties of plasma, immune complexes, toxic molecules and others. The therapeutic goal of plasma is to reduce circulating levels of these molecules to mitigate the underlying disease process. The vast majority of disorders successfully treated by plasmapheresis treatment involving the removal of IgG, as it has a longer half life and low rate of synthesis. Other factors removed as complement, coagulation proteins or inflammatory mediators contribute to a lesser extent the therapeutic benefit of plasmapheresis by its short half-life and high rate of synthesis.

Therapeutic plasma exchange has been used successfully in the treatment of many hematological, neurological, renal, and metabolic disorders, rheumatic and acute humoral rejection. This last is a condition that requires early diagnosis and intervention. Many groups have developed protocols for immunosuppression and immunomodulation that often include therapeutic plasma exchange.

Plasmapheresis therapy is successfully used in the treatment or prevention of rejection in solid organ transplantation. Although the cellular immune response is responsible for mediating most of the rejections of allografts, acute humoral rejection of the transplanted organ refers to a severe dysfunction associated with the presence of antibodies directed against the donor organ. This type of rejection is generally resistant to immunosuppressive and immunomodulatory therapies, occurs more frequently in patients with preexisting antibodies to the ABO system antigens or HLA expressed by the graft and is associated with a poor prognosis for graft survival. Numerous studies showed evidence of HLA antibodies decreased with plasmapheresis; in addition, patients with refractory acute rejection, the use of plasma exchange schemes and IVIG results in a better renal graft survival. The number of plasmapheresis sessions is greater the higher the antibody titer donor-specific. In addition, as soon as plasmapheresis stops, there is a rebound in the title antibody. Therefore, plasmapheresis is considered an additional technical assistance to other therapeutic procedures, particularly treatment with IVIG.

Extracorporeal immunoadsorption is other technique for the elimination of pathogenic antibodies and circulating immune complexes. Immunoadsorption is capable to eliminate huge amounts of immunoglobulins from the patient's circulation with a minimum of side effects (associated with the substitution of fresh frozen plasma or albumin or removal of other plasmatic factors to above 50%).

Most evidences about immunoadsorption are based on uncontrolled case series and individual observations. Indications for extracorporeal immunoadsorption are presently limited to HLA-pre-sensitised kidney recipients, rapidly progressive glomerulonephritis, haemolytic uraemic syndrome, life-threatening autoimmune diseases among others. Immunoadsorption devices can be subdivided into non-selective, semi-selective and highly selective adsorbers. In patients with acute vascular rejection after renal transplantation, immunoadsorption can be used to remove anti-HLA antibodies in combination with conventional anti-rejection therapy. It seems feasible to apply immunoadsorption instead of plasmapheresis for acute, vascular rejection although a controlled trial should demonstrate whether one or the other is more effective and associated with less adverse effects.

Immunoadsorption could also be successfully used for the reduction of anti-HLA antibody titre before transplantation for obtaining a negative cross match in highly sensitised patients. A median of plasma processed during the pre-transplant immunoadsorption session could be high and may not be achieved with the use of plasmapheresis due to a high likelihood of adverse reactions attributable to the administration of fresh frozen plasma or albumin. By contrast to plasmapheresis, immunoadsorption allows the treatment of higher plasma volumes with a greater reduction of immunoglobulins (immunoadsorption is capable of removing >85% of IgG during one session). In the future, immunoadsorption may replace plasmapheresis in the treatment of some but not all diseases, however, the high costs associated with immunoadsorption therapy must be taken into account. (Schwenger,& Morath,C, 2010).

3.1.13 Others agents in Phase I, II or III clinical trials

ISA247 (voclosporine), a cyclosporine analogue, has the advantage of inducing less postransplantation diabetes and reduced nephrotoxicity (Phase III study).

CP-690550, a specific inhibitor of the JAK3 protein kinase, has an effect comparable to tacrolimus on the acute rejection rate and kidney function. Orally is administered with basiliximab, mycophenolate and steroids. Initial results suggest that co-administration with mycophenolate involves excessive immunosuppression, with increased BK virus infection and cytomegalovirus.

Belatacept, is a humanized antibody that blocks the costimulatory signal by binding to CD80 and CD86 antigen presenting cells, thereby promoting anergy and apoptosis of T cells. Its efficacy is similar to that of cyclosporin A, but with a more favorable toxicity profile. The

need for intravenous injection and a slight increase in the development of lymphoproliferative disease in liver transplantation recipients with negative serology to Epstein-Barr virus could partially limit its use (Multiple Phase II and III trials).
Alefacept and Efaluzimab are humanized antibodies that inhibit T-cell adhesion and are in Phase I and II clinical trials.

3.2 Clinical evidences on desensitization therapy strategies in high immunological risk patients

In this section, we review the most relevant publications related to therapies in high immunologic risk patients, making emphasis on aspects such as incidence of acute rejection, long-term allograft survival and function, mortality and others. Highly sensitized transplant recipients, regardless of the desensitization protocol used, are at increased risk for AMR. Both desensitization and AMR are managed with the similar therapeutic arsenal; however protocols are center-specific and there are no consensus guidelines. The two desensitization protocols more frequently used are high-dose IVIG or low-dose IVIG with either plasmapheresis or immunoadsorption. Additionally, some transplant centers may add intravenous steroids, rabbit antithymocyte globulin, or rituximab. For variant of AMR where over 30% of infiltrating cells are mature plasma cells, which do not express CD20, several transplant centers have utilized bortezomib instead of rituximab.
Yuan XP et al (Yuan XP et al., 2010) evaluated the efficacy of plasmapheresis plus low-dose intravenous immunoglobulin in highly sensitized patients waiting for a deceased-donor renal transplant. In 25 patients (group 1), a positive T- and/or B-cell cytotoxicity crossmatch was rendered negative by plasmapheresis plus low-dose intravenous immunoglobulin treatment. During the same time, 32 highly sensitized patients (group 2), without desensitization, had a negative crossmatch and received deceased-donor renal transplants. Group 1 showed a numerically higher rate of acute rejection and antibody-mediated rejection, but the difference was not statistically significant. No differences in Kaplan-Meier graft survival were found between group 1 and group 2 after long-term follow-up. They conclude that desensitization with plasmapheresis, plus low-dose intravenous immunoglobulin enables successful deceased-donor renal transplant in highly sensitized patients with a positive crossmatch and achieve results similar to highly sensitized patients with negative crossmatch. Moreover, antibody-mediated rejection occurred predominantly in recipients with donor-specific antibodies of high titers. They used anti-thymocyte globulin for induction in both groups.
Loupy A, (Loupy A et al., 2010), combined posttransplant prophylactic intravenous immunoglobulin, rituximab and plasmapheresis in kidney recipients with preformed donor-specific antibodies. All patients had a concomitant evaluation of glomerular filtration rate, protocol biopsies, and DSA mean intensity of fluorescence (MFI) at 3 month and 1 year posttransplant. The first strategy combined posttransplant quadritherapy and intravenous immunoglobulin (group 1, n=36) and the second added to the above protocol rituximab and plasmapheresis (group 2, n=18). Peak and day-0 class-I or II DSA max-MFI were similar in both groups. The rate of acute antibody-mediated rejection (AMR) was similar in both groups (about 19.6% vs. 16.6%, respectively). At 1 year posttransplant, group 2 was characterized significantly by lower score microcirculation inflammation lesions, a lower rate of transplant glomerulopathy and a lower rate of chronic AMR. The decline in DSA-MFI from day 0 to 1 year was about 44% in group 1 compared with 80% in group 2 and the 1-year glomerular filtration rate was about 43 vs. 54 ml/min/1.73 m2, respectively. The

study raises the possibility that a more prophylactic immunosuppressive strategy at day 0 combining intravenous immunoglobulin/anti-CD20/plasmapheresis in high-risk population, is associated with significant differences in long-term function and chronic AMR rate, although similar rates of early acute clinical humoral rejection may be observed.

Vo A, et al (Vo AA et al., 2010, 2008) used high-dose intravenous immune globulin (2 g/kg x2 doses) and rituximab (2 doses) for desensitization of highly HLA-sensitized patients awaiting kidney transplantation. All patients received intravenous ganciclovir while staying at the hospital and valganciclovir for 6 months as outpatients, with dose adjustments for renal function. Both fungal and bacterial infection prophylaxis, including Pneumocystis carinii, was performed in all patients according to standard clinical practice. From July 2006 to February 2009, seventy-six treated patients (31 living donors, 45 deceased donors) were transplanted. For living donors (LD) and deceased donors (DD) recipients, significant reductions were seen in T-cell flow cytometry crossmatch from pretreatment to time of transplant. Patients received their kidney transplants when the complement-dependent cytotoxicity (CDC) T-cell crossmatch was negative at a 1:2 dilution of serum or the mean flow-channel shift in the T-cell flow-cytometric crossmatch was below 250. Time on wait list for DD recipients was reduced from a mean of 95 to 4.2 months after treatment; 37% experienced acute rejection but patient and graft survival up to 24 months was 95% and 84%, respectively. The mean serum creatinine, at 12 and 24 months were about 1.5 and 1.3 mg/dl, respectively. They concluded that IVIG and rituximab seems to offer significant benefits in reduction of anti-HLA antibodies allowing improved rates of transplantation for highly sensitized patients, especially those awaiting DD, with acceptable antibody-mediated rejection and survival rates at 24 months. All patients had reduced numbers of CD19+ cells after rituximab infusion. No patients developed neurologic symptoms suggestive of progressive multifocal leukoencephalopathy or required further hospitalization, and the rate of urinary tract infection was not greater than that among transplant recipients who were not highly sensitized. No other important infectious complications were noted.

Although 13 of 16 patients who received a kidney transplant had a persisting positive crossmatch at the time of transplantation (below the threshold given above), no hyperacute rejection episodes were noted. The same group developed an in vitro test system to predict whether intravenous immune globulin might reduce PRA or crossmatch positivity in individual patients. For patients who did not respond well in this test system or who had high antibody titers before desensitization, intravenous immune globulin and rituximab were considered not to be sufficient alone, and the patients received in addition plasmapheresis.

Vo AA, Jordan SC, et al (Vo AA; Jordan, SC. et al., 2008, 2009), analyzed the use of subcutaneous alemtuzumab induction therapy with intravenous immune globulin and rituximab in an uncontrolled study in 54 highly HLA-sensitized patients from 3/05 to 4/07. No patient developed acute injection-related reactions after alemtuzumab, however, bone marrow suppression was occasionally seen requiring reduction or elimination of mycophenolate mofetil approximately 1-2 months posttransplant. Patient and graft survival at 12 month was 98%/96%, respectively. Acute rejection episodes occurred in 35% with 20% being C4d+ acute rejection. Mean serum creatinine at 12 month was about 1.4 mg/dl. Infections occurred in eight patients (five with polyoma BK viremia, one CMV/PBK and two with CMV viremia). They concluded that induction therapy with alemtuzumab appears feasible and indeed promising, but awaits more definitive study.

Scemla A et al (Scemla A et al., 2010), revised the incidence of infectious complications in 38 highly sensitized renal transplant recipients treated by rituximab. They compared this population with 26 highly sensitized renal transplant recipients who received comparable

treatment but without rituximab. Mean posttransplant follow-up was 25.5±11.5 and 34.6±16.4 months in the rituximab and control groups, respectively. A total of 84 severe infectious episodes occurred in 39 patients (rituximab 55.3% vs. controls 69.2%, ns). Two patients died in each group. Three of these four deaths were related to infectious complications. Specifically, rituximab was not associated with an increased risk of infection.
Kamar N et al (Kamar N et al., 2010), revised the occurrence of infectious disease and its outcome after rituximab therapy (375 mg/m^2, 2-8 courses) in 77 kidney-transplant patients between April 2004 and August 2008. Their results were compared with a control group (n=902) who had received no rituximab. After a median follow-up of 16.5 months for rituximab patients and 60.9 months for control patients, the incidence of infectious disease was 45.45% and 53.9% (ns), respectively. The incidence of bacterial infection was similar between the two groups, whereas the viral-infection rate was significantly lower, and the rate of fungal infection was significantly higher in the rituximab group. Nine out of 77 patients died after rituximab therapy, of which seven deaths were related to an infectious disease, compared to 1.55% in the controls (p=0.0007). They concluded that in the whole population, the independent predictive factors for infection-induced death were the combined use of rituximab and antithymocyte-globulin given for induction or anti-rejection therapy, recipient age, and bacterial and fungal infections.
Flechner SM et al (Flechner SM et al., 2010), revised the role of proteasome inhibition with bortezomib in the treatment of antibody-mediated rejection in 20 patients. AMR was diagnosed about 19.8 months posttransplant. De novo class I DSA was detected in 55% and class II DSA in 90% recipients. Patients received intravenous corticosteroids followed by a 2-week cycle on days 1, 4, 8 and 11 of plasmapheresis and 1.3 mg/m^2 bortezomib; then 0.5 mg/kg intravenous immunoglobulin four times. Their results were a significantly decrement in peak-nadir dominant DSA. Patient survival was 100%, and graft survival 85% with a mean follow-up of 9.8 months. The treatment was generally well tolerated but caused fatigue, gastrointestinal complaints, fluid retention, and thrombocytopenia in a number of patients. The last follow-up estimated glomerular filtration rate was 41.9±16.8 ml/min, however, only 25% returned to their baseline renal function. They concluded that the bortezomib-containing regimen demonstrated activity in AMR but seems to be most effective before the onset of significant renal dysfunction or proteinuria and the use of bortezomib to treat AMR should be evaluated in controlled trials using dosing strategies that include longer courses or retreatment schedules.
Something similar was found by Raghavan R et al (Raghavan R et al, 2010), this author revised the use of bortezomib in kidney transplantation and said that the use of this biological agent in the field of transplantation may seem to show promise in the realm of transplant recipients desensitization and treatment of AMR, and will be defined better as more clinical data and trials become available.
Lonze BE et al (Lonze BE et al., 2010) review a 43-year-old patient with end-stage renal disease and 100% panel reactive antibody who was treated with desensitization protocol using two cycles of bortezomib undertaken after anti-CD20 and intravenous inmunoglobulins. A flow-positive, cytotoxic-negative cross-match live-donor kidney at the end of an eight-way multi-institution domino chain became available. The patient received three pretransplant plasmapheresis treatments. Intraoperatively, the superior mesenteric vein was the only identifiable patent target for venous drainage. Eculizumab was administered postoperatively in the setting of antibody-mediated rejection and an inability to perform additional plasmapheresis. Creatinine remains normal at 6 months

posttransplant and flow cross-match remained negative. In this report, they described the combined use of new agents (bortezomib and eculizumab) and modalities (nontraditional vascular access, splanchnic drainage of graft and domino paired donation) in a patient who would have died without transplantation.

Wahrmann M et al, (Wahrmann M et al., 2010), analized two sensitized hemodialysis patients that were selected to receive two subsequent bortezomib cycles (1.3 mg/m^2 on days 1, 4, 8, and 11). Dexamethasone was added to the second cycle to enhance treatment efficiency. During a half-year follow-up period, cytotoxic panel reactive antibody decreased from 87% to 80% (patient 1) and 37% to 13% (patient 2). Patient 1 showed a 40% reduction in binding intensities of identified Luminex HLA single antigen reactivities and, in parallel, slight reductions in ABO blood group antibody and total immunoglobulin levels. In patient 2, bortezomib did not affect circulating antibody levels in a meaningful way. Both patients showed a more than 50% reduction in the levels of anti-HLA antibody-triggered C4d deposition to Luminex beads. They concluded that, without additional immunosuppressive measures, bortezomib has modest effects on circulating antibodies against HLA or blood group antigens. Hovewer, the reduced levels of antibody-triggered complement fixation, imply potential clinical relevance of proteasome inhibition for recipient desensitization.

Sberro-Soussan R (Sberro-Soussan R, et al., 2010), evaluated the in vivo efficacy of one cycle of bortezomib (1.3 mg/m^2 x 4 doses), used as the sole desensitization therapy, in four renal transplant recipients experiencing subacute antibody-mediated rejection with persisting DSA (>2000 Mean Fluorescence Intensity, MFI). Bortezomib treatment did not significantly decrease DSA MFI within the 150-day posttreatment period in any patient. In addition, antivirus (HBV, VZV and HSV) antibody levels remained stable following treatment suggesting a lack of efficacy on long-lived plasma cells. They concluded that one cycle of bortezomib alone does not decrease DSA levels in sensitized kidney transplant recipients in the time period studied and need to evaluate this new desensitization agent properly in prospective, randomized and well-controlled studies.

Locke JE et al, (Locke JE et al., 2009) present a single case in which eculizumab was used combined with plasmapheresis e inmunoglobulins to salvage a kidney undergoing severe AMR. They showed a marked decrease in C5b-C9 (MAC) complex deposition in the kidney after the administration of eculizumab.

Stegall et al. recently reported on their results obtained in a first series of patients in whom the use of eculizumab was tested for the prevention of AMR in crossmatch-positive kidney transplantation. Sixteen crossmatch-positive kidney transplantations realized under the usage of eculizumab were compared to a historical control group of 51 transplantations where desensitization had been performed without eculizumab. Acute humoral rejection was found in only 6% of patients desensitized with eculizumab as compared to a 40% rate in the historical control group. However, 4 of 16 patients in the eculizumab group with persistent levels of high DSA after transplantation showed signs of chronic allograft injury, including endothelial cell activation and transplant glomerulopathy (Stegall,2010, as cited in C. Siisal & Morath C, 2011).

Thielke et al. reported that a negative crossmatch was successfully achieved in 51 of 57 positive-crossmatch patients treated with antithymocyte and anti-CD20 antibody induction therapy in addition to plasma exchange and low-dose intravenous immunoglobulin. The rate of allograft survival was 93% at 1 year and 81% at 2 years.

Glotz et al (Glotz et al., 2002) reported 15 patients with either a panel reactive antibody (PRA) of >50 percent or with a positive crossmatch to their potential living donor who were given 2 g/kg of IVIG monthly for three months. Thirteen of the 15 showed evidence of desensitization (reduction of PRA by at least 50 percent or a repeat negative crossmatch to the living donor) and underwent renal transplantation. The mean decrease in PRA for recipients was 80 percent and a post-IVIG administration NIH cytotoxicity crossmatch was negative prior to transplantation. The IVIG was repeated at the same dose on post-transplant day zero and one. Thymoglobulin was used for induction and maintenance immunosuppression consisted of mycophenolate, corticosteroids and tacrolimus. The IVIG was again repeated at post-transplant day 20 or 21 and 40 or 41. One graft was lost secondary to thrombosis and one graft was lost secondary to rejection. No other episodes of rejection were reported in the remaining allografts during follow-up of over one year.

Kaposztas et al. reported 2-year outcomes in their recent retrospective study looking at 54 patients treated for AMR. Group A had 26 patients who underwent treatment with plasmapheresis and rituximab, and group B had 28 patients who received plasmapheresis without rituximab. Patients who had low serum IgG levels also received IVIG. Two-year graft survival was significantly better in the group that received rituximab (90% vs 60%), with the difference attributed to rituximab. A trend toward improved graft survival was also seen in those who received IVIG. This retrospective study has one of the largest cohorts reported to date and supports the use of rituximab for treating AMR, with good short-term allograft survival; however, many patient variables were not consistent between the groups (Kaposztas et al, 2009, as cited in Jordan, S, 2010).

Gloor et al, (Gloor et al., 2003) described 14 patients with a positive cytotoxicity crossmatch to a potential living donor. Patients underwent plasmapheresis on days four, three, and one pretransplant, on the day of transplantation, and on day one and three post-transplantation. Intravenous immunoglobulin 100 mg/kg was administered after each plasmapheresis session. Rituximab at a dose of 375 mg/m^2 was given on post-transplant day four. Splenectomy was performed at the time of transplantation in those with an intact spleen (two had previously been splenectomized). Thymoglobulin was used for induction and tacrolimus, mycophenolate and corticosteroids were used for maintenance therapy. Patient survival at a mean follow-up of 15 months was 86 percent. Histologic evidence of AMR occurred in 43 percent. The risk of AMR was related to the baseline anti-HLA antibody titer. All four subclinical episodes responded to treatment and follow-up protocol biopsies showed no histologic evidence of rejection. Both episodes of rejection defined as clinically significant AMR demonstrated evidence of chronic allograft nephropathy on subsequent biopsies.

Stegall et al (Stegall et al, 2006, as cited in C. Siisal & Morath C, 2011) deigned one study to compare high dose IVIG (13 patients) with plasmapheresis/low dose IVIG protocols (32 patients) in renal transplant recipients with high DSA levels. Plasmapheresis plus low dose intravenous inmunoglobulins (IVIG) received also anti-CD20 antibody (32 patients), and 19 of the 32 patients in this group also underwent splenectomy; post-transplant plasmapheresis and low dose IVIG were continued on post-surgery days one to three for a total of two to three sessions. High single dose IVIG (13 patients), which is the high dose IVIG group. Plasmapheresis plus low dose IVIG plus anti-CD20 antibody plus pretransplant Thymoglobulin combined with post-transplant DSA monitoring (16 patients), was the plasmapheresis/monitoring group. Achieving a negative crossmatch was significantly more likely with both plasmapheresis protocols versus high dose IVIG (84, 88, and 38 percent respectively). Significantly lower humoral rejection rates were also reported with the plasmapheresis protocols (37, 29, and 80 percent, respectively), although none of the patients in the high single dose IVIG group received rituximab or post-transplant administration of

IVIG. Patients with low baseline antibody titers responding to high dose IVIG may do equally as well with further optimization of therapy. However, whether or not the administration of rituximab or the routine post-transplant administration of IVIG would be of benefit in reducing the incidence of acute rejection in a high dose IVIG protocol is unclear at this time as this study not included randomization and only participated a low numbers of patients.

4. Remarks and conclusions

The main goal of monitoring circulating antibodies is to measure PRA and identify specific antibodies in order to evaluate the patient's immunological risk and interpret a crossmatch. The introduction of HLA antibody characterization based on interactions between recipient serum and purified HLA antigens bound to solid-phase substrates has improved detection and quantification of donor-specific antibodies (DSAs).

Currently, few kidney transplant options exist for hypersensitive patients on the waiting list if they do not undergo previously to desensitising treatments or strong induction therapy. In this respect, high doses of intravenous immunoglobulins may reduce the level of circulating antibodies, but, many patients only respond partially, and the efficacy varies among patients. Plasmapheresis can decrease circulating antibodies, but there is normally a significant increase in their titre levels once the sessions have been completed. Therefore, this technique is now considered a complement to the use of immunoglobulins for decreasing antibody levels. Likewise, rituximab has also been shown to have a beneficial effect when combined with immunoglobulins and plasmapheresis to reduce anti-HLA antibodies rate and to treat antibody-mediated rejection. On the other hand, newer interventions aimed at the prevention of DSA-mediated allograft injury using complement blockade, or the inhibition of DSA synthesis using proteasome inhibitor-mediated plasma cell depletion are promising.

In any case, the best therapeutic strategy may be of combining these drugs, particularly when there is early detection of acute antibody-mediated rejection through histological or serological techniques. Whether long-term beneficial outcomes are achived with these drugs without life-threatening side-effects, remains to be elucidate.

According to our previous results, we tentatively propose the following desensitization and induction protocol:

Recipients with positive cytotoxicity crossmatch or retransplantation recipients with positive cytometry crossmatch and negative cytotoxicity crossmatch are potential candidates for pre-transplant desensitisation. For first transplant recipients with positive cytometry crossmatch but with negative cytotoxicity crossmatch, desensitisation may not be necessary. For patients who are only positive for virtual lymphocyte crosssmatch, with negative cytotoxicity and cytometry crossmatches, there are currently insufficient data that support the appropriateness of desensitisation. Patients on the waiting list more than 12 months and at least three studies quarterly permanently with PRA> 50-75% polyspecific, multiple previous positive crossmatch, and multiple HLA-antigens positive reactivity that makes transplantation highly unlikely, if they have absence of IgA deficiency and antibodies antiIgA, they could receive high dose of immunoglobulins, plus plasmapheresis and one or two doses of rituximab.

Requirements for performing kidney transplantation in these patients would be:

a. Pre-transplant negative cytotoxicity crossmatch, and
b. Negative virtual crossmatch test prior to the kidney transplant, i.e., abscense of all class I or II HLA antigens in the donor that have produced an alloresponse in the recipient at any time.

c. Induction therapy with thymoglobulin tacrolimus, mycophenolate, methylprednisolone.
d. Desensitisation treatment would consist in rituximab, various plasmapheresis sessions with IV immunoglobulin infusion following each session.
e. Monitorization of CD19+/CD20+ lymphocyte populations and checking for any appearance of opportunistic infections using a PCR assay for CMV, Epstein-Barr viral serology, B-19 parvovirus and polyomavirus BK are necessary.
f. Cytomegalovirus infection prophylaxis with gancyclovir/valgancyclovir 6 months, pneumocistis jirovecii prophylaxis with trimethoprim sulfamethoxazole and fungal infection prophylaxis with nystatin or oral fluconazole must be considered.
g. Monitoring PRA title every 15 days the first 3 months and then monthly during first year and before or after any deterioration of renal function. A rising DSA titter may suggests the need for intensification of therapy with potential modification of maintenance immunosuppression or initiating intensive therapy using IVIG and/or plasmapheresis.
h. Monitoring of neurological symptoms: progressive multifocal leukoencephalopathy, reactivation of polyoma JC virus also is very important.
i. In the case of immunoligal-mediated renal dysfunction, it is important perform a graft biopsy and C4d staining. Treatment for apparent AMR is essentially by combining metilprednisolone, plasmapheresis (or immunoadsorption) and IVIG, with a duration that will be dependent upon an improvement in renal function, decrease in the titter of DSA or improvement of biopsy findings. If there is no good response to treatment, individual assess whether repeated rescue therapies, such as rituximab or eculizumab. In the case of appearance of plasma cells in the renal graft biopsy, it should be assessed individually using bortezomib as salvage therapy. Subclinical rejection (as defined by positive C4d staining associated with histologic evidence of antibody mediated rejection) on protocol biopsies may be associated with future AMR or subsequent evidence of chronic allograft injury. Whether or not treatment of subclinical rejection in this setting has a benefit on long-term graft survival is unknown, however, given the high risk of acute rejection, most physicians would favor restarting plasmapheresis/IVIG or other treatment.
j. An additional critical issue is antibody development against allogeneic antigen systems on graft other than HLA that are not necessarily detected in routine antibody testing, like anti-major histocompatibility complex class I related A (anti-MICA), antiendothelial antibodies, antibody binding to angiotensin type-1 receptor and others. These antibodies have found a strong association with antibody-mediated rejection in recipients whose sera did not contain antibody to donor HLA, indicating that antibodies directed against non-HLA antigens also have a certain impact. These issues are not reasons for this chapter and may be addressed in future. More studies are required in this field to determine the frequency and magnitude of damage caused by non-HLA immunity.

5. References

Brennan,C.; Daller, JA.; Lake, KD.; Cibrik, D. & Del Castillo, D. (2006). Thymoglobulin Induction Study Group. Rabbit antithymocyte globulin versus basiliximab in renal transplantation. *N Engl J Med* Vol.355 No.9, (Nov 2010), pp. 1967-1977, ISSN 0028-4793

Ercilla, MG. & Martorell, J. (2010). Immunologic study of the donor-receptor couple. *Nefrologia,* Vol.30, suppl. 30, (Nov 2010), pp. 60-70, ISSN 2013-7575.

Everly, MJ.; Terasaki, PI.; Hopfield, J.; Trivedi, HL & Kaneku, H. (2010). Protective immunity remains intact after antibody removal by means of proteasome inhibition. *Transplantation,* Vol.90, No. 12, (Dec 2010), pp. 1493-1498, ISSN 1534-0608.

Flechner, SM.; Fatica, R.; Askar, M.; Stephany, BR.; Poggio, E.; Koo, A.; Banning, S.; Chiesa-Vottero, A. & Srinivas, T. (2010). The role of proteasome inhibition with bortezomib in the treatment of antibody-mediated rejection after kidney-only or kidney-combined organ transplantation. *Transplantation,* Vol 27. No 12, (Dec 2010), pp. 1486-1492, ISSN.

Gaber, AO.; Knight, RJ.; Patel, S. & Gaber, LW. (2010). A review of the evidence for use of thymoglobulin induction in renal transplantation. *Transplant Proc,* Vol.42, No. 5, (Jun 2010), pp. 1395-1400, ISSN 0041-1345

Gloor, JM.; DeGoey, SR.; Pineda, AA.; Moore, SB.; Prieto, M.; Nyberg, SL.; Larson, TS.; Griffin, MD.; Textor, SC.; Velosa, JA.; Schwab, TR.; Fix, LA. & Stegall, MD. Overcoming a positive crossmatch in living-donor kidney transplantation. *Am J Transplant,* Vol 3. No 8, (Aug 2003), pp. 1017-1023, ISSN 1600-6143.

Gloor, J. & Stegall, M. (2010). Sensitized renal transplant recipients: current protocols and future directions. *Nat. Rev. Nephrol,* Vol 6. (March 2010), pp. 297-306, ISSN 1759-5061,1759-507X.

Glotz, D.; Antoine, C.; Julia, P.; Suberbielle-Boissel, C.; Boudjeltia, S.; Fraoui, R.; Hacen, C.; Duboust, A. & Bariety J. (2002). Desensitization and subsequent kidney transplantation of patients using intravenous immunoglobulins (IVIg). *Am J Transplant,* Vol 2. No 8, (Sep 2002), pp. 758-760, ISSN 1600-6143.

Jordan, SC.; Peng, A. &Vo, AA. (2009). Therapeutic strategies in management of the highly HLA-sensitized and ABO-incompatible transplant recipients. *Contrib Nephrol,* Vol 162. (2009), pp. 13-26, ISSN 0302-5144 .

Jordan S, Reinsmoen, N,; Peng,A.; Lai, C.; Cao, K.; Villicana, R.; Toyoda,M.; Kahwaji, J & Ashley A. (2010). Advances in diagnosing and managing antibody-mediated rejection. *Pediatr Nephrol,* Vol.25, No.10, (Oct 2010), pp. 2035-2048, ISSN 0931-041X

Jordan, SC.; Toyoda, M.; Kahwaji, J. &Vo, AA. (2011). Clinical aspects of intravenous immunoglobulin use in solid organ transplant recipients. *Am J Transplant,* Vol 11. No 2, (Feb 2011), pp. 196-202, ISSN 1600-6143.

Kamar, N.; Milioto, O.; Puissant-Lubrano, B.; Esposito, L.; Pierre, MC.; Mohamed, AO.; Lavayssière, L.; Cointault, O.; Ribes, D.; Cardeau, I.; Nogier, MB.; Durand, D.; Abbal, M.; Blancher, A. & Rostaing, L. (2010). Incidence and predictive factors for infectious disease after rituximab therapy in kidney-transplant patients. *Am J Transplant,* Vol 10. No 1, (Jan 2010), pp. 89-98, ISSN 1600-6143.

Klein,C, Brennan,D (Sep2010). HLA and ABO sensitization and desensitization in renal transplantation, In: *Up to Date,* 9.2010, Avalaible from http://learn.uptodate.com/index.

Locke, JE.; Magro, CM.; Singer, AL.; Segev, DL.; Haas, M.; Hillel, AT.; King, KE.; Kraus, E.; Lees, LM.; Melancon, JK.; Stewart, ZA.; Warren, DS.; Zachary, AA. & Montgomery, RA. (2009). The use of antibody to complement protein C5 for salvage treatment of severe antibody-mediated rejection. *Am J Transplant,* Vol 9. No 1, (Jan 2009), pp. 231-235, ISSN 1600-6143.

Lonze, BE.; Dagher, NN.; Simpkins, CE.; Locke, JE.; Singer, AL.; Segev, DL.; Zachary, AA. & Montgomery, RA. (2010). Eculizumab, bortezomib and kidney paired donation facilitate transplantation of a highly sensitized patient without vascular access. *Am J Transplant,* Vol 10. No 9, (Sep 2010), pp. 2154-2160, ISSN 1600-6143.

Loupy, A.; Suberbielle-Boissel, C.; Zuber, J.; Anglicheau, D.; Timsit, MO.; Martinez, F.; Thervet, E.; Bruneval, P.; Charron, D.; Hill, GS,; Nochy, D, & Legendre, C. (2010). Combined posttransplant prophylactic IVIg/anti-CD 20/plasmapheresis in kidney recipients with preformed donor-specific antibodies: a pilot study. *Transplantation,* Vol. 15, No. 89, (Jun 2010), pp.1403-1410, ISSN 1534-0608

Nocera, A. (2009). Desensitization protocols in immunized living donor kidney transplant recipients. *G Ital Nefrol ,* Vol. 26, No. 4,(Jul-Aug 2009), pp. 499-515, ISSN.Oppenheimer, F.; Pascual, J. & Pallardo.L. (2010). Inmunosuppression in renal transplant, In: *Nefrología al día,* V. Lorenzo Sellares, J.M. López Gómez, ALM, de Francisco Hernandez & D. Hernandez Marrero, (Ed.), 731-747, Grupo Editorial Nefrología de la Sociedad Española de Nefrología, ISBN 978-84-96727-97-7, Barcelona, Spain.

Raghavan, R.; Jeroudi, A.; Achkar, K.; Gaber, AO.; Patel, SJ. & Abdellatif, A. (2010). Bortezomib in kidney transplantation. *J Transplant,* Vol 2010. (Sep 2010), pp. 1-6, ISSN.

Sberro-Soussan, R.; Zuber, J.; Suberbielle-Boissel, C.; Candon, S.; Martinez, F.; Snanoudj, R.; Rabant, M.; Pallet, N.; Nochy, D.; Anglicheau, D.; Leruez, M.; Loupy, A.; Thervet, E.; Hermine, O. & Legendre, C. (2010). Bortezomib as the sole post-renal transplantation desensitization agent does not decrease donor-specific anti-HLA antibodies. *Am J Transplant,* Vol 10. No 3, (Mar 2010), pp. 681-686, ISSN 1600-6143.

Scemla, A.; Loupy, A.; Candon, S.; Mamzer, MF.; Martinez, F.; Zuber, J.; Sberro, R.; Legendre, C. & Thervet, E. (2010). Incidence of infectious complications in highly sensitized renal transplant recipients treated by rituximab: a case-controlled study. *Transplantation,* Vol 90. No 11, (Dec 2010), pp. 1180-1184, ISSN 1534-0608.

Schwenger V & Morath,C. (2010). Immunoadsorption in nephrology and kidney transplantation. *Nephrol Dial. Transplant* Vol. 25, No 8, (May 2010) pp. 2407-2413. Online ISSN 1460-2385 - Print ISSN 0931-0509

Siisal, C & Morath, C. (2011). Current approaches to the management of highly sensitized kidney transplant patients. *Tissue Antigens,* Vol 77. No 3, (Mar 2011), pp. 177-186, ISSN 1399-0039.

Stegall, MD.; Gloor, J.; Winters, JL.; Moore, SB. & Degoey, S. (2006). A comparison of plasmapheresis versus high-dose IVIG desensitization in renal allograft recipients with high levels of donor specific alloantibody. *Am J Transplant* Vol 6. No 2, (Feb 2006), pp. 146-351, ISSN 1600-6143

Trivedi, HL.; Terasaki, PI.; Feroz, A.; Everly, MJ.; Vanikar, AV.; Shankar, V.; Trivedi, VB.; Kaneku, H.; Idica, AK.; Modi, PR.; Khemchandani, SI & Dave SD. (2009)Abrogation of anti-HLA antibodies via proteasome inhibition. *Transplantation,* Vol.87, No. 10, (May 2009), pp. 1555-1561, ISSN 1534-0608.

Vo, AA.; Wechsler, EA.; Wang, J.; Peng, A.; Toyoda, M.; Lukovsky, M.; Reinsmoen, & N, Jordan SC. (2008). Analysis of subcutaneous (SQ) alemtuzumab induction therapy in highly sensitized patients desensitized with IVIG and rituximab. *Am J Transplant,* Vol 8. No 1, (Jan 2008), pp. 144-149, ISSN 1600-6143.

Wahrmann, M.; Haidinger, M.; Körmöczi, GF.; Weichhart, T.; Säemann, MD.; Geyeregger, R.; Kikić, Z.; Prikoszovich, T.; Drach, J. & Böhmig, GA. (2010). Effect of the proteasome inhibitor bortezomib on humoral immunity in two presensitized renal transplant candidates. *Transplantation,* Vol 89. No 11, (Jun 2010), pp. 1385-1390, ISSN 1534-0608.

Yuan, XP; Wang, CX.; Gao, W. & Fu Q, He XS. (2010). Kidney transplant in highly sensitized patients after desensitization with plasmapheresis and low-dose intravenous immunoglobulin. *Exp Clin Transplant,* Vol. 2, No. 2, (Jun 2010), pp. 130-135, ISSN 1304-0855.

8

Combined Kidney-Islet Transplantation

Giuseppe Cavallari, Flavia Neri and Bruno Nardo
Department of General Surgery and Transplantation University of Bologna
Italy

1. Introduction

The possibility to transplant uniquely the endocrine part of the pancreas, islets of Langerhans, with the aim to recovery the endogenous insulin production in diabetic patients has always aroused attention from researches.

The initial experience of this procedure however was unsatisfying especially for what concerns the long term efficacy of the islet transplantation. The exciting results obtained by the Edmonton group in 2000, 100% of insulin independence in seven diabetic patients after 1 year from the islet transplant, encouraged several centers worldwide to approach this technique. Since then several programs of islet transplantation have been launched, and important multicentric clinical trials including an high number of patients were realized.

The Collaborative Islet Transplant Registry (CITR) collects data from 27 North American, 3 European and 2 Australian islet transplant centers and reported that a total of 412 patients underwent an islet transplantation in the time period between 1999-2009.

The global long-term results of CITR demonstrated an insulin independence after islet transplantation in a low percentage of cases but a partial function of the graft, and consequently important advantages for the patients, in the majority of these.

Actually islet transplantation is considered a valid therapeutic option only for selected patients affected by type 1 diabetes mellitus (DMT1). This limitation is a consequence of the benefit/cost ratio between improvement of the glycemic control and the necessity for transplant recipients to be treated with chronic immunosuppressive therapy which has, as well known, important side effects.

These considerations and the availability of new generation basal insulin and sophisticated micro insulin pumps lead the majority of European centers to perform islet transplantation almost exclusively in combination with kidney transplant in DMT1 patients candidate (simultaneous islets-kidney transplant), or just subjected (islet after kidney transplant), to a kidney transplantation for end-stage diabetic nephropathy. These patients therefore would anyway be treated with immunosuppressive drugs.

Even if the combined kidney-pancreas transplantation showed excellent results in DMT1 patients with end-stage diabetic nephropathy, the combined kidney-islet transplantation is considered a valid option in selected cases for this patient category.

2. History of islet transplantation: Past and current era

The history of the islet transplantation is long. The first transplant of fragments of the pancreatic gland in order to cure diabetes dates back even to the 20th December 1893, 28 years before the discovery of the insulin. Two English medical doctors from the Bristol Royal Infirmary Hospital, Dr. Watson-Williams and Dr. Harsant, harvested a pancreas from a deceased sheep and transplanted three pieces of the gland into the subcuticular tissue of a 15-years-old boy with uncontrollable diabetic ketoacidosis. Obviously, despite a temporary improvement of the clinical situation, the xenotransplant failed after three days for acute rejection.

After that first experiment almost one century passed before Paul Lacy and collegues in 1967 developed the technique of islet isolation in rats. Two important innovations made this procedure possible: the injection of digestion enzyme solution in the pancreatic duct and the centrifugation with different density gradients to separate the islets from the discarding tissue.

After few years the improvement of the glycemic control by intraperitoneal transplantation of islets was demonstred in diabetic rats (Younoszai et al., 1970) and subsequently the liver, using the same experimental model, was selected as preferable implantation site (Kemp et al., 1973). Actually the liver, by islets injection through the portal vein, is still the site preferably used for islet transplantation in the clinical setting.

The first clinical series of islet transplantations was reported in the late seventy using azathioprine and steroids as immunosuppressive therapy (Najarian et al., 1977). Although these first cases did not experience any complications the efficacy of the transplant was very limited. Seven patients over seven failed to reach the insulin independence after intraperitoneal or intraportal islet transplantation even though some of them reduced the need of exogenous insulin for a period.

Interestingly the first real clinical success in the field of islet transplantation was reported in one case of combined islet-kidney transplantation performed on a DMT1 uremic patient in Zurich in 1978. This patient reached the insulin independence and maintained it almost one year after the embolization in the spleen of fragments of donor pancreas (Largiader et al., 1979). In 1990 a series of nine islet transplantations was reported by the University of Pittsburgh. The patients underwent multivisceral resections for tumors and sequentially liver, kidney and small bowel transplantation: islets were injected in the portal vein at the liver reperfusion. More than 50% reached and mantained the insulin-indipendence until their death caused by neoplastic relapse (Tzakis et al., 1990). Subsequently other positive experiences were reported (Ricordi et al., 1992) but the global clinical results obtained by the Islet Transplant Registry from the total amount of islets transplantation performed between 1974 and 1999 were very disappointing with an insulin-indipendence presents in only about 10% of cases at one year from the transplant.

In 2000 the group of the University of Edmonton reported 100% of insulin indipendence at 1 year from islet transplantation in a series of 7 patients (Shapiro et al., 2000). Such extraordinary result was possible thanks to the employment of a protocol subsequently called the "Edmonton protocol". The key elements of this protocol were principally two. Firstly the recourse to two or more islets intrahepatic transplants in the same recipients provided an higher total number of transplanted islets (over 11000 IEQ/Kg of the patient body weight). Secondly the use of an immunosuppressive regimen without steroids and their hyperglycemic effect and consisting in interleukin-2 receptor blocking antibody daclizumab (Zenapax®) for induction therapy and sirolimus (Rapamune®) combined with low doses of tacrolimus (Prograf®) for chronic therapy.

Subsequently, with the aim to assess the applicability and reproducibility of the results obtained from the Edmonton group, a multicentric study started using the Edmonton protocol involving 9 transplant centers, 6 of which were American and 3 European.

The data from this study reported in 2006 did not confirm however the Edmonton results, showing an high variability in the outcome of the transplantation according to the isolation centre (Shapiro et al., 2006).
The critical passage in the procedure of islet transplantation is exactly the phase of organ processing in order to isolate the islets of Langerhans. These considerations lead to the development of several networks in which the isolation procedure is performed by few specialized and experienced centers and the islet transplantations are spread to several different centers even at long distance (Kempf et al., 2005).
In 2008 the Collaborative Islet Transplant Registry reported approximately a 30% of insulin independence by 3 years postoperatively over 325 adult recipients which were treated between 1999 and 2007 with an islet alone or a combined kidney-islet transplantations. However more than 75% of the recipients maintained a residual graft functionality detected by the endogenous secretion of C-peptide at 3 years from the transplantation.
This apparently disappointing outcome, showed anyway an important improvement in the quality of life of the patients reducing the episodes of severe hypoglycemia and the development of complications related to the diabetic disease (Alejandro et al., 2008).
In particular some studies have also focused on comparing the outcome of diabetic patients who underwent combined kidney-islet transplantation versus patient operated with kidney transplantation alone.
The group of Milan showed a decreased risk for micro and macroangiopathy, an improvement in the cardiovascular functionality and a reduced neuropathy also in cases of partial islet function after transplantation (Fiorina et al., 2003; Del Carro et al., 2007). Moreover the same authors showed that the improved glycemic control in patients with combined kidney-islet transplantation significantly increased also the kidney graft survival when compared to DMT1 patients with transplantation of the kidney alone (Fiorina et al., 2005).

3. Islets of Langerhans procurement

3.1 Pancreas harvest

The organs used for the islets isolation generally are pancreas previously proposed and not utilized or excluded for the whole pancreas transplantation. This strategy, adopted in order to decrease the competition between the two types of transplantation, allows in the case of pancreas for islets isolation the use of organs from donors with high BMI or >50 years old. Moreover, with the aim to expand the pool of donors, some authors reported positive experience of islet transplantation using donors after cardiac death (Saito et al., 2010).
The harvesting procedure of the gland is similar to the procedure for the whole pancreas transplantation. However, after perfusion with cold preserving solution, the pancreas is collected paying particular attention not to section the pancreatic capsule, event that may impair the enzymatic digestion while, obviously, the accuracy in the isolation and preservation of pancreatic vessels is not important as in case of the pancreas procurement for the transplantation of the whole gland.
The pancreas is harvested en bloc with a portion of duodenum and the spleen. After the pancreas is procured it is kept in cold preservation solution at 4°C. At the moment the pancreas preservation is obtained thanks to a double-layered system: the organ is placed within a superior layer of preservation solution and an inferior layer of perfluorocarbons (PFC) which are constantly oxygenated and help maintaining an high oxygen solubility

coefficient. This method allows the development of a highly oxygenated environment for the pancreas which is of great importance for the protection of the islets (Hering et al., 2002). The gland can be kept in this solution for several hours although it was reported that the best results were achieved when the cold ischemia time was < 16 hours at the beginning of the isolation procedure (Tsujimura et al., 2004).

3.2 Automated method for islets of Langerhans isolation

Before the beginning of the isolation procedure the spleen and the duodenum are removed from the pancreas and an accurate dissection and discard of the peripancretic fat, lymphonodes and vessels is performed (Fig. 1).

The procedure currently used to extract islets from human pancreas is the so called automated method for isolation of the islets of Langerhans, established in 1987 by Ricordi and collegues.

This procedure consists of two phases: digestion and purification phase. The digestion phase includes the digestion of the collagen scaffold of the pancreas releasing the esocrine and endocrine tissues within the gland. It includes a procedure of enzymatic and mechanical digestion. The phase of purification is aimed to obtain only the endocrine part of the gland, islets of Langerhans, separating them from the remain of the gland which is useless (acinar cells, ductal elements, fat tissue, lymph nodes, ganglia, etc).

Digestion phase: after the preparation of the pancreas the gland is devided at the isthmus and the pancreatic duct is cannulated in the proximal part (head and body) and in the distal part (body-tail) with two angiocatheters 18 gauge. The solution containing the digestion enzyme is injected in the Wirsung duct with a pressure of 180 mmHg slowly distending the two parts of the gland. The collagenase at warm temperature (37°C) is activated and starts the enzymatic digestion of the internal scaffold of the pancreas (Fig.2).

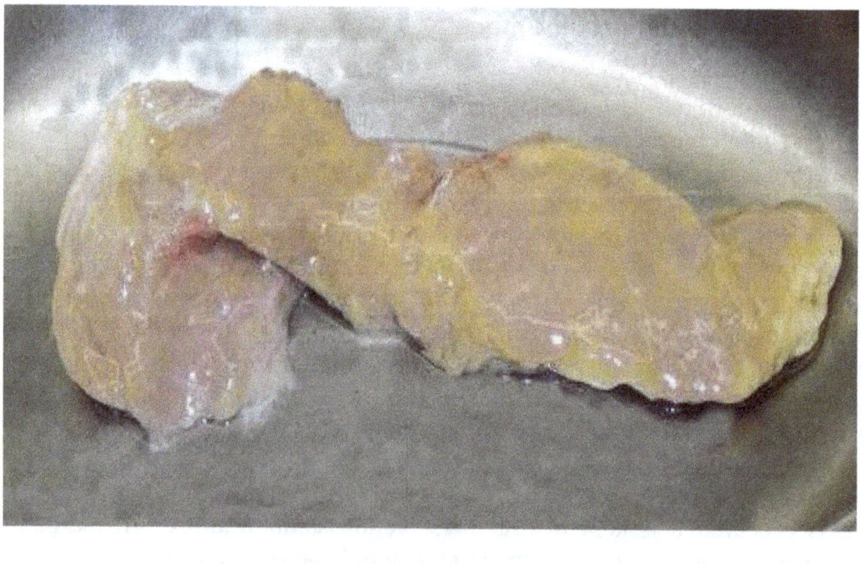

Fig. 1. Pancreas prepared for the isolation procedure.

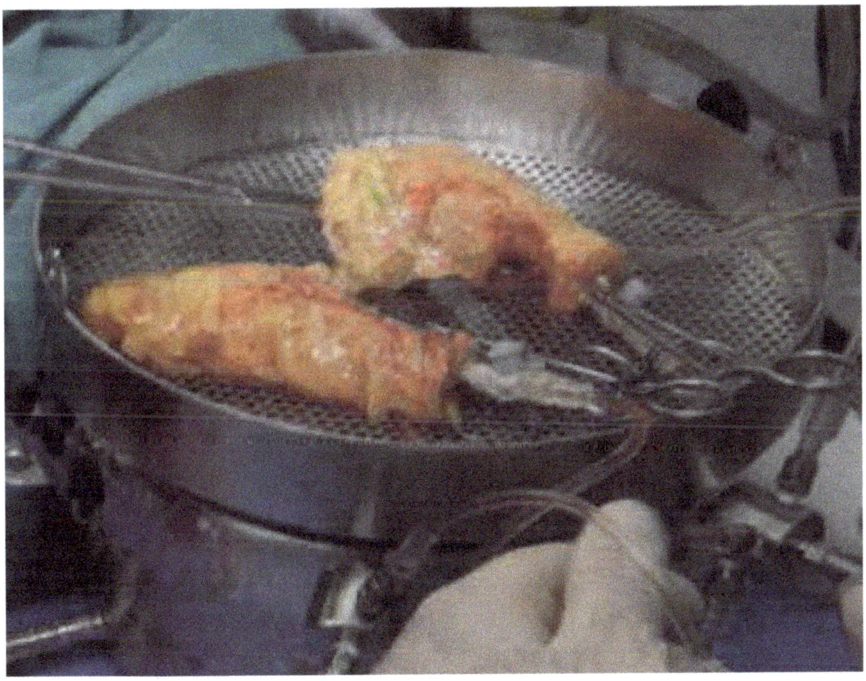

Fig. 2. Cannulation of the pancreatic duct and injection of the collagenase solution.

After some minutes the two portions of the pancreas are divided in smaller pieces and placed in a digestion chamber named "Ricordi chamber" after its inventor. This chamber is composed of a superior and an inferior part divided by a semi-permeable membrane which has holes of about 300 µm. Seven stainless steel balls together with the fragments of the pancreas are put into the inferior part, which is then filled with the digestion solution and closed together with the superior one. The chamber is connected to a mechanical arm with 10 cm excursion which is activated with a sussultory movement (300 oscillation/min) helping the complete mechanical digestion of the pancreas through the steel balls in the chamber. In the meantime a peristaltic pump connected to the system is activated creating a flow of 40 ml/min. The digestion runs in a closed circuit where warm Hank's solution is pumped in the inferior chamber and the tissue released in the solution passes in the superior chamber through the filter. The solution is collected in a cylinder passing in a refrigerator circuit at 4°C; at this temperature the activity of the enzyme and consequently the digestive process is stopped. Samples of the solution are collected from the circuit through a spigot every 2-3 minutes to monitor the progress of the digestion. When free islets are found in the samples the system is converted from closed to open: the solution is collected from the chamber into containers placed on ice. The procedure is stopped when no more islets are detected at samples (Fig 3).

Phase of purification: this includes the separation of the islets from the waste tissue through centrifugation cycles on different Ficoll density gradients. Islets which have a lower specific weight than the other structures, remain in the supernatant, the less dense part of the solution. Nowadays this procedure is generally performed using a COBE® 2991 cell processor system (Fig 4). At the end of the procedure samples of the islets preparation are collected and evaluated through a staining with dithizone (DTZ) which marks zinc in the insulin granules resulting in a characteristic red stain. Adding few drops of DTZ solution to a sample is possible easily evaluate the morphology and number of the isolated islets through a computerized digital analysis. Specific features of the final volume of islets are required in order to perform the islets transplantation, in particular purity (> 90% of the preparation composed by islets) and adequate number of islets (Fig.5).

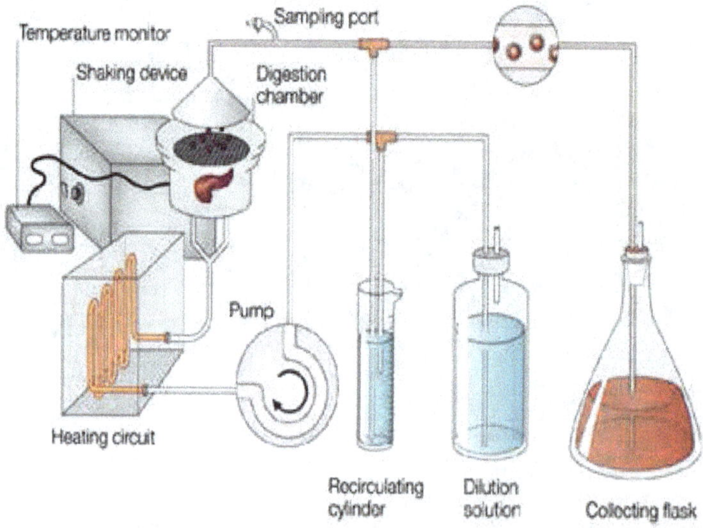

Fig. 3. Schematic representation of the automated method for islets of Langerhans isolation (modified from: Ricordi and Strom, *Nature Reviews Immunology* 2004).

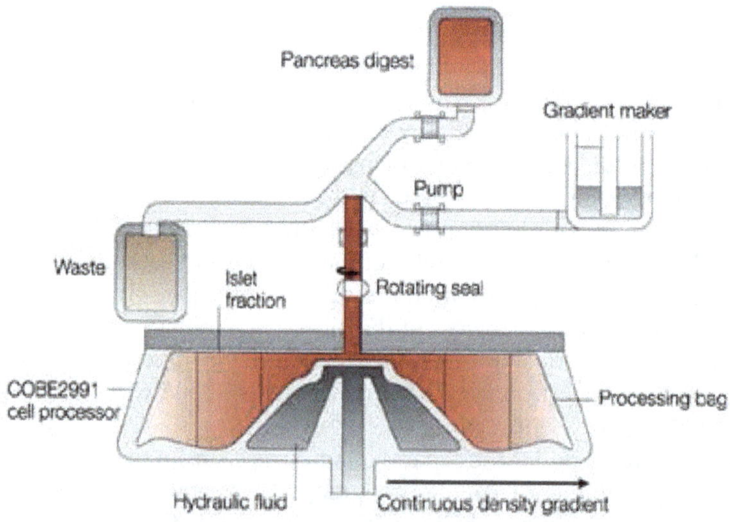

Fig. 4. Islets of Langerhans purification by density gradient separation (modified from: Ricordi and Strom, *Nature Reviews Immunology* 2004).

Although the procedure is quite standardized, only centers with the greatest experience in the field can count on an high percentage of procedures with a satisfactory purity and quantity of islets for the transplantation. Indeed the more the pancreas is manipulated in order to discard the exocrine part, the more islets are lost during this procedure. An additional important variable that reduces the reliability of the isolation process is the different enzyme lot used for the digestion procedure. The adequate amount of islets obtained is calculated with respect to the body weight of the recipient and resuspended immediately before the intrahepatic transplantation in 100 mL of adequate solution (45 mL of HBSS, 0.2 mL od HEPES 1M, 50 mL 20% Human Albumin and 2000 IE of heparin).

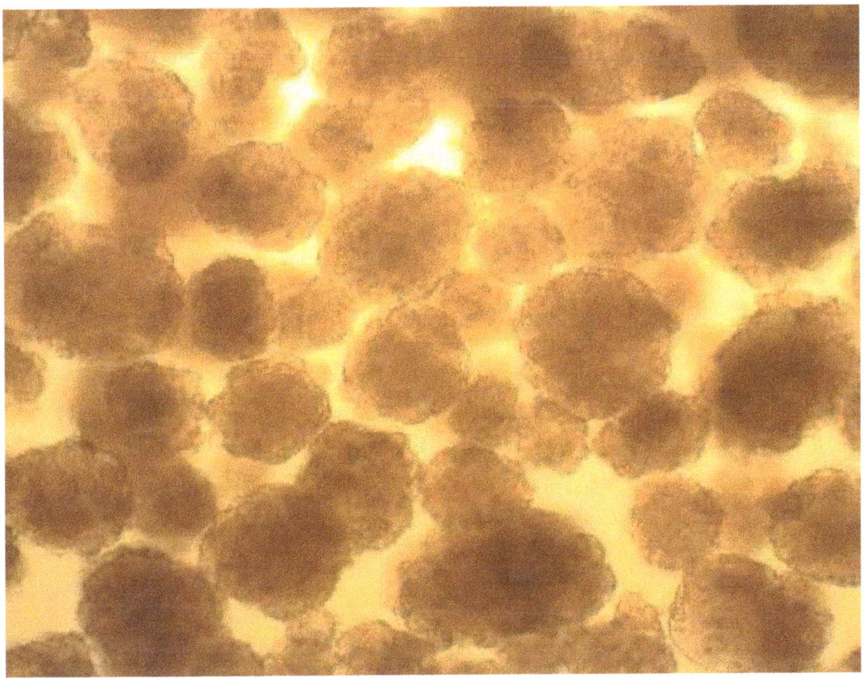

Fig. 5. Highly purified human islets of Langerhans at the end of the isolation procedure.

4. Islet transplantation procedure

The islet transplantation can be performed at the same time as the kidney transplantation (simultaneous islet-kidney transplantation) or in diabetic patients who had previously received a kidney transplant alone (islet after kidney transplantation). In both cases AB0 compatibility and a negative serum cross-match between the pancreas donor and the recipient are required. Obviously when a simultaneous kidney-islets transplantation is performed the pancreas which will undergo the isolation procedure is generally harvested from the same donor of the kidney.

As previously reported in recent years networks have developed connecting several islet transplant centers and single centers dedicated to the procedure of isolation.

The GRAGIL, Swiss-French Multicenter Network of Islet Transplantation, was organized as to send the pancreas to the Genève center for the procedure of isolation; and then distribute the islets obtained to different transplant centers in the south-east area of France.

By this network islet transplantations were performed also in centre at long distance provided that it would be done within 72 hours from the end of the isolation procedure (Langer et al., 2004). This organization allowed a cost decrease and an increase in the experience of the isolation center with a positive rebound on the percentage of successful isolations and consequently on the number of the transplants performed (Kempf et al., 2005). Further similar collaborations were created between north european centers (Nordic Network) and between american centers (Porrett et al., 2007).

In the case of simultaneous kidney-islets transplantation while the pancreas undergoes the procedure of isolation, generally the recipient contemporaneously undergoes kidney transplantation. Once the islets are received, they are infused through a surgical or, radiological procedure.

The implantation site is usually the hepatic parenchyma through the portal system of the recipient. Islets are infused by gravity into the portal circulation and flow with the portal blood to lodge in the hepatic sinusoids (Fig 6).

The surgical procedure is performed after the conclusion of the kidney transplant through injection of the islets in the portal system by opening the peritoneum and catheterization of an ileal vein.

The percutaneous approach is done by a minimally invasive procedure requiring interventional radiology technology. The portal vein is reached by a percutaneous catheter placed under ultrasound or angiographic guidance (Fig. 7).

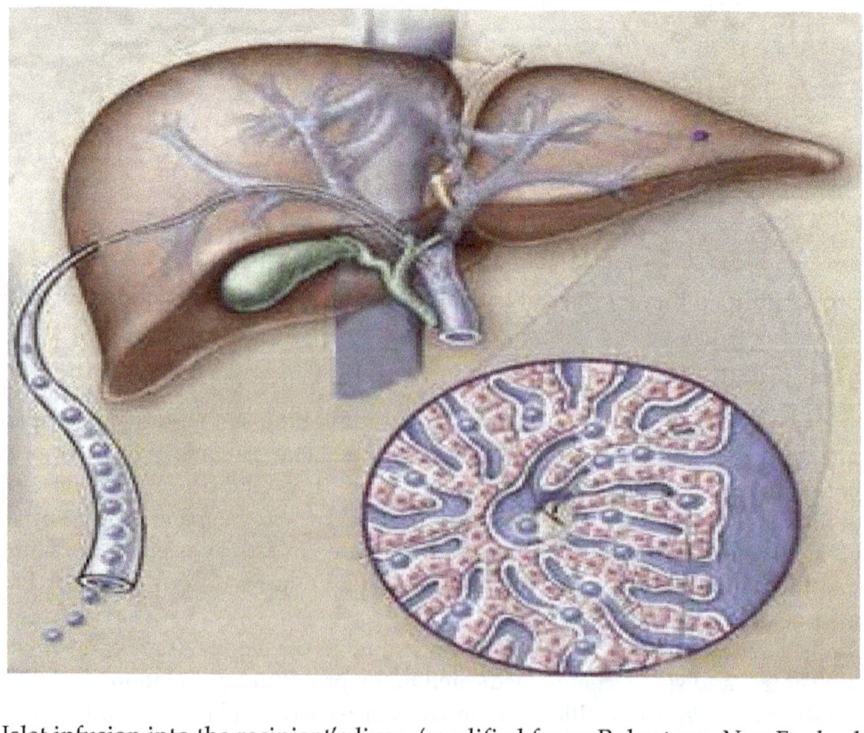

Fig. 6. Islet infusion into the recipient's liver (modified from: Robertson, *New England Journal of Medicine* 2004).

The radiological infusion of the islets can be performed few hours after the end of the kidney transplant or at long time after the operation, as for the islet after kidney transplant or in the case of subsequent islets infusions in patients just transplanted with islets.
Recently other implantation sites have been proposed in the clinical setting , like bone marrow (Cantarelli et al., 2009) or striated muscle (Christoffersson et al., 2010) which probably could show to be valid alternatives in a near future.

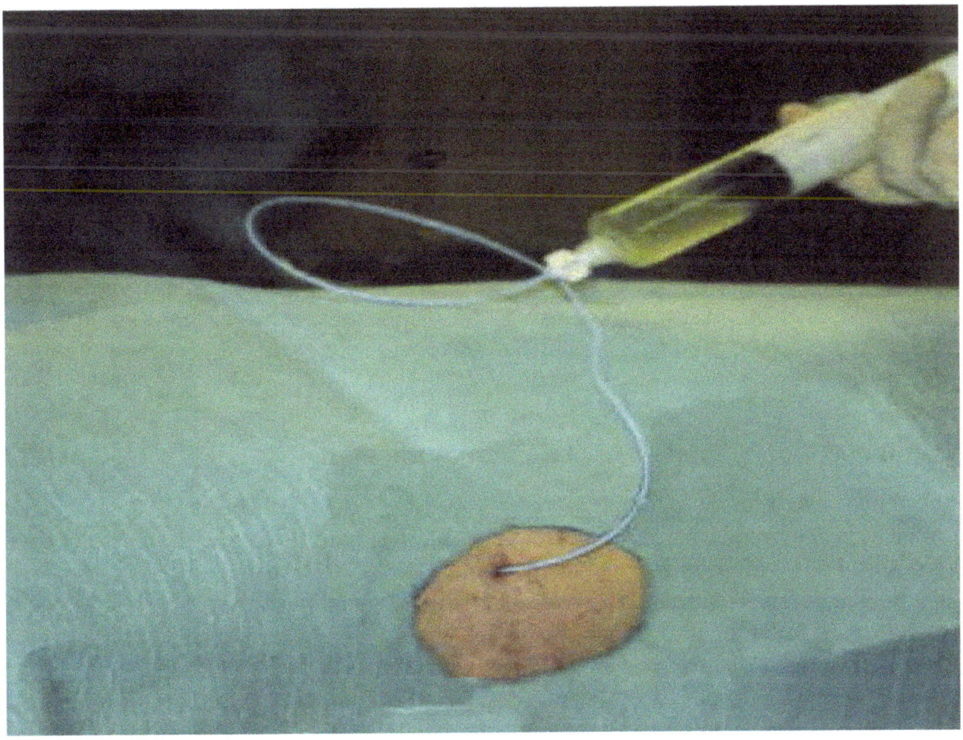

Fig. 7. Islet transplantation through a percutaneous catheter.

5. Complications related to islet transplantation

The procedure of islet transplantation proved to be very safe, especially when compared with the transplant of the whole pancreas. Data from CITR obtained from the analysis of more than 300 recipients showed that no complications occurred in case of injection by surgical approach and less than 10% of complications occurred in case of radiological infusion. Ower and collegues in 2003 showed that the most severe complications occurred in this case were intraperitoneal haemorrhages; anyway these were generally treated conservatively. The exact cause of bleeding in each case is often difficult to determine; however the peri-operative use of heparin to prevent portal thrombosis likely plays a role. The use of fibrin tissue sealant and embolization coils in the hepatic catheter tract seems to be effective in minimizing the bleeding risk.
Another complication related to the intrahepatic islet transplantation procedure is the insurgence of portal hypertension that can occur acutely during the islet infusion especially

in the case of subsequent infusions (Casey et al., 2002). The portal pressure however generally normalizes after the acute phase of the procedure.
Branch portal vein thrombosis was also frequently reported in the past; anyway this complication is generally limited and controlled with appropriate anticoagulation therapy. Actually the use of purer islet preparations, greater expertise in portal vein catheterization and new radiologic devices (catheters medicated for anticoagulation) will constantly reduce the risk of portal vein thrombosis although it will never be completely removed. A complication frequently reported is even the post-transplant elevation of liver enzymes but this is usually temporary and heals without further intervention.
In the past the appearance on magnetic resonance imaging (MRI) of intrahepatic periportal steatosis, occurring in a minority of islet recipients, has raised cautions. This finding is supposed to be due to the local effect of insulin produced by the transplanted islets on the hepatocyte metabolism and is reversible, since the complete resolution of MRI changes was reported in a patient after the graft function failed completely (Markmann et al., 2003). Successively the onset of focal steatosis in patient after islets transplantation was studied by sonogram (Maffi et al., 2005). These authors reported that signs of steatosis were often observed in patients after islet transplantation with total or partial function of the graft and normal liver function anyway was maintained in all of these. It was even proposed to consider the disappearance of this signs as a early marker of graft dysfunction.

6. Combined kidney-islet transplantation: Indications

The American Diabetes Association guidelines (http://www.diabetes.org/) remember that a combined kidney-pancreas transplantation should be always considered in case of uremic patient with DMT1 candidate to kidney transplantation. This recommendation is the result of the beneficial effects observed in terms of quality of life and survival after kidney-pancreas transplantation into patients suffering for DMT1 (Reddy et al., 2003). However since the procedure of pancreas transplantation has an high incidence of mortality and morbidity (Gruessner et al., 2004) it can be proposed only to selected population of patients candidate to kidney transplantation for diabetic nephropathy. In this the European Trial of Immunosuppression in Simultaneous Pancreas Kidney Transplantation (EUROSPK) study group reported that repeated laparotomies in the first 3 months after transplantation were performed in 35% of all the patients. Considering the much lower incidence of complication after islets transplantation several kidney-pancreas centers have also started programs of kidney-islets transplantation basing on the fact that these two procedures are complementary and suitable for patients with different features. Although the success of pancreas transplantation in term of graft survival is higher than islet transplantation with 80% of insulin-independency after 3 years (http://www.iptr.umn.edu/IPTR), some patients can be preferably directed towards a kidney-islet transplantation.
Actually the patient selection for either two therapeutic options is performed after a careful evaluation of possible advantages and disadvantages, with special regard to age and comorbidities. Patients at high risk of intraoperative complications are preferentially assigned to the less invasive procedure of islet transplantation, while younger and healthier patients are generally addressed to pancreas transplantation (Gerber et al., 2008).
In particular kidney-islets transplantation is preferred to kidney-pancreas for patients over 50 years of age or with severe macroangiopathy. Islet transplantation should also be

considered for all the patients who underwent kidney-pancreas tranplantation and have functioning pancreatic graft removed for complications as recidivant anastomotic leackage. In this case the possibility to use the removed pancreas for the islets isolation procedure has to be considered. The obtained islets could be then eventually transplanted in the same patient. The esecution of a combined kidney-islet transplantation is also a possibility for uremic patients with DMT1 and a good compliance to insulin therapy with lack motivation to undergo a combined kidney-pancreas transplant. These patients indeed may not accept the elevated peri-operative morbidity associated with kidney-pancreas transplant, which is much higher than with kidney alone transplant. The recipient's weight is also a key factor in the choice between pancreas or islet transplantation. Considering that the volume of islets necessary to obtain success after transplant is calculated with respect to the body weight of the recipient, patients with high weight are generally excluded from the procedure of islets transplantation and treated with a combined kidney-pancreas transplant.

The islet after kidney transplantation should be considered instead of the pancreas after kidney transplantation in patients over 45 years of age or with severe macroangiopathy if the creatinine blood levels are stable below 2 mg/dl at least six months after kidney transplantation and steroids discontinuation (Vantyghem et al., 2009).

Contraindications to the islets transplantion are severe heart diseases (as untreatable coronary artery diseases, severe dilated cardiomyopathy, previous stroke or recurrent transient ischemic attacks) and hepatic diseases as severe steatosis if the recipient liver is used as transplantation site.

In recent years positive experiences have been reported in the field of kidney-pancreas transplant in insulin-dependent patients with type 2 diabetes mellitus (Light et al., 2005). Nath and collegues in 2005 showed that these patients, as well as DMT1 patients, had an higher beneficial effect from a combined kidney-pancreas transplantation than a kidney transplantation alone. On the basis of the high percentage of DMT2 patients with end-stage renal disease and their characteristics, related to macrovascular degeneration, they are generally patients older and in worse clinical conditions than DMT1 patients likely the combined kidney-islet transplantation could be a valid therapeutical option to combined kidney-pancreas transplantation for these patients if they are lean and with low insulin-resistance.

7. Combined kidney-islet transplantation: Aims and results

As previously reported, the global results of the islet transplantations performed in the last decade showed a progressive decline in graft function in the months following the procedure which allows a long-term insulin-independence in a limited number of patients but a residual partial graft function in the majority of them.

In order to extend the period of insulin-independence after transplant several centers have adopted the strategy to perform two or more islet infusions in the same recipient using different pancreas donors. However it was observed that this strategy could increase the risk of sensitization of the patients and therefore jeopardize the possibility of an eventually kidney retransplantation (Campbell et al., 2007). On the basis of these considerations, nowadays the goal of islet in combination with kidney transplantation is not necessarily to arrive at the insulin-indipendence but the achievement of a good glycemic control by a single islet transplantation (Lehmann et al., 2008). A single infusion of functioning islets can reduce long term levels of HbA1c and consequently prevent the occurrence of severe asymptomatic episodes of hypoglycaemia and delay diabetes-related complications (Alejandro et al., 2008; Cure et al., 2008).

The group of Zurich (Gerber et al., 2008) reported their own experience in the field of combined kidney-islet and kidney-pancreas transplantation. They compared the long-term outcomes of diabetic patients subjected to kidney-islets transplantation and treated with immunosuppression carried out according with the Edmonton protocol versus patients subjected to kidney-pancreas transplant treated with conventional immunosuppression. In particular in the kidney-islet group induction therapy was performed with daclizumab and long-term therapy was carried out through levels of sirolimus and tacrolimus respectively of 7-10 µg/l and 3-6µg/l. In the kidney-pancreas group the induction therapy was performed with basiliximab and chronic immunosuppression was based on tacrolimus, mycophenolate mofetil and prednisone. The study demonstrated a similar kidney function and survival and an improvement of the blood glucose control in both groups.

Actually different protocols of immunosuppression are applied by different transplantation centers to patients trated with a combined kidney-islet transplantation. All of these protocols are steroid free and schedule different combinations beetween daclizumab or etanercept during the induction period plus mycophenolate mofetil or sirolimus and low-dose of tacrolimus or cyclosporine A. Since the number of the islets transplantation performed worldwide is low, a long period of time will be necessary in order to define which immunosuppressive protocol is the most favourable. Nowadays they seem all equally effective as long as steroids free (Alejandro et al., 2008).

As expected the Zurich group study reported a long-term insulin independence much lower in the group transplanted with kidney-islet than in the group transplanted with kidney-pancreas with a global result in line with the findings of the Edmonton trial group and a residual islet graft function sufficient to maintain glycemic control at a near-normal level. Interestingly it was showed that there was only a marginal benefit in terms of glucose control in those patients who received multiple islet infusions compared to patients who received only a single islet infusion. This finding and the not significant difference in glucose control between kidney-islet and kidney-pancreas patients despite much higher C- peptide levels and insulin independence in the latter group showed that even a minor residual beta cell function can significantly improve glycemic control, provided that patients are intensively treated with insulin. This consideration associate to the shortage of organs and the high risk of patient sensitization after multiple islet infusions reinforce the opinion that it preferable to undergo islet transplantation from a single pancreas donor. Moreover the cost is an additional important point in the context of repetitive islet transplantations. The same study reported that the cost of a combined kidney-islet transplantation is lower than the cost for a combined kidney-pancreas transplantation by about 10%, but exceeds in case two or more islet infusions have to be performed (Gerber et al., 2008).

8. Conclusions

The procedure of islet transplantation has made important progresses in the last decade, but the benefit/cost ratio between the improvement of glycemic control and the necessary chronic immunosuppressive therapy makes this option valid only for a restricted category of patients suffering from DMT1.

Actually the most frequent indication to islets transplantation is in combination with the kidney transplant in patients with end-stage diabetic nephropathy; patients therefore who will anyway undergo chronic immunosuppressive therapy.

The islet transplantation allows a long-term insulin independence in a limited number of patients. A residual partial graft function anyway leads to an improvement of the glycemic control, and consequently important advantages, in the majority of treated patients. In consideration of the low incidence of complications and the excellent kidney graft function results using immunosuppressive regimen avoiding steroids the combined kidney-islet transplantation procedure should be considered a valid alternative to kidney-pancreas transplantation for some patients categories.

Patient selection for either one of the two therapeutic options needs to be performed after a careful evaluation of possible advantages and disadvantages, with special regard to age and comorbidities. Patients older than 50 years or considered at higher risk of intraoperative complications were preferentially assigned to the less invasive procedure of kidney-islet transplantation, while younger and healthier patients could be preferentially assigned to kidney-pancreas transplantation.

Endogenous insulin production by transplanted islets combined with optimal insulin therapy is sufficient for maintenance of near-normal glucose levels that allows a delay of all diabetes-related complications and a strong reduction of the episodes of severe hypoglycemic episodes. Actually this should be considered the primary objective of the islet transplantation while the opportunity of increasing the periods of insulin-independence through multiple islets infusions is not commonly acceptable because of the high risk of sensitization to impair the possibility of a kidney retransplant.

In the face of organ shortage and cost procedure-related, these findings may lead to a new paradigm in islet transplantation, where the primary aim is not necessarily to achieve the same insulin-indipendence as in whole-organ transplantation but to improve the glycemic control of the patient through a much less invasive procedure.

Promising fields of research are nowadays focused on increasing the engraftment and survival of the islets after transplantation. If these studies will give positive results it will be possible in future to extend the actual indications of the combined kidney-islet transplantation procedure.

9. References

Alejandro R, Barton FB, Hering BJ et al. (2008). Update from the Collaborative Islet Transplant Registry *Transplantation* 2008 Dec 27;86(12):1783-8.

Campbell PM, Senior PA, Salam A et al. (2007). High risk of sensitization after failed islet transplantation. Am J Transplant 2007; 7: 2311–2317.

Cantarelli E, Melzi R, Mercalli A et al. (2009). Bone marrow as an alternative site for islet transplantation. *Blood* 2009 Nov 12;114(20):4566-74.

Casey JJ, Lakey JR, Ryan EA et al. (2002). Portal venous pressure changes after sequential clinical islet transplantation. *Transplantation* 2002, 74:913-915.

Christoffersson G, Henriksnäs J, Johansson L et al. (2010). Clinical and experimental pancreatic islet transplantation to striated muscle: establishment of a vascular system similar to that in native islets *Diabetes*. 2010 Oct, 59(10):2569-78.

Cure P, Pileggi A, Froud T, et al. (2008) Improved metabolic control and quality of life in seven patients with type 1 diabetes following islet after kidney transplantation. *Transplantation* 2008; 85:801–812

Del Carro U, Fiorina P, Amadio S et al. (2007). Evaluation of polyneuropathy markers in type 1 diabetic kidney transplant patients and effects of islet transplantation: neurophysiological and skin biopsy longitudinal analysis. *Diabetes Care* 2007, 30:3063–3069.

Fiorina P, Folli F, Bertuzzi F et al. (2003) Long-term beneficial effect of islet transplantation on diabetic macro-/microangiopathy in type 1 diabetic kidney transplanted patients. *Diabetes Care* 2003, 26:1129–1136.

Fiorina P, Folli F, Maffi P et al. (2005) Islet transplantation is associated with an improvement of cardiovascular function in type 1 diabetic kidney transplant patients. *Diabetes Care* 2005, 28:1358–1365.

Fiorina P, Venturini M, Folli F et al. (2005). Natural history of kidney graft survival, hypertrophy, and vascular function in end-stage renal disease type 1 diabetic kidney-transplanted patients: beneficial impact of pancreas and successful islet cotransplantation. *Diabetes Care,* 2005, 28: 1303–1310.

Gerber PA, Pavlicek V, Demartines N et al. (2008) Simultaneous islet–kidney vs pancreas–kidney transplantation in type 1 diabetes mellitus: a 5 year single centre follow-up. *Diabetologia,* 2008, 51:110–119.

Gruessner RW, Sutherland DE, Gruessner AC (2004) Mortality assessment for pancreas transplants. *American Journal of Transplantation,* 2004, 4:2018–2026.

Hering BJ, Matsumoto I, Sawada T et al. (2002). Impact of two-layer pancreas preservation on islet isolation and transplantation. *Transplantation,* 2002, 74:1813-1816.

Kaufman DB, Baker MS, Chen X et al. (2002). Sequential kidney/islet transplantation using prednisone-free immunosuppression. *American Journal of Transplantation,* 2002, 2:674-677

Kemp C, Knight M, Sharp D, et al (1973). Effect on transplantation site on the result of pancreatic islets isografts in diabetic rats. *Diabetologia,* 1973, 9:486-491

Kempf MC, Andres A, Morel P et al. (2005) Logistics and transplant coordination activity in the GRAGIL Swiss-French multicenter network of islet transplantation. *Transplantation.* 2005, 79(9):1200-5.

Lacy P, Kostianovsky M (1967) Method for the isolation of intact islets of Langerhans' from the rat pancreas. *Diabetes,* 1967,16:35-39.

Langer RM, Máthé Z, Doros A et al (2004) Successful islet after kidney transplantations in a distance over 1000 kilometres: Preliminary results of the Budapest-Geneva collaboration. *Transplant Proc.* 2004 Dec;36(10):3113-5.

Largiader F, Kolb E, Binswanger U, Illig R (1979). Succesful allotransplantation of an island of Langerhans. *Schweiz Med Wochenschr* 1979,109:1733-1736.

Lehmann R, Spinas GA, Moritz W, Weber M. (2008). Has Time Come for New Goals in Human Islet Transplantation? *American Journal of Transplantation* 2008, 8: 1096–110.

Light JA, Barhyte DY. (2005) Simultaneous pancreas– kidney transplants in type I and type II diabetic patients with end-stage renal disease: similar 10-year outcomes. *Transplant Proc* 2005, 37: 1283

Maffi P, Angeli E, Bertuzzi F et al. (2005). Minimal focal steatosis of liver after islet transplantation in humans: a long-term study. *Cell Transplantation*. 2005;14(10):727-33.

Markmann JF, Deng S, Desai NM et al. (2003). The use of non- heart-beating donors for isolated pancreatic islet transplantation. *Transplantation,* 2003, 75:1423-1429.

Markmann JF, Rosen M, Siegelman ES. (2003). Magnetic resonance-defined periportal steatosis following intraportal islet transplantation: a functional footprint of islet graft survival? *Diabetes* 2003, 52:1591-1594.

Najarian JS, Sutherland RL, Matas AJ, et al. Human islet transplantation: a preliminary report. *Tranplant Proc* 1977, 9:233-236.

Nath DS, Gruessner AC, Kandaswamy R et al. (2005) Outcomes of pancreas transplants for patients with type 2 diabetes mellitus. *Clin Transplant,* 2005, 19: 792.

Owen RJ, Ryan EA, O'Kelly K et al. (2003). Percutaneous transhepatic pancreatic islet cell transplantation in type 1 diabetes mellitus: radiologic aspects. *Radiology* 2003, 229:165-170.

Porrett PM, Yeh H, Frank A et al. (2007). Availability of suitable islet donors in the United States. *Transplantation* 2007, 84:280–282.

Reckard CR, Ziegler MM, Barker CF et al. (1973) Physiological and immunological consequences of transplanting isolated pancreatic islets. *Surgery,* 1973, 74:91-99.

Reddy KS, Stablein D, Taranto S et al (2003). Long-term survival following simultaneous kidney-pancreas transplantation versus kidney transplantation alone in patients with type 1 diabetes mellitus and renal failure. *Am J Kidney Dis.* 2003 Feb;41(2):464-70.

Ricordi C, Lacy P, Finke E et al. (1988) Automated method for isolation of human pancreatic islets. *Diabetes,* 1988, 37(4): 344-354.

Ricordi C, Tzakis AG, Carroll PB et al. (1992). Human islet isolation and allotransplantation in 22 consecutive cases. *Transplantation* 1992, 53:407-414.

Ricordi C and Strom TB (2004) Clinical islet transplantation: advances and immunological challenges. *Nature Reviews Immunology* 2004 April, 4, 259-268.

Robertson RP (2004) Islet transplantation as a treatment for diabetes - a work in progress. *New England Journal of Medicine* 2004 Feb. 12; 350-7:694-705.

Saito T, Gotoh M, Satomi S et al. (2010). Islet transplantation using donors after cardiac death: report of the Japan Islet Transplantation Registry. *Transplantation*. 2010, 90(7): 740-7.

Shapiro AM, Lakey JR, Ryan EA et al. (2000). Islet transplantation in seven patients with type 1 diabetes mellitus using a glucocorticoid-free immunosuppressive regimen. *N Engl J Med,* 2000, 343: 230–238.

Shapiro AM, Ricordi C, Hering BJ et al. (2006) International trial of the Edmonton protocol for islet transplantation. *N Engl J Med* 2006, 355: 1318–1330.

Tsujimura T, Kuroda Y, Avila JG et al. (2004). Influence of Pancreas Preservation on Human Islet Isolation Outcomes: Impact of the Two-Layer Method. *Transplantation,* 2004, 78(1): 96-100.

Tzakis AG, Ricordi C, Alejandro R et al. (1990). Pancreatic islet transplantation after upper abdominal exenteration and liver replacement. *Lancet* 1990, 336:402-405.

Vantyghem MC, Balavoine AS, Kerr-Conte J et al. (2009) Who should benefit from diabetes cell therapy? *Ann Endocrinol.* 2009, 70(6):443-8.

Younoszai R, Sorensen R, Lindall A et al. (1970). Homotransplantation of isolated pancreatic islets. *Diabetes*, 1970, 19:406-407.

9

The Transplantation Operation and its Surgical Complications

Junjie Zhao, Zhenli Gao and Ke Wang
Yantai YuHuangDing Hospital
China

1. Introduction

Over the past decades, the outcomes of kidney transplantation have improved markedly due to advancements in prevention and treatment of acute rejection episodes, management of posttransplant complications and better knowledge of immunosuppressive drugs. As a result, transplantation has become the mainstay and preferred treatment for patients of all ages with end-stage renal disease. However, the surgical technique for renal transplantation has changed little from the original pelvic operation described in 1951 by Küss et al. It seems the operation has been standardized and there is little need for further discussions over the topic. In fact, the argumentation on surgical technique has never ceased since its birth, for optimization of the surgical outcomes, many aspects of operative techniques have been modified and novel techniques have been invented. In modern immunosuppressive era, the pattern of surgical complications has evolved and gains some fresh features. In this chapter, we will review the standard operative procedures performed today and introduce the updated surgical techniques as well. Meanwhile, the characteristics of major surgical complications and the evolvement of their diagnosis and treatment will be expatiated on. After all, the surgical operation is invariably the key of a successful transplantation; surgical techniques are constantly related to the morbidity and mortality of the patients.

2. Standard surgical technique on kidney transplantation

The standard kidney transplant procedure is the pelvic operation originally used by French surgeons Küss, Dubost, and Servelle and their associates in 1951 and refined subsequently by Murray and Harrison for the first successful kidney transplantation in human history. The heterotopic pelvic approach has been widely accepted for its multiple advantages and considered a standard access. The classical surgical techniques of revascularization and urinary tract reconstruction have also been broadly used to this day. Each renal transplantation operation is a review of original historic work both in urological and vascular discipline.

2.1 Site

The operative site for standard kidney transplantation is pelvic fossa, however, there is always a disagreement on the criteria to select the appropriate side to accommodate the transplant. Initially, it is recommended that placing the donor kidney in the recipient's contralateral side to ensure the renal pelvis and ureter are anterior in case those future surgeries are required (John, 2002). Afterward, it is stated that the more important consideration is to avoid sites of previous transplants, other operations, or peritoneal dialysis catheters though the dissection on the right is slightly easier (James, 2004). Subsequently, suggestion from scholars is presented that each side of the recipient's pelvis is acceptable, however the right external iliac vessels are longer and more horizontal compared to the left side, which facilitates the vascular anastomoses (Stuart, 2008). With progresses of surgical technique and accumulation of clinical experience the concept of selecting the right pelvic fossa as the preferred site for the first transplantation has been universally accepted. However, the ipsilateral severe atherosclerotic vascular disease, venous disorders such as previous deep venous thromboses and femoral dialysis catheters should be routinely excluded. The peritoneal dialysis catheters and previous minor abdominal operation such as appendectomy, conventional herniorrhaphy are not absolute contraindications according to our experiences. It also elicits one issue for nephrologists that the initial peritoneal dialysis catheter or femoral dialysis catheter is properly intubated on the left side for the potential renal recipients. The standard Gibson incision can avoid most stoma of peritoneal dialysis catheters. On the other hand, the minor transperitoneal surgeries or small operations on abdominal wall usually yield limited adhesion at the place to accomplish the transplantation. But, the transplantation is strongly not recommended at the side where has a history of herniorrhaphy with propylene mesh or ipsilateral open operation of ureter and bladder. Because the propylene mesh results in inflammatory response and connective tissue proliferation conducing to fibrosis formation and a thick scar plate on the inner surface of lower abdominal wall, which make the dissection of bladder a formidable task. Previous ipsilateral pelvic surgeries generally preclude the sequent transplantation due to local inordinate anatomical features and severe perivesical tissue conglutination. Massively enlarged polycystic kidneys are challenges for urologists; one would choose the side of the smaller kidney. However, bilateral extremely enlarged polycystic kidneys would make the transplant surgery very difficult or impossible. In that occasion, right or bilateral native nephrectomy might be considered. Sequential and simultaneous laparoscopic bilateral native nephrectomies have all been testified safe and effective. For the second transplantation patients the kidney is implanted on the contralateral side, usually left side.

2.2 Incision and exposure

The kidney transplant operation can be performed via many different routes, however two important issues must be considered when deciding the incision for a renal transplant: a good access to the iliac fossa and bladder and a minimal rate of wound related morbidity. Historically, three classic incisions have been recommended for kidney transplant surgery: pelvic Gibson incision, the hockey stick incision and oblique incision. Curvilinear incision made in lower quadrant of the abdomen, known as the "pelvic Gibson incision", which affords relatively atraumatic and convenient access to the iliac fossa and bladder is mainly used for renal transplantation. Oblique incision and inverted J-shaped incision, known as the "hockey stick incision" are the other two frequently used incisions in some centers. Nanni and colleagues compared the two incisions with regard to the incidence of long-term complications, they concludes that the oblique surgical incision was better than the hockey-stick incision for lower incidence of hernia and abdominal wall relaxation and the more favorable cosmetic results (Nanni et al. 2005). Paramedian, midline incision and even transverse incision are lately introduced to the practice of living kidney transplantation for better cosmetic appearance, but these incisions are of same inherent drawback of difficult exposure of operative bed, which can be possible alternatives for special candidates.(Filocamo et al., 2007; Park et al., 2008).

When a Gibson incision is made, the external oblique muscle and fascia are divided in the line of the incision and split to the lateral extent of the wound. The internal oblique and transverse muscles are divided with cautery in the line of the incision, or in a more beneficial way to divide the two layers of muscles on the confluence of the oblique muscles and the rectus sheath, which avoids division of the internal oblique and transversus muscles. The latter method, most frequently used in our institute, has two major advantages both for patients and surgeons. Firstly it markedly reduces the blood loss resulting from capillary hemorrhage of muscle wound surface during the transplantation, which is usually underestimated by surgeons. Uraemic patients often have a bleeding diathesis at the time of surgery due to malfunctioned platelet, especially when being heparinized during pretransplant hematodialysis. In addition, the muscle fibers could disrupt during closure because of high tension of the wound covering the graft, particularly, if there is a large kidney for a small recipient. The pararectus division of muscles and aponeurosis facilitates the process of wound closure and diminishes the incidence of muscles collapse and wound complications.

The inferior epigastric vessels are ligated and divided, but if there are multiple renal arteries, the inferior epigastric vessels should be preserved in the beginning in case the inferior epigastric artery is required for anastomosis to a lower polar renal artery. Division of the spermatic cord has not been advocated during past decades for its drawback of inducing secondary testicular complications, but freed laterally and retracted medially. The round ligament can be divided for adequate exposure.

The exposure of iliac vessels seems to be an effortless process, but bearish expansion of the extraperitoneal space might cause the peritoneum injury and subsequent enterocele, a rare but potentially fetal surgical complication, described as "renal paratransplant hernia" in recent year. We have encountered three cases of the rare surgical complication in early years. In our opinion, in most, if not all cases, paratransplant hernia is an iatrogenic surgical complication as a result of an unnoticed defect of the peritoneum due to improper maneuvers during the transplantation. Meticulous dissection may help avoid this complication. And if a peritoneal defect is found, it should be closed immediately, regardless of its size to avoid the occurrence of a postoperative paratransplant hernia.

A self-retaining retractor is usually inserted to obtain optimal exposure, which allows the assistant to free both hands to assist the anastomoses. However, the position of the retractor should be checked carefully before fixing it because the inadvertent retractor injury was one of the causes to femoral neuropathy, an unusual complication after kidney transplantation, with major clinical features of reversible muscle weakness or paralysis of hip flexion. The lymphatics that course along and over the vessels must be ligated with a nonabsorbable suture and divided, rather than cauterized, to prevent the later occurrence of a lymphocele. The surgeon must be cautious not to mistake the genitofemoral nerve for a lymph vessel. The former lies on the medial edge of the psoas muscle, and a branch may cross the distal external iliac artery.

2.3 Vascular reconstruction

In general, it is preferable to do the end-to-side venous anastomosis first, and then the end-to-side arterial anastomosis. Some scholars argued that the arterial anastomosis should be done first if the renal artery is to be anastomosed to the internal iliac artery. Although end-to-side anstomosis to the external iliac vein and end-to-end anstomosis to the internal iliac artery is once the classical vascular anastomosis pattern, and also practiced in some centers now, many facts have revealed that the internal iliac artery is not a preferred option for the arterial anastomosis compared with external iliac artery. Firstly, dissection of the internal iliac artery is not as straightforward as that of the external iliac artery. Meanwhile, a mobilization of a length of the external and common iliac arteries is also needed when the internal iliac artery is considered as the candidate of arterial anastomosis because of the application of vascular clamps and prevention of kinking of artery when being rotated laterally for anastomosis, which increases the operative time and risk of surgical complications. Furthermore, it is an intractable problem to handle if the concomitant internal iliac vein is inadvertently damaged during the dissection. Moreover, the risk of anastomosis site stenosis and erectile dysfunction is much higher than that of external iliac artery following the transplantation. Lastly, the short internal iliac artery and variation are common. Therefore, the routine end-to-end anstomosis to the internal iliac artery is not recommended.

Since Carrel described a 3-point anastomosis technique for an end-to-end allograft arterial anastomosis in 1902, transplant surgeons have invented different techniques for arterial and venous anastomoses. Most efforts have been made to decrease ischemic time and promote the quality of anastomosis. The classical and universally used technique is the 2-point anastomosis, with initial sutures placed at either end of the venotomy or arteriotomy. Sometimes, an anchor suture is placed at the midpoint of the lateral wall to prevent posterior or anterior wall being caught up in the suture line. Another running anastomoses fashion, so called "1-suture, 1-knot technique", which does not need to turn the kidney medial and lateral, has showed some advantages especially in obese patients and recipients with deep iliac fossa. Mital and associates, in 1996, performed arterial and venous anastomoses using 4-stay sutures and several vascular clips for each anastomosis, without a continuous vascular suture. (Mital et al, 1996). Afterwards, sutureless vascular anastomosis technique using vascular clips or titanium ring pin staplers have been described and suggested safe and time-saving in small series (Jones, 1998; Ye, 2006). However, these sutureless techniques seem not to be popularized, and their long-time outcomes need further observation.

2.3.1 Venous anastomosis

The renal vein is anastomosed end-to-side, usually to the external iliac vein using a continuous 5-0 monofilament vascular suture following an appropriate venotomy performed in the external iliac vein. In rare conditions such as thrombosis or hypoplasia of both iliac veins, the renal vein has to be anastomosed to other site. Anastomosis to the inferior vena cava is the most common alternative, usually associated with a native nephrectomy. The usage of infra-renal inferior vena cava or infra-hepatic inferior vena cava has been described in the literature. Otherwise, portal venous drainage system, inferior mesenteric vein, superior mesenteric vein, even venous collaterals with large caliber secondary to thrombosis of the inferior vena cava and iliac veins such as a presacral collateral vein and the left ovarian vein have been utilized for renal transplantation with satisfactory results (Wong et al, 2008).

Short right renal vein, particularly from living donors, represent a technical challenge to the transplant surgeon. Usually, the satisfactory anastomosis can be achieved by thorough mobilization of the recipient common and external iliac veins. Sometimes, the techniques of donor vein elongation are needed especially in obese recipients. Right renal vein extension using the inferior vena cava is an excellent option and frequently used in deceased kidney transplantation, but is not suitable to living donors. A variety of techniques have been developed to elongate the short live donor vein, and extension techniques using saphenous, gonadal vein or superficial femoral vein grafts or a polytetrafluoroethylene graft have demonstrated nice results. Extensively elongation of renal vein should be avoided either in live or deceased transplantation for prophylaxis of occurrence of renal vein thrombosis.

2.3.2 Arterial anastomosis

The end-to-side arterial anastomosis is generally placed more proximally than the vein, usually performed using an appropriately trimmed cuff of aorta attached to the renal artery with a continuous 5-0 or 6-0 monofilament vascular suture after a suitable arteriotomy placed in the external iliac artery. The arterial clamps should be applied with great care to avoid the disruption of vascular calcified plaque. Endarterectomy is usually unnecessary. An opening of proper caliber created with artery puncher in the external iliac artery may facilitate the anastomosis of renal arteries from live donors in the absence of "Carrel patch". Careful suture performance is absolutely crucial for the allograft to maintain normal arterial blood flow and function. Appropriate full-thickness suture of arterial wall must be achieved in each stitch, particularly in patients with arteriosclerosis.

Kidney with multiple arteries is a challenge before artery anastomosis. There are various anastomosis patterns for this situation. How best to manage multiple arteries depending on the characteristics of multiple arteries and individual transplant surgeon's preference. Anastomosis of two arteries close together on an aortic patch of a left-sided deceased donor kidney is comparatively straightforward. If they are more than 2 cm apart, consideration could be given to perform two separate anastomoses. Dual arteries to a right-sided kidney often make positioning of the kidney difficult without kinking one or the other artery, sometimes the arteries have to be shortened to fulfill two separate anastomoses. Most complicated cases are encountered in live transplant setting, cuff of aorta is impossible, multiple and short arteries are common with the increasing popularity of laparoscopic living donor nephrectomy. For double arteries, two separate anastomoses are recommended in most occasions. Double parallel anastomoses to the external iliac artery are most common pattern. Sometimes the lower hilar artery or lower polar artery can anastomose to internal iliac artery or inferior epigastric artery in an end-to-end manner. Very small accessory renal arteries, particularly at the upper pole, can be ligated without problems. Arteries reconstruction on the back table operation before revascularization is an effective way suggested by many authors. The advantages of ex vivo reconstruction techniques are that they preserve the small accessory renal arteries by an end-to-side or conjoined anastomosis to renal artery stem and reduce the operative time by simplifying the anastomosis. Multiple short arteries or arteries with other vascular anomalies can also be salvaged. Theoretically, the incidence of vascular complications may be higher using complicated reconstruction techniques on back table. It is necessary to consult the vascular surgeons to achieve the difficult reconstruction under magnification.

2.4 Urinary tract reconstruction

Reconstruction of urinary tract begins following a successful revascularization. The type of urinary tract reconstruction is various. The standard and usual form of urinary tract reconstruction is ureteroneocystostomy. But the classical status of ureteroneocystostomy has

been challenged recently. Pyeloureterostomy and ureteroureterostomy conventionally is considered salvage procedures when the transplant ureter's blood supply seems to be compromised or the urinary bladder is difficult to identify. Nie and associates recently compared the overall incidence of urological complications between ureteroureterostomy and ureteroneocystostomy in kidney transplantation, no difference was found, moreover, ureteroureterostomy decreased the incidence of urine leakage and therefore was advocated a good first option for urinary tract reconstruction with a greater possibility of resolving a ureteral stenosis with endourology and no risk of reflux (Nie et al, 2010). Timsi and collages compared results in 151 consecutive kidney transplantations with routine pyeloureterostomy and that in 129 procedures with extravesical anti-reflux ureteroneocystostomy, the outcomes from routine pyeloureterostomy group were even better and also had the similar advantages as the ureteroureterostomy's (Timsit et al, 2010).
However, ureteroneocystostomy is still the preferred selection of urinary tract reconstruction for most surgeons because of its various advantages. ureteroneocystostomy is a familiar technique we often applied in general urological surgeries. Deep dissection of native ureter and native nephrectomy are unnecessary. It can be performed regardless of the quality or presence of the native ureter and retains the possibility of conversion to an ureteroureterostomy or pyeloureterostomy if the implant fails. The location of ureteroneocystostomy is usually several centimeters away from the vascular anastomoses, which facilitate the examination and correction of a possible urinary complication during the reinterventions.

2.4.1 Ureteroneocystostomy

There are a variety of techniques for ureteroneocystostomy, which in general can be categorized into transvesical or extravesical and antireflux or non-antireflux. The Leadbetter-Politano (LP) technique is the classic transvesical ureteroneocystostomy described by Murray et al in 1954 for the first successful renal transplant. This technique utilizes one cystostomy to access the interior of the bladder and another cystostomy to recreate a new ureteric orifice in a normal anatomic position. The ureter is tunneled in the submucosal space to prevent reflux. The extravesical ureteroneocystostomy was first described by Witzel in 1896, then again by Gregoir in April 1961, and soon thereafter by Lich et al, who published the technique in November 1961. The Lich-Gregoir (LG) technique was designed to avoid a second cystostomy, yet retain an antireflux mechanism. It creates a 2-3 cm submucosal tunnel with muscle backing of the ureter to provide a valve effect. In addition to the avoidance of a separate cystostomy, other comparative advantages were less bladder dissection, a shorter ureteral length, and no interference with native ureteral function. Additionally, the LG was noted to be rapid and technically easier to perform than the LP technique. Several variations of the LG implantation have been described, such as the use of running instead of interrupted sutures to create the ureteral mucosal anastomosis, performance of a tunnel by submucosal blunt dissection instead of muscular imbrication, placement of a single horizontal Halsted stitch at the proximal apex of the bladder incision to the ureter to prevent tension at the acute angle of the anastomosis, placement of an anchor stitch on the distal ureteral tip to the full thickness of the bladder, folding back the tip of the ureter to make a terminal cuff, incorporation of the muscular layer with the mucosal layer of the bladder in the anastomosis and the parallel-incision technique with a submucosal tunnel created between the two parallel incisions in the lateral bladder. All of these so-called modified Lich ureteroneocystostomies include extravesicular access, the formation of an antireflux tunnel, and an urothelial anastomosis (Kayler et al, 2010).

Another extravesical approach to ureteroneocystostomy that also includes an antireflux tunnel but lacks an urothelial anastomosis, called the U-stitch technique. By elimination of the urothelial anastomosis, this technique was demonstrated to shorten operative times even further than that of the LG technique. But this technique is associated with an increased risk of a urinary complication and abandoned at our center, and being against by many other institutions.

The techniques without an antireflux mechanism are least often described. Althrougt early comparative analyses have failed to show significant differences between reflux and antireflux techniques, but most non-antireflux techniques have been marginalized and abandoned.

The management of double ureters is something like management of dual arteries to some extent. If there is a common part, a straightforward ureteroneocystostomy can be done as a single ureter. Two separate ureteroneocystostomy using L-G technique is preferred in our center when two ureters are not in one common sheath. The dual ureters can also be reconstructed on back table conjoining them into one common stem to anastomose with bladder or native ureter

2.4.2 Other alternatives

There are some unusual forms of urinary tract reconstruction technique using in special conditions, such as pyelopyelostomy in orthotopic renal transplantation, ureteroenterostomy into an intestinal conduit or an intestinal pouch and pyelovesicostomy when the native ureter and the renal transplant ureter are unsuitable for urinary tract reconstruction. No matter what method is used, a tension-free and watertight anastomosis is most important.

2.5 Closure

There are three aspects should be taken into consideration before closing the wound: Haemostasis, reexamination and placement of drains. Careful haemostasis is necessary for every surgery especially for a uremic patient. The special attention should be paid to the vascular anastomosis site and renal pedicle area in case there is active bleeding from an unrecognized leak or an unligated vessel, which is a cause of emergent reoperation during the very early postoperative period even before leaving the operating room. The significance of reexamination is to find if there are some grave technique faults and correct them before the closure. Vessels are always the emphasis for checking, besides the bleeding the strength of renal artery pulsation and the vascular tension of renal vein should be sensed gently using fingers, adjusting the position of graft if there is a kinking or compression of long vessels. In the mean time, the ureter should be tension free and burden free from adjacent structures after the graft is properly placed. No urine leak is permitted. Drain placement is a very important step that can not be ignored, the related issues we will discuss soon.

The value of obtaining a baseline biopsy specimen before closure remains controversial, but it is the fact that it incurs some unnecessary biopsy-induced vascular complications for some grafts with perfect function. A capsulotomy of the transplanted kidney before closure basically has been abandoned in adult transplantation because it is of no use on the whole.

The process of closure is not as easy as incision making. Muscular tension often higher either from an additional graft or descending effect of muscle relaxant. A running #1 polydioxanone suture (PDS) provide a convenient choice for closure, some centers routinely close muscles and aponeurosis with single-layer PDS suture (Nanni et al. 2005), which reduce the closing time but is also a risk factor of wound complications. Our experience is to close the wound with two-layer PDS suture plus five to six interrupted anchor stitches in muscle layers with nonabsorbable sutures, which has been proved an appropriate method. Otherwise, attention should also be paid to avoid injuring the peritoneum when closing the incision, for one careless stitch can tear the peritoneum leading to a defect and the paratransplant hernia especially in patients with obesity and ascites. The vaulted transplanted ureter under the muscle layer should not be involved by suture when closing. Furthermore, excessive tension on the suture may lead to compression of the kidney or lead to defects resulting in wound complications, a mesh could be used to achieve a tension free closure.

2.6 Stent, catheter and drains

The debate about the three types of tube has never stopped. The viewpoints varies too much, some of disputes are swordplay. Double J stent is an object full of controversy since its introduction to urology. Its function in renal transplants to significantly reduce ureteric complications is broadly accepted. One meta-analysis has addressed the prophylactic routine stenting in renal transplants is cost-effective (Mangus et al, 2004). The minor flaw such as an increased risk of urinary tract infection, an additional cystoscopy and patient discomfort from bladder spasm is relatively unimportant and controllable, can not counteract its contribution to a markedly lowered incidence of ureteric complications, which sometimes can be a cause of graft loss. The optimal duration of prophylactic stenting has also not been determined. Based on local center preference, it is usually 2 to 6 weeks. In our center, stent is removed during an office visit 4 weeks after tranplantation, accompanying with a routine general checkup.

A dwelling catheter is necessary for every kidney transplantation patients, it is important to maintain the catheter in an unobstructed condition during the early postoperative period. The reported duration time usually is 5 to 7 days, our experience is 7 days. Seven-day is a proper compromise to prevent urine leak in the absence of an increasing incidence of urinary tract infection. What's more, acute vascular rejection usually occurs one week after transplantation, a dwelling catheter is helpful for the patients to detect the early sharp reduction of urine output, a usual signal of acute rejection.

There always remains considerable controversy over the necessity and duration of perigraft drains. Some authors suggested non-drains closure if the heamostasis is satisfactory because drain tubes increase the infection risk in immunosuppressive patients. But most others support placing a closed suction retroperitoneal drain at the time of transplant and a considerable majority of them suggest removal of drains in 48 hours in case of infection. However some authors argue the rationality of prolonged drainage, as reported, the median day of drain removal was 18 days in individual center. (Tiong et al, 2009). Based on our preference, we suggest a "two-drain policy" routinely for every transplant patients. The incidence of postoperative hematomas and lymphoceles in renal transplantation is dramatically higher than general urological surgeries' for various reasons. So the principle of drain placing can not simply mimic the pattern of general surgery. In the early posttransplant period, bleeding is commonly from the operative bed, it is usual to record 100 to 200 mL of heavily blood-stained drainage in the first few hours of transplantation. After that, even a week later, the spontaneous bleeding of graft can also develop a problematic hematoma. Moreover, most lymphoceles formations and urine leak occur approximately one week after transplantation, too early removal of drains increase the risk. The reason of two drains is based on the fact that there are two isolated dead space created by the allograft, over the upper pole and under the lower pole of the transplant kidney; one lower drain often can not drain the bleeding from the upper pole. We place one additional drain onto the upper pole of graft and the other one down to prevesical space, centimeters away from the renal vessels and ureter. The upper drain usually is removed 4 to 5 days posttransplant or until drainage is less than 20 mL daily, the lower drain is routinely removed one day after the catheter removal if there is no evidence of urine leak or lymphorrhea, which significantly diminishes the incidence of postoperative hematomas, lymphoceles and urinomas compared with our early experiences with one-drain policy, but no increase of wound related infection.

3. Surgical considerations in pediatric recipient

In children, the standard surgical approach in adult carries two disadvantages. First, there is a size mismatch between the available extraperitoneal space and the adult sized donor kidney. Secondly, the recipient artery may be small compared with the artery of the graft that make the vascular anastomosis more difficult and may jeopardize the blood pressure and blood flow which is required for the donor kidney to survive. The conventional view is that the transplant procedure is same as for adults if their weight is more than 20 kg. If weight less than 20 kg, the right Gibson incision can be carried up to the costal margin to increase exposure of the right extraperitoneal space or using a transperitoneal approach. Some centers usually perform transperitoneal kidney transplantation in children below 5 years. However some advocated extraperitoneal renal transplantation technique in children who weigh less than 15 kg, which limits potential gastrointestinal complications and allows the confinement of potential surgical complications, such as bleeding and urinary leakage (Furness et al, 2001). When a transperitoneal approach used, it is generally done through a midline incision from the xyphoid to the pubis, the posterior peritoneum is incised lateral to the ascending colon. Ligating and dividing two to three lumbar veins posteriorly is often necessary to facilitate the application of vascular occluding clamp. The terminal aorta is dissected free at its junction with the right or left common iliac artery. The donor artery is either anastomosed to the distal aorta to obtain the best arterial inflow, or with one of the common iliac arteries in an end-to-side fashion using 5-0 or 6-0 monofilament vascular suture. The selection of common iliac artery avoids a complete occlusion of the aorta which is associated with temporary acidosis of both lower extremities (van Heurn et al, 2009). The donor vessels are often amputated and may be spatulated to ensure a wide anastomosis and to avoid kinking which may lead to impaired blood flow. An aortic punch is basically used to prevent renal artery occlusion if significant hypotension occurs. The ureter of an adult size kidney is usually long and wide enough to obtain a tension free ureteroneocystostomy. The problem is the too long ureter is easy to be kinked and twisted, even causing internal hernia (Sánchez et al, 2005); therefore, sometimes the long ureter should be shortened to obtain best result. Temporary ureteral stenting is beneficial to prevent urological complications, but special care should be taken for the removing technique because standard cystoscopy in adults is not suitable for a very young child. It is a smart way to attach the stent with the indwelling bladder or reservoir catheter and removing it as the catheter is withdrawn. An antireflux procedure is imperative for pediatric patients. Because a large number of recipients are a result of obstructive uropathy due to outflow obstruction, small capacity or poor function of the bladder, which all predisposes to vesicoureteral reflux of the transplanted kidney.

4. Dual kidney transplantation

As a result of the shortage of kidneys for transplantation and the increasing demand for transplantable grafts, the option for using organs from expanded criteria donors has become widely accepted. One option for using organs from donors with a suboptimal nephron mass is dual kidney transplantation (DKT). Dual kidney transplantation is the deceased renal transplantation using two marginal kidneys simultaneously either from the donors older than 60 years old, or from solitary pediatric donors age younger than 5 years or small (< 21 kg). The paired kidneys from solitary pediatric donors are recovered and transplanted as en bloc, known as "en bloc kidney (EBK)". The double kidneys from old donors can be also used as en bloc, but mostly in a split individual implantation technique, bilaterally or ipsilateral. Clinical kidney transplants using solitary paired deceased donor kidneys were reported in the early 1960s, followed by increasing interest in the use of paired pediatric deceased donor kidneys as en bloc with the first case to a pediatric recipient and thereafter, to adult recipients showing possible advantage of more renal reserve and technical feasibility. One recent report shows EBK pediatric donor transplants had the best long-term outcomes among deceased donor transplants (Bhayana et al, 2010). Various strategies have improved the outcome of EBK pediatric donor transplants, including changes in techniques.

For an adult recipient, the paired kidneys usually also placed extraperitoneally in the iliac fossa via a Gibson incision. Commonly, the aorta and the inferior vena cava of EBK are anastomosed to the external iliac artery and vein with 5-0 or 6-0 monofilament vascular suture in an end-to-side technique. Sometimes, the end-to-side anastomosis is applied to the aorta and inferior vena cava to prevent kinking of renal vessels and ureters. For the same purpose, the upper pole of the grafts sometimes fixes to the iliopsoas muscle. Double ureteroneocystostomies of the native contracted bladder are performed separately, or the ends of the two ureters are reconstructed into a conjoined ureter and then one ureteroneocystostomy is performed. Sometimes ureteroureterostomies are performed. Kato and collages, in 2008, developed the urinary tract reconstruction technique with a vascularized "bladder patch" including the vesical trigone from the same donor, which precludes the challenging ureteral reconstruction and ureteroneocystostomy, and excludes the risk of anastomotic strictures and postoperative reflux, significantly reduces the incidence of urine leak. In the mean time, the donor bladder wall served a purpose of bladder augmentation as well. (Kato et al, 2008).

Since first report of DKT from an adult deceased donor in the United States was revealed in 1996, many centers now perform DKT using various organ selection criteria and surgical techniques, including the extra- or intraperitoneal bilateral placement of the two kidneys through two separate Gibson incisions or one midline incision. In 1998, Masson et al. were the first to transplant both adult donor kidneys unilaterally into the same iliac fossa. Their reasoning was that this would reduce the surgical trauma and thus facilitate the immediate postoperative recovery of the patient, and also leave the contralateral iliac fossa intact for a further transplantation procedure in the event of graft loss. However, extraperitoneal unilateral placement through a single Gibson incision presents several technical hurdles, such as more extensive vessel dissection and a higher risk of renal vein thrombosis due to compression by the two kidneys. A comparison between 29 unilateral and 29 bilateral DKT procedures in an initial series has showed both techniques are safe, with no differences in surgical complication rates. In brief, the procedure begins with the classic Gibson incision, preferably on the right side. After creating an adequate extraperitoneal space, the right donor kidney is preferably placed superiorly because its renal vein can be lengthened by a segment of inferior vena cava. Another reason to position the right kidney superolaterally in the right flank is because the right kidney has a longer artery. If necessary, the internal iliac vein is dissected to mobilize the external iliac vein and thus facilitate renal vein anastomoses to the external iliac vein of the recipient. The extended renal vein and renal artery of the right kidney are anastomosed end-to-side to the iliac vessels of the recipient; these anastomoses are often to the external iliac vessels. After revascularization of the right kidney, vascular clamps are placed immediately below the venous and arterial anastomoses. The left donor kidney is transplanted distally, allowing the transplanted right kidney to continue to be perfused. The left kidney is positioned inferomedially to the right kidney. The renal artery and vein of the left kidney are anastomosed end-to-side to the external iliac vessels. Extravesical ureteroneocystostomies are performed separately, with a double J stent for each ureter, leaving the ureter of the upper transplanted kidney lateral to the lower one.

5. Orthotopic kidney transplantation

Orthotopic kidney transplantation (OKT) is seldom performed due to its complicated procedure and high related morbidity. However an increasing percentage of patients with end-stage renal disease currently are not candidates for a heterotopic kidney transplant because of associated severe vascular pathology, obesity, or retained iliac fossae from a former graft. In such situations, where heterotopic transplant is not appropriate, an orthotopic kidney transplant is an alternative.

The surgical technique consists of a retroperitoneal approach to the splenic hilus via lumbotomy. To preserve its entire length, the vein is ligated close to the renal parenchyma including its bifurcation. The renal artery is often narrow and cannot be used in most cases. The recipient's urinary tract is always carefully dissected and preserved. In most of the reported cases, renal graft revascularization was performed using the recipient's splenic artery and left renal vein. Types of artery revascularization include end-to-end anastomoses between graft renal artery and native splenic artery, renal artery or inferior mesenteric artery or end-to-side anastomoses between graft renal artery and Aorta. Types of vein revascularization include end-to-end anastomoses between graft renal vein and native renal vein or splenic vein or end-to-side anastomoses between graft renal vein and inferior vena cava. The excretory system is reconstructed using pyelo-pyelic anastomoses in most cases, and uretero-ureteral anastomoses, uretero-pyelic anastomoses, ureterocalicostomy in the others.

The reported overall vascular complication rate is about 5.4%, and total urological complication rate is about 8.1%. Musquera et al. in their recent report demonstrated that no statistically significant differences are observed between orthotopic and heterotopic transplant series when comparing overall patients and graft survival. OKT is a feasible alternative for selected patients who are considered unsuitable for heterotopic kidney transplant.

6. Minimally invasive kidney transplantation

During the past decade, the use of minimally invasive surgical procedures has increased in popularity among surgeons and patients. The introduction of minimally invasive techniques in the transplant field is expanding the number of living-related donor nephrectomies. The minimally invasive approach allows a significant reduction of postoperative pain, decreased length of hospital stay, shorter recovery time, and enhanced cosmesis, representing a significant advantage for the patient. However, the renal transplant surgery is always the forbidden zone of minimally invasive techniques because of the formidable technical barriers. The pioneers initially attempted the laparoscopic techniques in the renal autotransplantation of experimental animals, establishing the basis for clinical performance of autotransplantation and other complex urologic vascular procedures laparoscopically. Then the laparoscopic autotransplantation for patients with ureteral lesions or renovasular hypertension have been reported in few cases. In 2002, Hoznek and associates presented their initial experience on robotic assisted kidney transplantation, Operative time was 178 minutes. Robotic assistance made anastomosis possible by its unique ability of stereoscopic magnification and ultra-precise suturing techniques due to the flexibility of the robotic wristed instruments. Renal perfusion was excellent with immediate diuresis. The study demonstrates that robotic assisted kidney transplantation is feasible. However, technical and cost hindrances limit the routine use of robots. Until 2010, another robotic transabdominal kidney transplantation has been reported in a morbidly obese patient (BMI 41Kg/m^2) with 4 trocars and a 7 cm midline incision. The operative time was 223 min, and the blood loss was less than 50 ml. The kidney had immediate graft function. No perioperative complications were observed, and the patient was discharged on postoperative day 5 with normal kidney function. In 2011 the first European case of robotic renal transplantation was accomplished using 3 trocars and a 7 cm suprapubic incision. The suprapubic incision used for introduction of the kidney and also the uretero-vescical anastomosis. Besides the robotic renal transplantation, Rosales et al presented the first laparoscopic renal transplantation, without robotic assistance, using 4 trocars, a hand-access device and a 7 cm Pfannenstiel incision. In this case the ureterovesical reimplantation was done laparoscopically using a modified Taguchi technique. In view of the rapid progresses in laparoscopic vascular and urological reconstruction technique, we have reason to believe that minimally invasive kidney transplantation would have a bright future.

7. Surgical complications of kidney transplantation

Surgical complications of kidney transplantations have always been received considerable attention in the literature, because they can lead to morbidity, graft loss and mortality. As with other surgical cases, postoperative hemorrhage, wound complication may be seen in kidney transplant operation. However, there are some transplant-related surgical complications are special issues unique to kidney transplantation recipients, which can be categorized as vascular, urologic or lymphatic.

7.1 Wound complications

As with other types of surgery, wound complications are probably the most common surgical complication after a kidney transplant, with an approximate incidence of 5%. The general risk factors of wound complications is similar to other sorts of surgery, including systemic factors (e.g. increased age, obesity, diabetes and malnutrition), wound features (e.g. hematoma and dead space) and operative characteristics (e.g. poor surgical technique, lengthy operation (>2 h) and intraoperative contamination). In the transplant setting, the graft creates two natural dead spaces at the either pole of the kidney, and the formation of hematoma and lymphoceles is more frequent than general urological procedure.

Furthermore, the inevitable immunocompromising medications have significant adverse effect on wound healing and resistance to infection. Besides the well-known impairment of steroids on wound healing, the commonly used immunosuppressant, mycophenolate mofetil (MMF), has been defined as a significant risk factor of wound complications. Recently, the mammalian target of rapamycin (mTOR) inhibitors, sirolimus and everolimus, believed not to be nephrotoxic, have showed the strong association with problematic lymphoceles and impaired wound healing attributed to their powerful antiproliferative, anti-inflammatory, antiangiogenesis and antilymphangiogenic activity, which are essential for the healing and repair of wounds. Interestingly, although patients undergoing transplantation are at an elevated risk for poor wound healing and infection, the incidence of wound complications are not significantly higher in kidney recipients compared with that in nontransplant patients undergoing similar types of surgery. But wound complication often incurs patient dissatisfaction and increasing cost, moreover, in certain situations, wound complications may also be associated with graft loss and mortality. In general, wound complications can be broadly categorized into infectious and noninfectious complications.

7.1.1 Wound Infections

Wound infections can be divided into superficial wound infections and deep wound infections.

Superficial wound infections: Diagnosed within 30 d of operation, limited to skin or subcutaneous tissue, and at least one of the following should be present:

a. purulent drainage from the superficial incision;
b. a sign or symptom of infection, such as pain, tenderness, heat, or swelling, and the incision is deliberately left open by a surgeon, unless culture becomes negative;
c. the diagnosis of superficial wound infection is confirmed by the surgeon.

Deep wound infections: Diagnosed within 30 d of operation, involvement of the fascial or muscular layers, and at least one of the following should be present:

a. purulent drainage from the deep incision;
b. spontaneous dehiscence while the patient has fever (>38℃), localized pain, or tenderness;
c. An abscess is found on direct examination, on reoperation, or by radiologic examination; the content contains pus, and the culture yielded one or more micro-organisms;
d. the diagnosis of deep incisional infection is confirmed by the surgeon.

The treatment of wound infections should follow the universal principals of general surgery including application of broad-spectrum antibiotic and surgical care, such as opening the wound, evacuating pus, cleansing the wound and dressing changes. But for kidney transplant patients, the aggressively higher doses of immunosuppressors in recipients should be lowered; the sirolimus-based immunosuppressive regimen might be converted to tacrolimus or cyclosporine-based scheme according to conditions of surgical site. On the other hand, the timing and dosage of broad-spectrum antibiotic should be investigated systematically for prolonged duration of antibiotic administration in immunocompromised patients usually incurs opportunistic infection.

7.1.2 Noninfectious wound complications

Noninfectious wound complications generally refer to all of the wound problems except infections including wound dehiscence, perigraft sterile fluid collection and incisional hernias. Although noninfectious, each of them is important risk factor of wound infections. Perigraft sterile fluid collections mainly involve the seroma and lymphocele, which we will expatiate on later. Herein, we chiefly discuss the clinical characteristics of wound dehiscence and incisional hernias.

Wound dehiscence is defined as an incision prematurely bursting open or splitting along surgical suture lines in the absence of documented infection. Similarly, it can be categorized into superficial and deep wound dehiscence. Incisional hernias refer to a protrusion of a portion of an organ or tissue through the incision, which is a result of deep wound dehiscence. The majority of incisional hernias developed in the first three months after kidney transplantation.

Generally, superficial wound dehiscences are treated as superficial wound infection excluding antibiotic therapy. For an anergic wound the healing process can be electively stimulated with the vacuum sealing method, which has shown promising results. Conversely, deep wound dehiscence, as well as symptomatic incisional hernias, requires operative repair. The open surgical procedure varies according to the surgeon's preference. Routinely, small defects undergo primary fascial repair, and large or recurrent defects are repaired with mesh.

7.2 Vascular complications

Vascular complications during and after kidney transplantation are usually uncommon with an incidence of less 10%. But they are important causes of graft dysfunction. According to the location of affected vessels, vascular complications can be grouped into graft vessels complications and recipient vessels complications. Actually, the lesion often affected the both.

7.2.1 Graft vessels complications

7.2.1.1 Renal Artery Thrombosis

Occlusion of renal artery by thrombus is a rare event occurring in 0.2-3.5% of renal transplantations. Though uncommon, it is a transplant emergency that often results in graft loss. The exact cause of renal artery thrombosis has remained obscure. The aetiology is multifactorial. Technical factors are the important causes, but not always. Other possible contributory factors may be concluded as thrombophilic state, history of previous thrombosis, lupus anticoagulants, atherosclerosis, poor cardiac output, ATN or acute rejection. Vessel kinking, torsion, intimal injuries are the frequently reported technique errors resulting in renal artery thrombosis, which should be avoided. Adequate training on techniques of vascular anastomosis and graft recovery is essential, to reduce the occurrence of repeated reanastomosis and iatrogenic vascular injury. Renal artery thrombosis can occur at any time, but commonly occurs in the early postoperative period. The typical clinical presentation is a sudden onset of oliguria or anuria with deterioration of graft function, usually painless, which demands a differential diagnosis with acute rejection and urologic complications. Helical computerized tomography (CT) may be more diagnostic than ultrasound for that it can directly depict renal artery thrombosis when ultrasound studies are inconclusive. Angiography is warranted in confusing cases. Prompt reoperation is crucial to salvage such a graft when diagnosis is suspected, because irreversible cortical necrosis can occur within minutes. That is why it could be responsible for more than one-third of early graft losses. Actually, transplant nephrectomy is usually the rule. Since the extremely bad prognosis of graft survival, prevention is of utmost importance especially in high-risk patients.

7.2.1.2 Renal Vein Thrombosis

Renal vein thrombosis (RVT) is an unusual but disastrous complication, reported to occur with an incidence of 0.3-3%, more frequent than renal artery thrombosis. Pathogenesis of RVT is still controversial, the multiple factors conducing to renal artery thrombosis discussed earlier also contribute here, moreover, technique reasons seem to play an invariable role. A long renal vein is considered a contributory thrombogenic factor by some studies, some center even routinely shorten the left renal vein at the time of surgery to prevent thrombosis. So an immoderately prolonged right renal vein using the inferior vena cuff should be avoided during the back table preparation. Small vein and multiple veins may also predispose to thrombosis. Unlike artery, wall of vein is subtle and fragile, more inclined to be damaged, compressed and twisted, meticulous surgical techniques on renal retrieval, renal vein repair and anastomosis and positioning of kidney may prevent most avoidable occurrence of RVT. In contrast to the renal artery thrombosis, the clinical presentation of RVT is more evident and perilous, sometimes, life-threatening. Majority of RVT occurs during the early period after transplantation, particularly due to technique problems. Rare late RVT even occurring years after operation mainly results from thrombophilic states, secondary thrombosis from ipsilateral DVT or de novo nephropathy. For most early acute cases, besides the typical sudden onset of oliguria or anuria with deterioration of graft function, severe pain and swelling over the graft is definite, an unstable haemodynamics status and decreasing concentration of haemoglobin is present if incurring rupture of graft. Clinical presentation of late RVT may be gentle, especially for the kidneys with partial occlusion of the renal vein, sometimes, only present a deteriorating dysfunctional graft. On Ultrasound images, the allograft may appear swollen and hypoechoic. At Doppler ultrasound examination, venous flow is absent, and the arterial waveform shows reversed, plateauing diastolic flow. A perinephric fluid collection or huge hematoma can be seen if graft rupture occurs.

After an early diagnosis is made by clinical presentation and ultrasound examination, patient should be underwent emergent exploration as soon as possible, which is the sole chance to salvage the graft. There are two ways to save the allograft, thrombectomy or retransplantation. Firstly, patient needs to be heparinized before any procedure, if no obvious evidence of technique error, a thrombectomy of renal vein may be attempted, fresh clot should be removed and flushed out completely, and the transplant renal artery might be clamped to control the bleeding if the graft is ruptured, accompanying with a repair of rupture. A routine vein tissue biopsy is essential to identify the cause. Removal of the kidney and reperfusion with preservation solution may be the last option especially if encountering the short right renal vein from live donor. The iliac vein has to be mobilized to a maximal extent to facilitate the reanastomosis. Besides the open surgical technique, percutaneous chemical and mechanical thrombolysis has been showed a feasible method but with a risk of leading to pulmonary embolism. It may be possible to treat a partial RVT with heparin. We have been associated with three cases of late partial RVT, revascularization of renal vein in all three cases has been achieved by subcutaneous low molecular weight heparin injection combing with intravenous infusion of thrombolytics for 2-3 weeks, no graft loss occurs.

7.2.1.3 Transplant Renal Artery Pseudoaneurysm and Transplant Renal Artery Rupture

Transplant renal artery pseudoaneurysm and transplant renal artery rupture are two extremely rare but potentially devastating vascular complications after kidney transplantations, with an incidence rate of less than 1%. Transplant renal artery pseudoaneurysm is a major risk factor of transplant renal artery rupture. Related data are limited in isolated case reports, but some essentials can be concluded from them. Transplant renal artery pseudoaneurysm can be extra-renal or intra-renal. Extra-renal pseudoaneurysm are usually located at the anastomotic site, and are commonly caused by poor surgical technique, vessel wall ischemia or arterial dehiscence caused by perivascular infection, especially fungi infection. Patients with pseudoaneurysm after their renal transplant are usually asymptomatic and diagnosed incidentally. Few are reported to present with fever, anemia, hypertension, functional impairment, graft loss and life-threatening hemorrhage due to acute rupture. From the review of literature, there are no specific physical findings to predict the risk of rupture. Ultrasound doppler and scanning can readily recognize them. CT angiography, Magnetic resonance (MR) angiography or catheter directed conventional angiography can be used to confirm the diagnosis. The indications for repair of pseudoaneurysm and management options remain controversial. Life-threatening hemorrhage due to acute rupture needs an urgent intervention, the allograft is definitely jeopardized and transplant nephrectomy might inevitably be needed. Recent reports advocate that symptomatic false aneurysms, large size (larger than 2.5 cm), presence of infection, progressive enlargement and impending rupture are indications for repair. Some authors suggest positive surgical repair so long as the pseudoaneurysm is found regardless of if it is symptomatic. Asymptomatic small pseudoaneurysms can be managed conservatively with regular monitoring, but with a risk of acute transplant renal artery rupture. Open surgical repair, endovascular repair and ultrasound-guided percutaneous thrombin injection are the current reported treatment options for managing extra-renal pseudoaneurysm complicating renal transplantation.

7.2.1.4 Transplant Renal Artery Stenosis

Transplant renal artery stenosis (TRAS) is the most common vascular complication following renal transplantation. Depending upon the criteria used for diagnosis its incidence varies from 1 to 23%. It accounts for approximately 1 to 5% of cases of posttransplant hypertension and at least 75% of all posttransplant vascular complications. TRAS is a potentially curable cause of refractory posttransplant hypertension and graft dysfunction. There are three main types of renal transplant artery stenosis: (1) stenosis at the anastomosis; (2) localized stenosis, and (3) multiple or diffuse stenoses. It can occur at any times, usually becomes apparent between 3 mo and 2 yr after renal transplantation. Different locations and timings of disease onset may reflect different etiologies. The most common causes of stenosis are technical resaons. The stenosis due to defective surgical technique, usually located at the anastomosis and especially at the end-to-end anastomosis. The other technical causes reported were vessel lesions during preservation or intimal trauma due to vascular clamps and torsion, kinking or angulation of the artery. Stenosis can be also a result of donor or recipient atherosclerosis. Immunological injury is also proposed as the possible cause, especially in diffuse and multiple stenoses. TRAS resulting from technical resaons usually arises early after transplantation. Stenoses occurring later, sometimes several years posttransplant, usually reflect atherosclerotic disease either of the transplant renal artery or of the adjacent proximal iliac artery. In subtle TRAS postglomerular resistances are usually increased to sustain intracapillary pressure despite the low renal perfusion pressure. Thus, the glomerular filtration rate may be normal or only slightly depressed. When hemodynamically significant stenoses occur, hypertension and progressive kidney dysfunction are common, without treatment, irreversible graft loss is the rule. TRAS is usually manifested as intractable hypertension, with deterioration of renal function. A vascular murmur in the iliac fossa can often be present but significant stenosis can also occur in the absence of the audible bruit. The gold standard for diagnosing TRAS still remains renal angiography, but it is only electively indicated when a stenosis is suspected on the basis of non-invasive tests. Doppler ultrasound, with many advantages has become the imaging modality to enable the diagnosis and follow-up of TRAS.

A TRAS could be treated conservatively or by revascularization. Stenosis can be treated successfully pharmacologically provided that allograft perfusion is not jeopardized. Revascularization can be by percutaneous transluminal angioplasty (PTA) or by surgical correction. PTA is the preferred initial mode of therapy. Technical success has been reported at greater than 80% with clinical success, the restenosis rates are reported to be 10% to 60%. Surgical techniques include resection and revision of the anastomosis, saphenous vein bypass graft of the stenotic segment, patch graft, or localized endarterectomy. The success rate ranges from 63 to 92%, and the recurrence rate is close to 12%. A prompt intervention is mandatory in stenosis exceeding 70%.

7.2.2 The recipient vessels complications

7.2.2.1 Iliac Artery Stenosis

Iliac artery stenosis is a rare complication after renal transplantation, though unusual it can be the cause of hypertension and renal dysfunction. The stenosis can occur at proximal or distal to the anastomosis site or both, also can be bilateral or multilevel occlusive disease. Usually the lesion is located proximal to the transplant anastomosis site, known as" stenosis of the iliac segment proximal to the transplant renal artery (Prox-TRAS)". The incidence for Prox-TRAS was reported to be 2.4%. The causes inducing TRAS are also predisposing factors of iliac artery stenosis, such as technical errors and atherosclerosis. The iliac artery stenosis is usually suspected by the clinical manifestations including bruits, lower extremity claudication, hypertension and renal allograft dysfunction. But it may be asymptomatic and discovered incidently. Surgeons have paid much more attention to Prox-TRAS not only because of the higher incidence but it can cause ischemia of allograft and ipsilateral lower extremity at the same time compared with the distal stenosis. The diagnosis is established based on direct and indirect evidences, because visualization of the stenosis proximal to the transplant artery could not be achieved with the duplex sonography method in all the patients due to the depth of the common iliac artery or an unfavorable angle of the Doppler beam. The criteria for diagnosing isolated Prox-TRAS are summarized as follows (Voiculescu et al, 2003):

1. Decrease in low pulsatility index when compared with data obtained before
2. Low low pulsatility index (<1.0)
3. Pulsus parvus et tardus
4. No TRAS
5. V max within the iliac artery proximal to the graft greater than 200 cm/sec
6. Monophasic flow profile within the iliac artery distal from the transplant artery

PTA with stents for short iliac artery occlusions or stenosis has showed profitable short- and long-term outcomes in most patients. In patients with multilevel occlusive or bilateral lesions, particularly with atherosclerotic disease, endarterectomy or bypass surgery could be taken into consideration.

7.2.2.2 External iliac Artery Pseudoaneurysms

External iliac artery pseudoaneurysms following renal transplantation are very uncommon, with an incidence rate of <1%. Its etiology is similar with that of the transplant renal artery pseudoaneurysm, usually a result of vascular injury due to defective surgical technique or perivascular infection. On ultrasound the diagnosis is straightforward. However, the surgical management is somewhere different. Besides the transplant nephrectomy and pseudoaneurysm excision, arterial reconstruction is recommended to prevent lower limb ischemia. During the past decade, endovascular repair has become the first-choice treatment of posttransplant iliac pseudoaneurysms even in emergent setting in some centers. As the end-to-side arterial anastomosis has been becoming the standard fashion, the incidence of internal iliac artery pseudoaneurysms is exceedingly rare regardless of the biopsy-induced complications.

7.2.2.3 Deep Venous Thrombosis

Deep venous thrombosis (DVT) is a well-recognized complication in patients undergoing any type of surgery. Its occurrence after general surgical procedures is well characterized. However, the real incidence of DVT after kidney transplantation is uncertain, varying from 0.8% to 25%. In our center the incidence of symptomatic posttransplant DVT is less than 1%. Some authors feel it occurs with greater frequency, comparing with patients underwent other types of major surgery. Possible resaons include a pelvic dissection, venous anastomosis with clamping of the vein, decreased venous emptying secondary to the position of the kidney, mechanical compression by hematoma or lymphoceles, and the higher proportion of diabetic patients. The opponents advocate the reasons of a decreased risk of DVT, including bleeding tendency of uremic patients and lower hematocrit levels. Theoretically, the position of the graft adjacent to the iliac vein could affect venous outflow from the lower limb. But in previous studies, no statistically significant difference of posttransplant DVT was found on the side of the graft versus the contralateral side. One study suggested the recipients with severe early renal insufficiency should be regarded as high risk patients for late DVT after renal transplantation. Other well defined risk factors of DVT, such as age >40 years, obesity, history of venous thromboembolism, bed rest >5 days also contribute to DVT after kidney transplantation. Purely clinical signs and symptoms of pain, swelling and calf tenderness cannot be used to diagnose DVT, but they alert one to obtain further testing to exclude or confirm the diagnosis. Actually, majority of the DVT patients are asymptomatic and some present as acute pulmonary embolism alone, a potentially fatal complication. In rare occasion, DVT can be a cause of renal allograft loss due to proximal extension of ileofemoral deep venous thrombosis. Duplex ultrasonography has now replaced venography as the most widely used diagnostic test for an acute DVT with excellent sensitivity and specificity of 97% and 94% respectively, CT pulmonary angiography can be performed when excluding pulmonary embolism.

Therapeutic anticoagulation is imperative for a symptomatic posttransplant DVT patient to prevent clot extension, fatal and non-fatal pulmonary embolism and to reduce the risk of recurrent thrombosis. The current options include unfractionated heparin, warfarin and low molecular weight heparin. Graduated compression stockings should be used immediately to reduce pain and swelling and decreases the incidence of the post-thrombotic syndrome. The role and timing of venous thrombectomy for ilio-femoral vein thrombosis is pendent, especially for kidney transplant patients. Early clot removal is achieved by either mechanical thrombectomy using an open or endovascular approach, or catheterdirected thrombolysis. Permanent or retrievable inferior vena caval filters could be placed for the patients at highest risk of pulmonary embolism. The usual principles and measures of DVT prophylaxis, such as early ambulation, calf exercises or fitting of graduated compression stockings, are also important for kidney transplant patients, in particular, the high risk patients. Subcutaneous injection of low molecular weight heparin can be added for higher risk patients, such as an obese patient with a history of DVT. Of course, the corresponding bleeding risk should be taken into account as well.

7.3 Urological complications

Urological complications are quite common following renal transplant procedure associated with significant morbidity and sometimes a compromising graft function. In general, the urological complications involve any postoperative morbidity related to urinary system and male genital system, whereas the surgical complications are undoubtedly the most important, to some extent, may be prevented. Other urologic complications discussed in the literatures such as hematuria and urinary tract infection, are often a portion of symptoms or results of surgical complications; and some overlaps the surgical aspects but not the whole, for instance, urinary calculi and erectile dysfunction. Four major surgical urological complications discusses here are urine leak, ureteral obstruction, vesicoureteral reflux, and renal allograft rupture.

7.3.1 Urine leak

Urine leaks can be pyelic, vesical or ureteral in origin with a reported incidence of 1% to 4.3%. Pyelic leak is often a result of unrecognized surgical laceration of the renal pelvis during the back table preparation or transplantation. The occurrence of vesical leak is dramatically low after L-G technique fundamentally replaced the conventional transvesical ureteroneocystostomy due to escape from an additional cystic incision. But ureteral leak is constantly considered for its high incidence because the transplant ureter is by nature prone to ischemia, which is one of the two key contributing factors to ureteral leak. The blood supply of the transplant ureter only derives from the small branches of renal artery of allograft in the subtle periureteral fat and sometimes from the end arterial branches of a lower pole renal artery; thereby the more distal ureter is the more tendencies to be ischemic, which partially interprets the fact that most ureteral leak originate from the ureterovesical junction. The ischemia can be aggravated by immune injury during the course of acute rejection. The other key causative factor of leakage is surgical technical problems, most of which are technical errors that should be avoided. The leading technical error is the failure to achieve a watertight and tension-free anastomosis. Dehiscence of anastomotic site due to a full bladder from blocked Foley catheter or undetected electrocautery injury to ureter is occasionally encountered. Ureter ischemia and perforation caused by a malposed double J ureteral stent is the rare cause. The clinical presentation of ureteral leaks can be apparent or mild. Timetable of obvious symptoms have a few diagnostic significance. Leaks due to technical errors like misplacement of ureteral sutures often occur within the first 4 days, whereas leaks from necrosis usually occur within the first 14 days. The symptoms are various typically with a significant reduction of urine output but volume of perigraft drain increases dramatically, however it is not always the case. Sometimes the urine leak can not be drained due to displacement of drains or drain tubes have been removed, the urine would flow into retroperitoneal cavity or out of the wound, or even be reabsorbed into the peritoneal cavity under high pressure or from an unrecognized hole made in the transplant procedure, developing into urine ascites. Evident manifestations include lower abdominal bulge, a swollen, tender scrotum or edema of labia, abdominal and/or back pain. Fever is a frequent signs even no evidence of infection. Graft function is compromised when large volume urine leak compress the collecting system or vessels. The diagnosis can be established if the urine output recovers and collections decrease immediately after the reinsertion of catheter into the bladder. However, generally a creatinine value mensuration of collections is needed to differentiate urine from the lymphorrhea or seroma. Creatinine in lymph and serum are almost identical, whereas that in urine is prominently high. Various imaging modalities may be used to assist the diagnosis. Ultrasonography often may be applied first for its advantages of convenient and atraumatic, urinary extravasation can be found but usually impossible to identify the origin. Intravenous pyelography might have a positive finding if the graft function is normal and a cystogram may show the leak especially when it is situated at the anastomotic site. Radionuclide imaging can be diagnostic if a confusing case is presented.

Most ureteral leak may be cured simply by prolonged catheterization for at least 2 weeks if there is an indwelling ureteral stent. If there is no ureteral stent conservative treatment is still recommended as the initial management and quite a few leakages can be resolved. If conservative method fails, surgery is indicated. Endoscopic technique is fascinating but technically challenging, the ectopic ureteral orifice and unfixed irregular position of the ureter usually make the retrograde placement of ureteral stent a mission impossible. Percutaneous nephrostomy tube placement might be more practical if there is a hydronephosis as a result of the secondary ureteral obstruction. Therefore open surgery is recommended by many authors as a preferred management. Difficulty in locating the leak is often beyond our imagination due to the presence of extensive tissue edema. Filling and emptying the bladder intermittently, sometimes using the methylthioninium chloride, a dye, can help to identify the leak. Based on our experience, we do not recommend simple repair of the leak even if it is clear at the ureterovesical junction because ureteral stent can not be placed, more important, most leaks are a result of necrosis. Reimplantation of the ureter over a stent is a good option. If the visible necrosis is found, the transplant ureter should be cut back to where it is clearly healthy. After the removal of the necrotic part of ureter, if a tension-free anastomosis can be achieved reimplantation of the transplant ureter is usually sufficient, if not there are multiple options available to solve the problem. Above all native urinary tract should be considered, and ureteroureterostomy with the ipsilateral native ureter may be the best choice with many advantages. Boari bladder flaps are also useful if native ureter is unavailable. Boari bladder flaps have been used to bridge a loss of total ischemic ureter with a satisfactory result. But this technique reduces the bladder volume and should be selected cautiously for the "small bladder" patient from any reason. Sometimes, the bladder can be anastomosed directly to the kidney capsule with a nephrostomy tube for several weeks, but pyelovesicostomy often fail to perform due to an inability to mobilize the transplant kidney or bladder sufficiently. If the native urothelium can not be reached ileal substitution is a feasible alternative and has been reported successfully to salvage difficult and recurrent transplant urinary fistulae when native urinary tract could not be used. Appendix has been reported to replace complete necrotic ureter of pediatric recipient successfully. Recently a new minimally invasive technique of total ureteral replacement, initially described for the palliative treatment of ureteral obstructions has been introduced as an alternative to an open procedure to treat ureteral necrosis after renal transplantation. This technique is based on the use of a silicone-polytetrafluoroethylene -bonded tube tunnelled underneath the skin to bypass the graft and bladder.

7.3.2 Ureteral obstruction

The obstruction of the transplant ureter is another most common urological complication; the incidence would be probably 3% to 7%. Causes of the obstruction are miscellaneous, which can be broadly divided into extraureteral, ureteral and intraureteral. Extraureteral factors include compression from lymphocele, hematoma, urinoma, spermatic cord or adhesive band. Ureteral cause means a ureteral twist, ureteral narrowing from ischemia, infarction or fibrosis due to rejection or infection, an anastomotic site stenosis, congenital ureteropelvic junction obstruction in the donor ureter, or in exceptional condition, a ureteral inguinal hernia. Intraureteral factors involve stone, clot, sloughed renal papilla, fungal ball or foreign body. The clinical presentation of ureteral obstruction can occur in early postoperative period or years after the transplant depending on different causes, the symptoms commonly subtle, whereas the obstruction symptoms associated with a technical error usually occur early and obvious with a symptom of acute or subacute upper urinary tract obstruction and a climbing creatinine level. Hydronephrosis on ultrasound may be seen or not according to the extent of obstruction and timing of detection.

The emergent exploration should be considered if the symptoms are apparent and advancing. The original incision can be reopened, and some possible technique faults should be taken into consideration. One rare but serious fault is that the anterior transplant ureter is angulated by a careless stitch during closing the wound, in that situation, the suture should be removed and injured ureter should be repaired carefully. A redundant and twisted ureter usually needs correction by another ureteroneocystostomy. More frequently, the problem arises from the ureterovesical junction due to overtight muscular tunnel by an aggressive anti-reflux anastomosis. We prefer reimplantaion of the transplant ureter instead of simple loosen the suture over the seromuscular layer because the local edema and inflammation may proceed. Spermatic cord should be divided if it is suspected a cause of obstruction. Late ureteral stenosis is usually asymptomatic but gradual; the reason is complicated, and some of them have little relation to the surgery but most of the obstruction usually need surgical intervention for better long-term graft survival. Endoscopic technique is above all considered, unlike the urine leak, late ureteral stenosis basically accompany a hydronephrotic transplant kidney, the stricture can be diagnosed and managed in an antegrade fashion and approximately half of the patients can be cured. Balloon dilation, incision with a holmium:YAG laser or knife have been reported effective in treating transplant ureter stricture. Recurrent stricture is the main barrier for the technique as other percutaneous dilation surgery. A long-term stent is a compromise between redilation and open surgery. Open surgery is the standard way to manage the recurrent strictures, but painstaking and dangerous course is inevitable. A sufficient preparation is essential to identify the location of the stenosis, a preoperative temporary percutaneous ureteral stent is very benenifical for the assistance of locating the ureter. After finding and removing the unhealthy part of transplant ureter, the various reconstruction techniques discussed earlier can be used.

7.3.3 Vesicoureteral reflux

The exact incidence of posttranspant vesicoureteral reflux (VUR) is not known since most patients with VUR are asymptomatic and the gold standard for diagnosis, voiding cystourethrograms (VCUG), is not a routine item. When routinely checked in transplant patients in some series, the frequency of VUR varies from 1% to 86%; such a large variation can be attributed to different surgical techniques, time when VUR was tested, methods used to detect VUR, underlying urological condition, and selection criteria of the study groups. Surgical techniques are vital and controllable factors to reduce the occurrence of posttranspant VUR, therefore the non-antireflux techniques have been nearly abandoned in most of institutions. The association between VUR and urinary tract infection and reflux nephropathy has been well established in pediatric patients with native kidneys. However, the clinical significance of posttranspant VUR in the kidney transplant patients and the impact of postoperative VUR on short-term and long-term graft survival still remain controversial. Early, it was argued that VUR might be a cause of late deterioration in function, mimicking chronic rejection. Shortly after that, however, researchers suggested VUR is not a frequent cause of late renal allograft failure. A recent report has showed posttransplant VUR did not negatively affect graft function during short-term period after kidney transplantation. More recently, other authors described the presence of low-grade VUR did not affect long-term graft function in patients with late urinary tract infections. Therefore it is not necessary to screen the posttransplant VUR routinely. Positive management is only taken into account for a symptomatic posttransplant VUR. A VCUG is indicated if recurrent pyelonephritis or urinary tract infections are present, which show a symptomatic posttransplant VUR incidence of approximately 1%.
Administration of appropriate antibiotics is the primary and crucial treatment. Long-term continuous prophylaxis was sufficient in most cases. Surgical intervention is only considered for intractable cases because randomized trials of antibiotic prophylaxis versus surgical therapy plus antibiotic prophylaxis have not shown a difference in development of nonfebrile urinary tract infection in primay VUR studies. The surgery indications are recurrent febrile graft pyelonephritis or urinary tract infections refractory to antibiotic therapy and severe reflux (grade IV ~V) resulting in renal scarring or a compromising graft function. Open surgery is the standard approach to solve the problem. Reimplantation of the transplant ureter using the L-G technique has been proved to be effective and provides excellent long-term results for patients with VUR in combination with recurrent urinary tract infections after kidney transplantation. Endoscopic treatment has developed rapidly over the past decade along with the advancement of minimally invasive technique in the treatment of primary VUR. Endoscopic techniques mainly involve injection of a bulking substance into the muscular posterior wall of the ureterovesical junction. The resulting bulking effect compresses the ureteral lumen and provides a substitute for the normal muscular backing of the transmural ureter. However the overall success rates are lower than those reported for primary reflux or for open reconstruction.

7.3.4 Renal allograft rupture

Renal allograft rupture (RAR) was first described by Murray et al. in 1968. The reported incidence varies from 0.3 and 9.6%, although uncommon, it is an emergent and dangerous urological complication, potentially threatens graft and patient survival. The acute rejection is the most frequent cause of graft rapture. Acute tubular necrosis has been revealed another important risk factor comparable to severe acute rejection. Uncommon causes of RAR include renal vein thrombosis, ureteric obstruction, renal biopsy, heparin therapy, complete lymphatic legation, trauma, nephrostomy tubes and renal cell cancer development. RAR usually develops within 2-3 weeks after transplantation, however, the longest reported interval between clinical renal transplantation and renal allograft rupture was 4 years. Timing of the onset often indicated etiologies; rupture emerging in very early posttransplant period usually a result of renal vein thrombosis due to technique errors, for instance, twisting and kinking of the vein or intima tear; whereas rupture occurs later when caused by rejection. Clinical manifestations are commonly similar, presenting a sudden pain and swelling over the graft area, oliguria or anuria with hypotension and a drop in haematoglobin. Sometimes bleeding from the incision or haematuria can be found, fever is not uncommon. Clinical diagnosis may be confirmed by ultrasound or CT scan. On ultrasound a perinephric fluid collection or crescent of clot along the convex margin of the kidney usually can be revealed, sometimes, associated with extensive renal vein thrombosis. At the emergent exploration, a huge hematoma surrounding the convexity of the graft can usually be found, the rupture can occur along the convex border or at either renal pole. Do not hesitate to perform a prompt graft nephrectomy if there is an unsteady hemodynamic status. In other situations, the immediate decision of transplant nephrectomy is mainly depending on the condition of graft and experience of surgeon. Nephrectomy is almost the definite treatment for RAR in early age; however, surgical conservative treatment has been advocated by more authors over the past two decades, with a amazing reported salvage rate varying from 40~ 100%. Mattress suture of parenchyma over haemostyptic material as well as electrocautery haemostasis are the most commonly used and efficacious salvage techniques. The additional application of a mesh (Polyglactin absorbable mesh, lyophilized dura, fascia) wrapping the graft can improve the haemostasis and prevents the expansion and fragmentation of the parenchyma. In our opinion, transplant-preserving management could be attempted but not recommended when there is irreversible concomitant rejection, or a second RAR.

7.4 Lymphorrhea and lymphoceles

Lymphorrhea, also known as lymphorrhagia, is the large volume collection of lymph that drains from perigraft drainage tubes, which may develop into a lymphocele when the collection accumulates in the postoperative dead space. The clinical incidence of lymphorrhea and lymphocele is uncertain in large series varying from 0.6% to 18.1%, however, the actual rate of occurrence is unexpected high up to approximately 50% owing to the advent of ultrasound for routine graft surveillance, for that the majority of lymphatic collections are asymptomatic or subclinical. The major origin of the lymphorrhea has been identified by lymphangiography and radionuclide imaging as extravasation of the lymph from the lymphatics adjacent to the iliac vessels of the recipient due to an excessive dissection of lymphatic vessels and a failure to occlude all of the lymphatic vessels divided during the preparation of the operative bed. It still remains unexplained why unligated lymphatic vessels from the renal hilum and capsule of the graft contribute so little to the formation of a lymphocele. Despite of unavoidable dissection of lymphatics overlying the iliac vessels and potential dead space the allograft create the high occurrence of lymphocele after kidney transplantation is also closely related to the immunosuppressive regimen. Steroids adversely affected macrophage function, and more important, the mTOR inhibitors such as sirolimus and everolimus have a direct antilymphangiogenic effect and powerful antifibroblastic activity, which could prevent the healing of dissected lymph channels around the host iliac vessels. Another important contributing factor is acute cellular rejection. Obesity has been reported an independent risk factor for lymphocele formation. Low molecular weight heparin and excessive use of diuretics also have been implicated as contributing factors to lymphocele formation. Most lymphorrhea and lymphoceles are clinically silent and resolve spontaneously over time, but the clinical presentation can also be clinically evident, even presenting as 'acute abdomen'. Symptoms usually emerge at 2 weeks to 6 months after transplantation with the peak incidence at 6th week posttranplant. Symptoms may be primary or secondary, primary symptoms result from mechanical compression of lymphoceles to the adjacent strcutures such as abdominal bulging or mass, painless leg edema due to compression of ipsilateral iliofemoral vein, hydronephrosis as a result of compression of the ureter, urinary frequency or retention due to compression of the bladder neck. Secondary symptoms may be local or systematic, frequently misleading, such as ipsilateral DVT, deterioration of renal function, weight gain, hypertension and fever, even compartment syndrome. Ultrasonography is crucial to diagnosis, simple and effective. On ultrasound, lymphoceles appear as mostly anechoic or hypoechoic, rounded, perigraft fluid collections, they can have septations and multiple in number, Most noninfectious lymphoceles can be distinguished from hematomas and abscesses in term of distinctive homogeneity. Urinomas, usually around the ureter, have the similar appearance to a lymphocele, and may be distinguished by the irregular and indistinct margins owing to the lack of true wall. The accurate differential method is to measure the creatinine concentration of the liquid accommodating in the cysts by ultrasound-guided aspiration, also a way of treatment. This measure can also be used to differentiate lymphorrhea and urine leak when large volume of clear, weak yellow liquid collections appearing in perigraft drainage bag. Other adjunctive procedures such as CT, MR and intravenous pyelography are not routine diagnostic modality unless complicated cases happens or in preparation for a surgery.

It is unnecessary to deal with the small and asymptomatic collections for that most of them may resolve spontaneously; on the contrary, if large or symptomatic, an intervention may be necessary. The modality of treatment may be simple aspiration, percutaneous drainage placement, sclerotherapy and surgery. Percutaneous aspiration or drainage alone is sometimes curative, however, frequently the therapeutic effect is counteracted by the high recurrence rates and infection incurred. Because of the trait prone to recurrence, percutaneous aspiration or drainage combining the injection of sclerosants have been advocated by more authors as a simple, safe and efficacious minimally invasive method to manage the majority of lymphoceles due to a significantly fall of recurrence rates. Povidone-iodine is the classic and effective sclerosant, with which many novel sclerosants compare the therapeutic efficacy. Other potent sclerosants suggested in the literatures include the ethanol, diatrizoate and octreotide. Surgery is only indicated for refractory cases, the main purpose of surgery is to drain the lymph collections into the peritoneal cavity, known as "unroofing" or "fenestration". The procedure can be performed using either open or laparoscopic surgical techniques depending on its relationship with the allograft. If the cysts locate adjacent to peritoneal cavity, laparoscopic unroofing is an agreeable option. Surgeons can reach the lymphocele via transperitoneal approach; during the surgery the lymphocele wall is excised a 5cm disc and sutured to the peritoneum to keep the window open, a simultaneous omentoplasty has been recommended for a better resolvable effect. Laparoscopic procedures are least invasive but should be done meticulously to prevent the inadvertent lesions of the urinary tract to promote the advantages of laparoscopy. Open surgery is considered when the lymphoceles situates an improper position especially deep in pelvic beside vessels of graft, usually via a lower midline abdominal incision and a transperitoneal approach. In some conditions, previous transplant incision may be reopened for better access. It is important to ensure the lymphocele cavity is full and the bladder is empty before the operation. Intraoperative ultrasound is beneficial for localization when the operative finding is dubious.

8. Conclusion

Surgical operation is the first, critical step of a successful kidney transplant. A good few graft loss result from severe surgical complications, which are frequently associated with technique errors. Meticulous surgical technique during transplantation may help avoid majority of preventable surgical complications and related morbidity and mortality.

9. References

Bhayana, S.; Kuo, YF.; Madan, P.; Mandaym, S.; Thomas, PG.; Lappin, JA.; Rice, JC. & Ishihara, K. (2010). Pediatric en bloc kidney transplantation to adult recipients: more than suboptimal? *Transplantation*, Vol.90, No.3 (August 2010), pp. (248-254), ISSN 0041-1337

Boggi, U.; Vistoli, F.; Signori, S.; D'Imporzano, S; Amorese, G.; Consani, G.; Guarracino, F.; Melfi, F.; Mussi, A. & Mosca, F. (2011). Robotic renal transplantation: first European case. *Transplant International*, Vol.24, No.2 (February 2011), pp. (213-218), ISSN 0934-0874

Filocamo, MT.; Zanazzi, M.; Li Marzi, V.; Marzocco, M.; Guidoni, L.; Dattolo, E. & Nicita G. (2007). The approach by midline incision for extraperitoneal kidney transplantation. *Transplantation Proceedings*, Vol. 39, No. 10, (December 2007), pp. (3077-3080), ISSN 0041-1345

Furness, PD 3rd.; Houston, JB.; Grampsas, SA.; Karrer, FM; Firlit, CF. & Koyle, MA. (2001). Extraperitoneal placement of renal allografts in children weighing less than 15 kg. *Journal of Urology*, Vol.166, No.3 (September 2001), pp. (1042-1045), ISSN 0022-5347

Giulianotti, P.; Gorodner, V.; Sbrana, F.; Tzvetanov, I.; Jeon, H.; Bianco, F.; Kinzer, K.; Oberholzer, J. & Benedetti, E. (2010). Robotic transabdominal kidney transplantation in a morbidly obese patient. *American Journal of Transplantation*, Vol.10, No.6 (June 2010), pp. (1478-1482), ISSN 1600-6135

Hoznek, A.; Zaki, SK.; Samadi, DB.; Salomon, L.; Lobontiu, A.; Lang, P. & Abbou, CC. (2002). Robotic assisted kidney transplantation: an initial experience. *Journal of Urology*, Vol.167, No.4 (April 2002), pp. (1604-1606), ISSN 0022-5347

James, F. (2004). Transplantation of Abdominal Organs, In: *Sabiston Textbook of Surgery*, Seventeenth Edition, pp. (708-709), Elsevier, ISBN 0-7216-0409-9, Philadelphia, Pennsylvania, USA

John, M. (2002). Renal Transplantation, In: *Campbell's Urology*, Eighth Edition, pp. (358-359), Elsevier Science, ISBN 0–7216–9058–0, Philadelphia, Pennsylvania, USA

Jones JW. (1998). A new anastomotic technique in renal transplants reduces warm ischemia time. *Clinical Transplantation*, Vol. 12, No. 1, (February 1998), pp. (70-72), ISSN 0902-0063

Kato, T.; Selvaggi, G.; Burke, G.; Ciancio, G.; Zilleruelo, G.; Hattori, M.; Gosalbez, R. & Tzakis, A. (2008). Partial bladder transplantation with en bloc kidney transplant--the first case report of a 'bladder patch technique' in a human. *American Journal of Transplantation*, Vol.8, No.5 (May 2008), pp. (1060-1063), ISSN 1600-6135

Kayler, L.; Kang, D.; Molmenti, E.& Howard, R. (2010). Kidney transplant ureteroneocystostomy techniques and complications: review of the literature. *Transplantation Proceedings,* Vol.42, No. 5 (June 2010), pp. (1413-1420), ISSN 0041-1345

Mangus, RS.; Haag, BW.& Carter, CB. (2004). Stented Lich-Gregoir ureteroneocystostomy: case series report and cost-effectiveness analysis. *Transplantation Proceedings,* Vol.36, No.10 (May 2004), pp. (2959-2961), ISSN 0041-1345

Mital, D.; Foster, PF.; Jensik, SC.; del Rio, JV.; Sankary, HN.; McChesney, LP.& Williams, JW. (1996). Renal transplantation without sutures using the vascular clipping system for renal artery and vein anastomosis--a new technique. *Transplantation,* Vol. 62, No. 8, (October 1996), pp. (1171-1173), ISSN 0041-1337

Nanni, G.; Tondolo, V.; Citterio, F.; Romagnoli, J.; Borgetti, M.; Boldrini, G.& Castagneto, M. (2005). Comparison of oblique versus hockey-stick surgical incision for kidney transplantation. Transplantation Proceedings, Vol. 37, No. 6, (August 2005), pp. (2479-2481), ISSN 0041-1345

Nie, Z.; Zhang, K.; Huo, W.; Li, Q.; Zhu, F.& Jin, F. (2010). Comparison of urological complications with primary ureteroureterostomy versus conventional ureteroneocystostomy. *Clinical Transplantation,* Vol.24, No. 5 (October 2010), pp. (615-619), ISSN 0902-0063

Park, SC.; Kim, SD.; Kim, JI. & Moon IS. (2008). Minimal skin incision in living kidney transplantation. *Transplantation Proceedings,* Vol. 40, No. 7, (September 2008), pp. (2347-2348), ISSN 0041-1345

Sánchez, AS.; Tebar, JC.; Martín, MS.; Bachs, JM.; Moreno, MJ.; Navarro, HP. & Rodríguez, JA. (2005). Obstructive uropathy secondary to ureteral herniation in a pediatric en bloc renal graft. *American Journal of Transplantation,* Vol.5, No.8 (August 2005), pp. (2074-2077), ISSN 1600-6135

Stuart, M. (2008). Renal Transplantation, In: *Smith's general Urology,* Seventeenth Edition, pp. (547-548), Lange Medical Publication, ISBN 0-07-145737-2, New York, USA

Timsit, MO.; Lalloué, F.; Bayramov, A.; Taylor, M.; Billaut, C.; Legendre, C.; Kreis, H.; Badet, L.& Méjean, A. (2010). Should routine pyeloureterostomy be advocated in adult kidney transplantation? A prospective study of 283 recipients. *Journal of Urology,* Vol.184, No. 5 (September 2010), pp. (2043-2048), ISSN 0022-5347

Tiong, HY.; Flechner, SM.; Zhou, L.; Wee, A.; Mastroianni, B.; Savas, K.; Goldfarb, D.; Derweesh, I.& Modlin, C. (2009). A systematic approach to minimizing wound problems for de novo sirolimus-treated kidney transplant recipients. *Transplantation,* Vol.87, No.2 (January 2009), pp. (296-302), ISSN 0041-1337

Voiculescu, A.; Hollenbeck, M.; Plum, J.; Hetzel, GR.; Mödder, U.; Pfeiffer, T.; Sandmann, W& Grabensee, B. (2003). Iliac artery stenosis proximal to a kidney transplant: clinical findings, duplex-sonographic criteria, treatment, and outcome. *Transplantation,* Vol.76, No.2 (July 2003), pp. (332-339), ISSN 0041-1337

van Heurn, E & de Vries, EE. (2009). Kidney transplantation and donation in children. *Pediatric Surgery International,* Vol.25, No.5 (May 2009), pp. (385-393), ISSN 0179-0358

Wong, VK.; Baker, R.; Patel, J.; Menon, K. & Ahmad N. (2008). Renal transplantation to the ovarian vein: a case report. *American Journal of Transplantation,* Vol. 8, No. 5 (May 2008), pp. (1064-1066), ISSN 1600-6135

Ye, G.; Mo, HG.; Wang, ZH.; Yi, SH.; Wang, XW. & Zhang YF. (2006). Arterial anastomosis without sutures using ring pin stapler for clinical renal transplantation: comparison with suture anastomosis. *Journal of Urology,* Vol. 175, No. 2, (February 2006), pp. (636-640), ISSN 0022-5347

10

Preemptive Kidney Transplantation

Burak Sayin
Baskent University Faculty of Medicine, Ankara
Turkey

1. Introduction

End-stage renal disease (ESRD) is a severe health problem with high mortality and morbidity rates and growing incidence worldwide. Recently, two main renal replacement therapy modalities have been used for ESRD patients: Dialysis and kidney transplantation. It is undoubtedly clear that transplantation is the best choise for long term survival and every transplantation candidate is also a preemptive transplantation candidate.

Preemptive kidney transplantation(PKT) may be summarized as transplantation before the commencement of dialysis in ESRD patients. Preemptive transplantation confers a significant benefit in terms of both patient and allograft survival. The benefit thought to be the result of avoidence of cardiovascular adverse effects of long term dialysis. Current opinion allows ESRD patients to receive PKT when their GFR is 20 mL per minute or less and preparation for transplantation should be started at the time of the diagnosing chronic renal disease.

Kidney transplantation should be the choise of therapy in ESRD patients not only because of improving graft and patient survival and also preventing dialysis related comorbidities and lower cost in the long term(1,2,3). New and more effective immunsupressive drugs, growing experience in transplantation surgery are making kidney transplantation a more common and safe option.

Although there are studies showing nephrologists have the same opinion that preemptive transplantation is the best treatment modality for eligible ESRD patients, that has been convincingly shown to improve posttransplant graft and patient survival. Unfortunately, while PKT is much more beneficial over transplantation, preemptive kidney transplantation seems to be underutilized specially as a result of late referral of the patients to a nephrologist and transplantation center. Only 2% of ESRD patients receive PKT while one forth of transplantation procedures are preemptive in children in the USA. Of course, there are other difficulties for PKT such as poor health status, lack of compliance, comorbidities, older patients, longer waiting time for deceased kidney donors and lack of social insurance.

Ideally, preparation for transplantation should be initiated as soon as progressive chronic kidney disease (CKD) is recognized because cardiovascular morbidity and mortality rates increases while CKD progresses. Early referral to a nephrologist has a vital importance in this situation. Unfortunately, just about 50% of CKD patients come upon a nephrologist in end stage of chronic renal disease. Early referral not only allows careful preparation for PKT and also evaluation of potential living donor candidates and selecting the exact time for transplantation. Because the course of CKD varies according to the primary disease, earliest referral is synonymous to early preparation and beter outcome for transplantation.

GFR 20 mL per minute or less is widely accepted to be the time for preemptive kidney transplantation regardless of the etiology of the kidney disease. Diabetic CKD patients should also be evaluated for pancreatic islet cell transplantation. Kidney biopsy may be helpful for potentially recurring primary kidney diseases after transplantation. A living kidney donor enhances the chance for PKT but deceased kidney donor may be an alternative that should not be failed to remember and all patients should be added to waiting list when GFR decreases under 20 mL per minute. Previously transplantated patients may also be candidates for another PKT.

Recent studies show that preemptive transplantation has better outcomes than non-preemptive transplantation. Lower infection, lower hypertension and less acute rejection episode rates in preemptive transplant patients may be the main reasons for these results. PKT allows preventing from complications during hemodialysis, higher hemoglobin levels before transplantation, lower cardiovascular disease and coronary artery calcification rates, better consistency to immunsuppressive therapy and beter life-quality. Long term graft and patient survival are two major motivators for PKT.

Although kidney transplantation has many advantages against other therapeutic approaches, has its own problems. While kidney transplantation becomes more prevalent, post transplant problems growing as well and transplant recipients becomes a "special patient group". Minimazing the problems of this "special patient group" is a significant target and may only be achieved by proper choise of recipients, appropriate preparation and finally exact timing of transplantation.

Is preemptive kidney transplantation exact time of transplantation? Until mid 80's preemptive transplantation has been thought to have worse results than non preemptive (4,5). But after 90's more recent studies referred just the opposite (6,7). Currently, the question stil remains controversial for nephrologists.

Both in Turkey and in the world, widening of transplantation centers and experienced surgeons and nephrologists PKT has become a more common option. Specially in stage 3 and stage 4 CKD patients early referral to a transplantation center carries a high importance for long term survival.

In USA, PKT constitude 25% of living donor transplantations and 10% of deceased donor transplantations, while the rates are 34% and 14% for chidren recipients respectively(8,9). PKT in children has beter percentages because of family relationships, easier to find a donor for children and probably more doubt of adult nephrologist for PKT (10).

PKT offers preventing dialysis related co-morbidities. Approximately 20% of hemodialysis patients have been hospitalized for vascular access problems and 50% has cateter infections per year. In addition prolonging of hemodialysis process results irreversible cardiovascular problem even after transplantation (7,11). PKT has beter outcomes for both post transplant graft and patient survival and also co-morbidities happening during a dialysis period (10,11).

Mange et al showed improved graft survival of PKT in 8481 living donor transplantation with 52% decrease for graft loss for PKT over non preemptive (12). Kasiske et al found similar results for both living and deceased donor transplantation(13). Chronic allograft nephropathy rates are lower for PKT (14). Some investigators suggest that improved graft survival in PKT patients is a natural result of beter patient survival of selected patients for PKT. Besides other factors for graft survival are similar (15).

It is clear that prolongation of dialysis period in non-preemptive transplantation may result irreversible complications such as cardiovascular disease, renal allograft vascular disease, malnutrition, chronic inlammation,impaired immunologic functions and inadequate clearence in ESRD patients (16,17). Immun system impairment may cause unavoidable infections during dialysis period (18,19,20). Non-preemptive transplantation patients expose to dialysis membranes that may cause activations in immun system which may even cause acute rejection (21,22,23). Hypertensionand left ventricular hypertrophy are more common in nonpreemptive group because of the interdialytic weight gain.

Kidney transplantation should be the first choise in ESRD patients. PKT may be termed as *créme de la créme* and should never be underestimated. Preparation for transplantation should be initiated at the time CKD has been diagnosed and every CKD patient should be accepted as a candidate for PKT for better survival and life-quality.

2. Results and offers

Every CRD patient is a candidate for PKT.

PKT is an important alternative to avoid from dialysis related co-morbidities and complications.

PKT has improved graft and patient survival rates over non preemptive KT.

Early referral to a transplantation center allows proper choise of recipients, appropriate preparation and finally exact timing of transplantation.

PKT offers lower infection rates, lower cardiovascular disease and better life quality.

Every transplantation candidate is also a preemptive transplantation candidate.

3. References

Meier-Kriesche HU, Kaplan B. Waiting time on dialysis as the strongest modifiable renal transplant outcomes: a paired donor kidney analysis. Transplantation 74: 1377- 1381, 2002.

Wolfe RA, Ashby VB, Milford EL. Comparison of mortality in all patients on dialysis, patients on dialysis awaiting transplantation, and recipientss of a first cadaveric transplant. N Engl J Med 341: 1725, 1999.

Evans R. Cost effectiveness analysis of transplantation. Sug Clin North Am 66: 603-608, 1986.

Jacobs C, Brunner FP, Chantler C. Combined report on regular dialysis and transplantation in Europe. Proc Eur Dial Transplant Assoc 14: 3-9, 1977.

Kramer P, Broyer M, Brunner FP. Combined report of regular dialysis in Europe. Proc Dial Transplant Assoc 19: 4-8, 1981.

Migliori RJ, Simmons RL, Payne WD. Renal transplantation done safely without prior chronic dialysis therapy. Transplantation 43: 51-56, 1987.

Katz SM, Kerman RH, Golden D. Preemptive transplantation. An analysis of benefits and hazards in 85 patients. Transplantation 51: 351-355, 1991.

John AG, Rao M, Jacob CK. Pre-emptive live-related renal transplantation. Transplantation 66:204-209, 1998.

Papalois VE, Moss A, Gillingham KJ. Preemptive transplant for patients with renal failure. Arguments against waiting until dialysis. Transplantation 70(4): 625-631, 2000.

Mange K, Joffe MM, Feldman HI. Effect of the use or nonuse of long term dialysis on the subsequent survival of renal transplants on living donors. N Eng J Med 8: 726- 731, 2001.

Vats A, Donaldson L, Fine R. Pretransplant dialysis status and outcome of renal transplantation in north american children: a NAPRTCS study. Transplantation 69: 1414-1419, 2000.

Mange K, Weir M. Preemptive renal transplantation: Why not? Am J Transplant 3: 1336- 1340, 2003.

Wali RKGW, Bellimokunda L, Blahut S. What happens to patients with CHF due to left ventricular sistolic dysfunction defined as left ventricular ejection fraction (LVEF) of less than 40% (congestive cardiomyopathy in uremia) in dialysis dependent patients after successful renal transplantation? Am J Transplant 3(S5): 313, 2003.

Kasiske BL, SJ.Matas AJ, Ellison MD. Preemptive kidney transplantation: the advantage and the advantaged. J Am Soc Nephrol 13: 1358-1364, 2002.

Innocenti GR, Wadei HM, Prieto M. Preemptive living donor kidney transplantation: Do benefits extend to all recipients? Transplantation 83: 144-149, 2007.

Gill JS, Tonello M, Johnson N. Why do preemptive kidney transplant recipients have an allograft survival advantage? Transplantation 78: 873-879, 2004.

Wolfe RA, Ashby VB, Daugirdas JT. Body size, dose of hemodialysis, and mortality. Am J Kidney Dis 35: 80-88, 2000.

Drukker A, Schlesinger M. The Immune system in uremia. Child Nephrol Urol 10: 61- 64, 1990.

Meier-Kriesche HU, Port FK, Ojo A. Effect of waiting time on renal transplant outcome. Kidney Int 58: 1311-1317, 2000.

Nishimoto A, Matsumoto Y. Increase of periferal natural killer T cells in hemodialysis patients. Clin Nephrol 55: 121, 2001.

Kaul H, Girndt M, Sester U. Initiation of hemodialysis treatment leads to improvement of T-cell activation in patients with end stage renal disease. Am J Kidney Dis 35: 611, 2000.

Cooper AC, Mikhail A, Lethbridge MW. Increased expression of erytropoiesis inhibiting cytokines (IFN-gamma, TNF-alpha, IL-10, IL-13) by T cells in patients excibiting poor responce to erytropoietin therapy. J Am Soc Nephrol 14: 1776, 2003.

Joo KW, Shin SJ, Lee JW. Preemptive transplantation and long term outcome in living donor kidney transplantation, single center experience. Trans Proceed 39: 3061- 3064, 2007.

11

Augmentation Cystoplasty in Pretransplant Recepients

Ashraf Abou-Elela
Cairo University,
Egypt

1. Introduction

Augmentation cystoplasty is performed to increase bladder capacity and compliance. The primary use of augmentation cystoplasty is to protect renal function, to achieve urinary continence, and often to facilitate urinary tract reconstruction [1]. The most common problems necessitating bladder augmentation are neurogenic bladder dysfunction secondary to myelodysplasia, extrophy of the bladder, and posterior urethral valves. However, many other conditions may require bladder augmentation including tuberculosis, interstitial cystitis, multiple surgeries, chemotherapy and radiation therapy.

Not all patients undergoing augmentation cystoplasty, especially in the pediatric population, can achieve complete emptying of their bladder by spontaneous voiding. It was the success and wide spread acceptance of clean intermittent catheterization (CIC) in the mid-1970s that made augmentation cystoplasty and continent urinary diversion possible especially in children [2].

Conventional enterocystoplasty employs the use of detubularized segments of small or large bowel. Ileum, sigmoid and cecum have all been used; several studies have confirmed the reliability of these segments [3, 4].

Despite the functional success of enterocystoplasty, clinical experience has demonstrated that there are numerous complications that can result from the incorporation of small and large bowel and their heterotropic epithelium into the urinary tract. To avoid some of the deleterious side effects of enterocystoplasty, several procedures have been developed to augment the bladder without the use of the bowel. These include gastrocystoplasty, the use of dilated ureter (either naturally dilated or balloon dilated), autoaugmentation and seromuscular enterocystoplasty [5, 6, 7, 8, 9].

Autoaugmentation involves the excision of the detrusor muscle from the dome of the bladder allowing the epithelium to form a large diverticulum which may or may not be covered with a seromuscular gastric or sigmoid patch as a backing. In addition, recent advances in tissue engineering substrates and biomaterials have enhanced our abilities to possibly regenerate bladder tissue that is clinically useful for augmentation purposes. Generally, three classes of biomaterials have been used for engineering of genitourinary tissues; naturally derived materials, such as collagen and alginate, cellular tissue matrices such as bladder and small intestinal submucosa (SIS) and synthetic polymers such as polyglycolic acid (PGA) and polylactic acid (PLA) [10, 11, 12, 13].

At this time, even so, there are significant potential problems with the use intestinal segments in the lower urinary tract; gastrointestinal (GI) segments remain the gold standard for increasing bladder capacity and improving compliance. These problems include: hyperchloremic metabolic acidosis, hyokalemia, hypocalcemia, ammoniagenic encephalopathy, bone demineralization, vitamin B_{12} deficiency, malabsorption, drug absorption toxicities, growth retardation, mucus secretion, urinary tract infection, urinary calculi and tumor formation. Gastrocystoplasty may be complicated with hypochloremic metabolic alkalosis and hematuria-dysuria syndrome (14).

Therefore augmentation cystoplasty should be offered only after medical intervention such as anticholinergic medications and intermittent catheterization fail to achieve dryness or to improve bladder compliance sufficiently.

The majority of children who undergo augmentation cystoplasty will require intermittent catheterization (1). The commitment and capacity of both child and the family to comply with catheterization must be assessed carefully. All potential complications should be discussed in details with adult patients and with the family of the child.

Conditions that may require bladder augmentation

Neurogenic Bladder
- Myelodysplasia
- Sacral agenesis
- Caudal regression
- Spinal tumors, vascular malformation
- Myelitis
- Idiopathic

Congenital
- Exstrophy (cloacal, classic, epispadias)
- Posterior urethral valves

Cloaca
- Urogenital sinus
- Bilateral single ectopic ureters
- Infantile bladder syndrome
- Ureterocele
- Prune-belly syndrome

Other
- Infection (tuberculosis, viral cystitis, bacterial cystitis)
- Interstitial cystitis
- Iatrogenic (multiple surgeries)
- Chemotherapy
- Radiation therapy
- Tumor (rhabdomyosarcoma, neurofibromatosis)

2. Augmentation cystoplasty using bowel segments (enteroplasty)

2.1 General principles

The initial approach to augmentation cystoplasty is similar regardless of the bowel segments to be used. Cystoscopy should be performed preoperatively to avoid any unsuspected anatomic abnormalities that may affect the surgery. In augmentation cystoplasty, the two critical aspects of the surgery are the preparation of the bladder and the augmentation segment chosen.

2.2 Preparation of the native bladder

In augmentation cystoplasty, the bladder usually is addressed first. Most commonly, a midline incision is used to expose the abdomen & pelvis. If possible, the peritoneum is not entered until the bladder has been prepared for augmentation and other associated procedures such as ureteral reimplantation or bladder neck reconstruction have been performed. This minimizes third space fluid loss. The bladder is then bivalved through a sagittal incision from near the bladder neck anteriorly to near the trigone posteriorly, thus forming a "clam-shell" configuration. This maneuver is extremely important because the bladder must be opened fully to prevent the augmentation segment from acting as a diverticulum with the formation of an "hour-glass" deformity. Such an incision allows a technically easier anastomosis of the bowel segment and leaves the native bladder wings to add to the overall capacity. The bladder wings may also be used for implantation of a continent catheterizable channel (e.g. Mitrofanoff) or ureteral reimplantation.
Supratrigonal cystectomy is generally not recommended. The remaining cuff of the bladder is a relatively small area for anastomosis to the intestinal segment; therefore most of the bowel is approximated to itself which could result in the augmentation segment behaving as a diverticulum [1,15]. Nevertheless, other surgeons have recommended that the majority of the "diseased" bladder be excised in preparation for augmentation. A greater circumference for the anastomosis can sometimes be provided by opening the bladder in a stellate fashion with a second transverse incision into the two bladder halves [15].

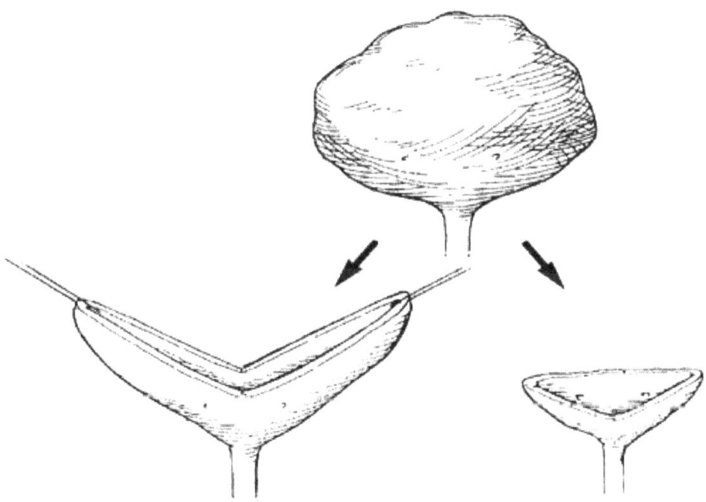

The dysfunctional bladder is opened in the sagittal plane from the bladder neck to the trigone [1].

2.3 Harvesting the augmentation segment

The size and configuration of the augmentation segment are probably more important than the type of bowel used.

Hinman (1988) and Koff (1988) have clearly demonstrated the advantages of opening bowel segments on their antimesenteric border, thereby allowing detubularization and reconfiguration of these segments. Detubularization and reconfiguration maximizes the added surface area to the bladder and thus the benefit of a given segment. Furthermore, the intrinsic innervation is disrupted and peristalsis is decreased significantly (16, 17).

Reconfiguration into a spherical shape provides multiple advantages that improve the overall capacity and compliance. Spherical configuration, by geometry, maximizes the volume achieved for a given bladder wall area. In addition, the spherical configuration also maximizes the radius of curvature, thereby increasing surface tension for a given bladder pressure, which tends to lead to further bladder expansion. This is the relationship of Laplace's law (T = k RP), where T is wall tension, k is a constant dependant on elasticity and wall characteristics, R is the radius of curvature, and P is the luminal pressure.

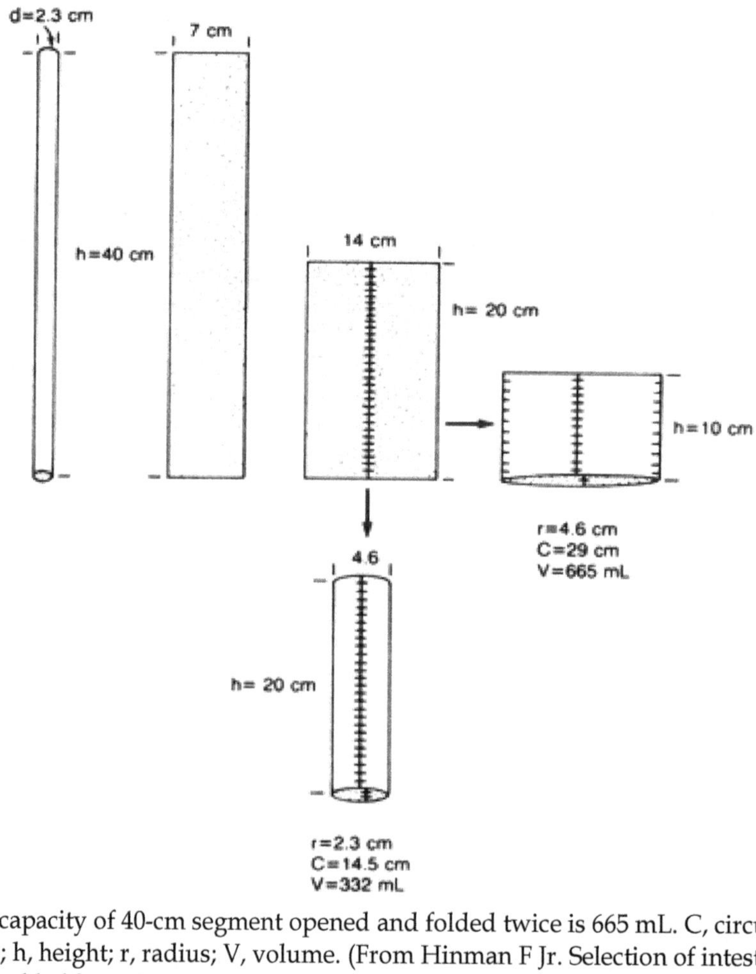

Calculated capacity of 40-cm segment opened and folded twice is 665 mL. C, circumference; d, diameter; h, height; r, radius; V, volume. (From Hinman F Jr. Selection of intestinal segments for bladder substitution: physiological characteristics. *J Urol* 1988;139:521)

The length of the segment used depends on: a) the radius of the bowel used; therefore a larger segment of small bowel usually is required; b) patient's age; c)the size of the pelvis; d) the volume of the native bladder being augmented; if the cystoplasty is being done on a bladder of moderate volume that generates high pressure by uninhibited contractions, less bowel is necessary than for a bladder that is tiny in capacity; e) patient's urinary volumes; patients with upper tract damage, particularly with concentrating ability, may make huge volumes of urine and require a larger capacity.

Depending on the volume needed, 15 to 40 cm of ileum and approximately 20 cm of colon is usually used for cystoplasty. If a segment of stomach is to be used as the augmentation segment, a wedge of at least one-third of the stomach is harvested (19). The gastric wedge requires no reconfiguration as it fits well onto the bivalved bladder. If the ureter is to be used as an augmentation segment, there must be significant dilation and it should likewise be detubularized before being anastomosed to the bladder (20).

The choice of the augmentation segment needs to be tailored individually to each patient. For example, patients with a short ileal mesentery may require the use of the sigmoid to allow for a tension-free anastomosis. Patients with a short gut, renal insufficiency, or a history of pelvic radiation may be better served with a gastrocystoplasty. Patients with myelomeningocele or imperforate anus theoretically could develop diarrhea if the ileocecal valve is taken from their gastrointestinal (GI) tract (21, 22). Other factors to consider include the need for ureteral reimplantation and the need for a continent catheterizable channel. Therefore, it is important to consider each patient individually when selecting the appropriate augmentation segment.

Cystoplasty	Mean	Mean	Mean	Mean Value	First Contraction	Max. Contraction		
	Age (yr)	F/U (mo)	Cap (mL)	At 300 mL cm H_2O	Mean Vol (mL)	Mean P cm H_2O	Mean Vol (mL)	Mean P cm H_2O
Tubular right colon	17.5	9.7	630	18.6	139	37	467	63
Detubularized right colon	28.5	5.1	641	9.4	329	24	596	42
Tubular ileum	66.8	7.0	311	36	110	60	218	81
Detubularized ileum	20.0	5.7	403	14.4	197	22	265	28

From Goldwasser B, et al. Cystometric properties of ileum and right colon after bladder augmentation, substitution or replacement. *J Urol* 1997; 138(2):1007.

Effect of detubularization of colon and ileum on cystoplasty compliance and contraction

3. Types and techniques of enterocystoplasty

3.1 Ileocystoplasty

3.1.1 Technical considerations

Goodwin and colleagues (1959) were among the first to demonstrate the numerous ways of anastomosing a patch of ileum to the native bladder. Virtually all surgeons recognize that ileum should be detubularized and reconfigured to achieve the most spherical shape possible (Q.15).

A segment of ileum at least 15 to 20 cm proximal to the ileocecal valve should be selected. The distal portion of terminal ileum is unique from a physiologic standpoint and should be avoided. The isolated segment should be 15 to 40 cm in length, depending on patient's size, native bladder capacity, type of reconfiguration and desired final capacity. With short ureters, an extra tail of isoperistaltic ileum can be useful to reach the foreshortened ureters. This requires creation of an ileonipple valve to prevent reflux, as in the Kock or hemi-Kock pouch. This type of construction may require up to 60 cm of small intestine.
The segment to be used should have an adequate mesentery to reach the native bladder without tension. After selecting the appropriate segment, the mesentery is cleared from the bowel at either end for a short distance to create a window. The bowel is divided at these ends, and a handsewn ileoileostomy or stapled anastomosis performed. The harvested ileal segment is irrigated clear with 0.25% neomycin solution and opened on its antimesenteric border. The ileum is most commonly folded in a U shape, although longer segments can be folded further into an S or W configuration. The ileum is then anastomosed to itself with running absorbable sutures. The suture line should approximate the full thickness of ileum to ileum while inverting the mucosa. If not opened previously, the bladder is incised in a sagittal plane. The anastomosis of the ileum to the native bivalved bladder is easily done when started posteriorly. The anastomosis may be done in a one-or two-layer fashion, always with absorbable suture. Permanent suture should never be used for any cystoplasty because it may serve as a nidus for stone formation. The mesenteric window at the bowel anastomosis is closed to prevent internal herniation.

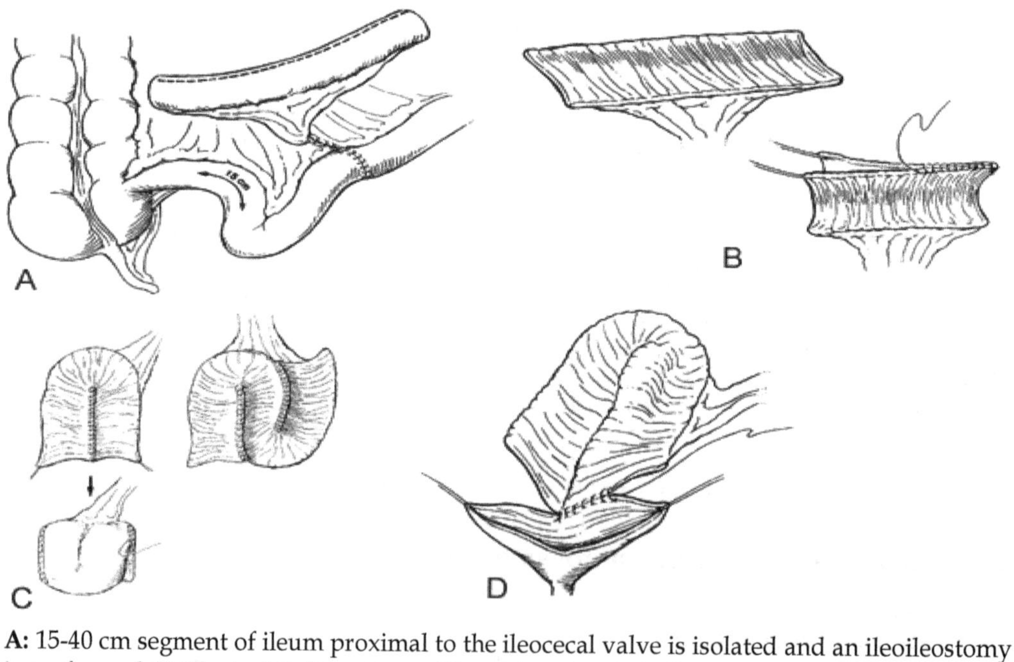

A: 15-40 cm segment of ileum proximal to the ileocecal valve is isolated and an ileoileostomy is performed. **B:** The isolated segment of ileum is opened along the antimesenteric border. The opened segment is then folded and the edges are sutured together. **C:** The opened segment is reconfigured to increase the surface volume. **D:** The reconfigured ileum is anastomosed to the opened bladder beginning at the posterior apex (1).

Ileum does not allow for standard reimplantation of the ureters or the creation of a continent catheterizable channel (i.e., Mitrofanoff), but newer techniques such as the seromuscular trough, as described by Abol-Enein and Ghoneim (22) do allow the use of ileum, should these procedures be required. However, because of its muscle backing, native bladder (or a gastric flap) is still the primary choice for ureteral reimplantation or the construction of a Mitrofanoff valve.
Although the jejunum can be used for urinary reconstruction, yet the high incidence of metabolic complications (hyponatremic, hypochloremic and hyperkalemic acidosis) associated with use of this segment make it less desirable and thus rarely used.

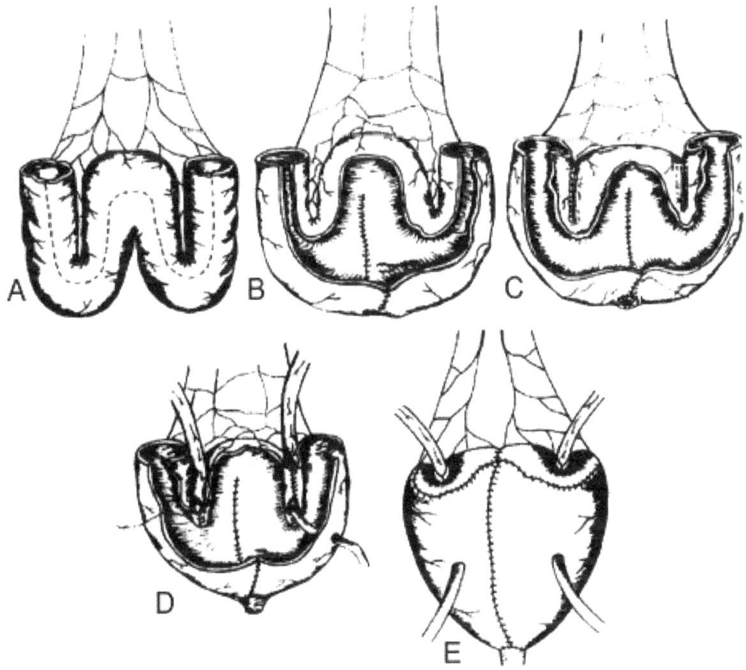

The seromuscular trough formed by anastomosing the edges of the ileum together allows for nonrefluxing ureteral reimplantation into the ileum (22).

3.1.2 Advantages

Ileum is the most commonly used bowel segment for bladder augmentation, as it is:'1) available in large quantity, 2) ease in handling and reconfiguration, 3) has a predictable and abundant blood supply, 4) most compliant segment of bowel, 5) produces moderate mucus compared to colon, 6) causes less severe metabolic complications than colon or stomach, 7) has fewer GI complications than cecum,

3.1.3 Disadvantages

The disadvantages in using ileum include: 1) occasional short mesentery that cannot reach the pelvis, 2) possible development of diarrhea and vitamin B_{12} deficiency, 3) difficulty with creation of submucosal tunnels, 4) hyperchloremic, hypokalemic melabolic acidosis, 5) bowel obstruction, 6) stone formation, 7) mucus production, 8) urinary tract infections, 9) tumor formation which is a risk with large bowel segments as well (14).

3.2 Sigmoid cystoplasty

3.2.1 Technical considerations

Use of the sigmoid colon for augmentation cystoplasty was first reported by Lemoine in 1912 (Q.15) and until nowadays continues to be used commonly.

Because of the strong unit contractions of the sigmoid, it is imperative to detubularize and reconfigure the segment used to provide maximal compliance and disruption of contractions. Fifteen to 20 cm of sigmoid colon is identified and mobilized. Its mesentery is transilluminated to identify the vascular arcade, after which the surgeon must ensure that the segment can reach the bladder without tension. If so, the bowel segment is divided between clamps and a colocolostomy perfomed. Detubularization and reconfiguration is done in a fashion determined by the surgeon's preference. The sigmoid patch is anastomosed to the bivalved bladder.

Sigmoid colon segments are usually reconfigured in one of two ways. Mitchell (1986) suggested closing the two ends and then opening the segment longitudinally opposite its blood supply (23). The segment easily fits on the bivalved bladder. The bowel segment may fit better in either the sagittal or the coronal plane. More radical reconfiguration, and perhaps breakup of unit contractions, may be achieved by folding the sigmoid segment in a U-Shape.

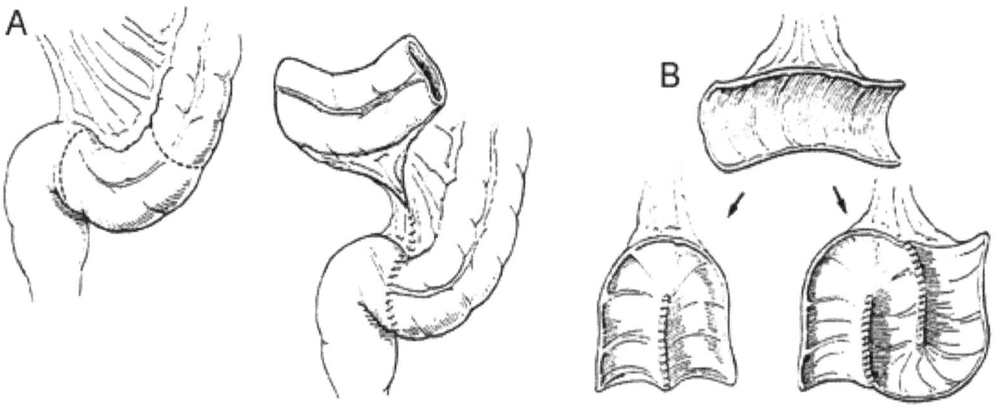

A: A segment of the sigmoid is resected and bowel continuity is reestablished. **B:** The isolated segment of sigmoid is opened on its antimesenteric border and then reconfigured before being anastomosed to the bladder (4).

3.2.2 Advantages

The major advantage of the use of sigmoid colon is the redundancy that is present especially in the spina bifida population. The mobile portion of the sigmoid is so redundant in these children that it often lays in the right lower quadrant. It can be easily opened and reconfigured into a U-shape to increase compliance. The thicker muscle can be used for an antirefluxing ureteral anastomosis as well as for placement of a tunneled continent catheterizable.

3.2.3 Disadvantages

The major disadvantage of the use of the sigmoid colon is the lessened ability to create a large capacity, compliant reservoir. The diameter of the sigmoid may be only similar to the ileum. In certain circumstance, at least a 20 to 30 cm segment of colon is required to create a large enough reservoir. This amount of sigmoid colon can occasionally be difficult to obtain in the non-spina bifida population. In the Indiana series, the highest spontaneous perforation rate occurred among those with sigmoid cystoplasties (19). However, this has not been observed in other large series. Finally hyperchloremic acidosis is more common when the sigmoid colon is employed, compared to other bowel segments. Frequently, these patients will need lifelong alkalinizing agents but this can also be true after ceco or ileocystoplasty as well (24).

3.3 Cecocystoplasty and ileocecocystoplasty

3.3.1 Technical considerations

Couvelair described the use of the cecum for augmentation cystoplasty in 1950 (Q.15). Numerous reports of simple cecocystoplasty have appeared since then. Presently, cecocystoplasty is an uncommon operative procedure; it has largely been replaced by various forms of ileocecocystoplasty.

With the ileocecocystoplasty technique, the cecum is opened, reconfigured, and used to augment the bladder alone, leaving a segment of ileum to reach the ureters or to create a continent abdominal wall stoma based on imbrication of the ileocecal valve and proximal ileum. Conversely, the ileal segment can be opened and used as a patch on the cecal segment before augmentation cystoplasty. Many modifications of the technique exist, but all start with mobilization of the cecum and right colon by incising the peritoneum along the white line of Toldt up to the hepatic flexure. Approximately 15 to 30 cm of the terminal ileum is used. The length of the ileal segment depends on the technique employed. As with all intestinal cystoplasties, before division of the bowel segment, it should be certain that it will reach the bladder without tension.

The isolated ileocecal segment is irrigated clear with neomycin solution and opened on its antimesenteric border through the ileocecal valve for its entire length. In the typical ileocecal augmentation, the ileal and cecal segments are of equivalent length such that the borders of the open segment can be anastomosed and then folded on themselves to form a cup cystoplasty. The anastomosis of the reconfigured segments is done in a one-or two-layer closure with absorbable suture. The opening should be left large enough to provide a wide anastomosis to the bivalved bladder. If more volume is necessary, the ileal segment can be significantly lenghtened, allowing it to be folded before anastomosis to the cecum. The Mainz ileocystoplasty uses an ileal segment twice the length of the cecal segment. The opened edge of the cecal portion is anastomosed to the first portion of the ileal segment. The first and second portions of the ileal segment are next approximated. The compound ileocecal patch is then anastomosed to the bladder.

The ileocecal segment has been used extensively for reconstruction and bladder replacement in the adult population. It has been used less frequently in children because most of the patients undergoing augmentation cystoplasty are doing so because of neurovesical dysfunction. Those patients usually have neuropraxic bowel dysfunction as well. Removal of the ileocecal valve in such children can result in intractable diarrhea (24, 25). Use of the ileocecal valve in such patients should be avoided unless other advantages of the segment outweigh the risk of diarrhea and fecal incontinence.

3.3.2 Advantages

One potential advantage of ileocecocystoplasy is the presence of the appendix. Particularly in children, the appendix is useful in the creation of a reliable continent abdominal wall

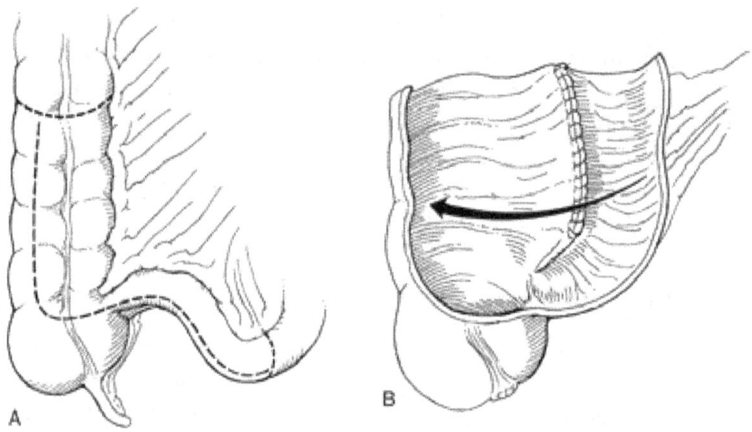

Ileocecocystoplasty. *A)*. An ileocecal segment is selected. The length of segment chosen depends on the technique employed. After removal, it is opened on the antimesenteric border *(dashed lines)*. *B*). The opened ileal and cecal segments are anastomosed to form a cup in the standard ileocecocystoplasty [(15)].

stoma. The appendix may be removed with a small cuff of cecal wall and tunneled into the native bladder or a tenia of the cecal segment to provide a continent mechanism. Likewise, it may be left in situ and the base safely tunneled by creating a window in the mesoappendix. If the appendix is not to be used, an appendectomy is performed with the standard ileocecocystoplasy.

There are further advantages to the use of the ileocecal segment. Antireflux tunnels can easily be made into the tenia of the cecum when necessary. Again, for the short ureter, a tail of ileum can be left intact to bridge the gap, with the imbricated ileocecal valve used for antireflux. The same imbrication technique can be used to create a continent abdominal wall stoma as with the appendix. Cain and Husmann (1994) and Cain et al (1999) have proposed using the ileocecal segment for augmentation with the plicated ileal segment brought to the abdominal wall as a catheterizable stoma, as in the Indiana pouch [(26,27)]. Another major advantage of these segments is the use of a portion of bowel that has a large diameter resulting in a capacious and compliant reservoir that often fits the bladder base rather nicely. It also has a well-defined reliable blood supply.

3.3.3 Disadvantages

The major disadvantage to the use of the ileocecal segment is related to the loss of the ilieocecal valve. Patients with neurologic disorders or short gut often have an increased incidence of diarrhea and difficulty with fecal continence. In addition, this segment is not available in the cloacal exstrophy population who has little to no hindgut. The ileocecal segment also reabsorbs urinary wastes which may result in hyperchloremic acidosis. Finally, cecum usually produces more mucus than the ileum which can lead to increased infections and stone formation.

3.3.4 Summary

Through the early 1980s, the cecum and sigmoid colon were more commonly used than ileum for enterocystoplasy. However, because of the shorter mesenteries, increased mucus production, and difficulty with configuration that is associated with large bowel, ileum has come to be the preferred segment of bowel for enterocystopasty for most surgeons. However, detubulairzed large bowel is still used for simple bladder augmentation in select patients [14].

3.4 Gastrocystoplasty

3.4.1 Technical considerations

Two basic techniques exist for the use of stomach in bladder augmentation. Leong and Ong (1972) described the use of the entire gastric antrum with a small rim of body for bladder replacement. With their technique, the left gastroepiploic artery is always used as a vascular pedicle. If the right gastroepiploic artery is dominant and the left vessel ends high on the greater curvature, a strip of body along the greater curvature from the left gastroepiploic artery to the antrum is maintained and provides adequate blood supply. Continuity of the upper gastrointestinal tract is restored by a Billroth I gastroduodenostomy [28].

In the second type of gastrocystoplasly, a gastric wedge based on the midportion of the greater curvature is used [29]. The gastric segment used in this technique is made up mainly of body and consequently has a higher concentration of acid-producing cells. The right or left gastroepiploic artery may be used as a vascular pedicle to this segment. The right artery is commonly dominant and therefore is more frequently used. The wedge-shaped segment of stomach includes both anterior and posterior wall. The segment used may be 10 to 20 cm along the greater curvature, depending on patient age and size as well as the needed volume.

The incision into the stomach is stopped just short of the lesser curvature to avoid injury to branches of the vagus nerve that control the gastric outlet. Branches of the left gastric artery just cephalad to the apex of this incision are suture ligated in situ before incision to avoid significant bleeding. Parallel atraumatic bowel clamps are placed on either side of the gastric incisions to avoid excessive bleeding or spillage of gastric contents. Alternatively, the stomach may be incised using a gastrointestinal stapling device that places a double row of staples, on each side of the incision [30]. The staple lines, however, must be excised. The native stomach is closed in two layers using permanent sutures on the outer seromuscular layer.

The short gastric branches of the gastroepiploic artery to the antrum on the right or to the high corpus on the left are divided to provide mobilization of the gastroepiploic pedicle leaving the short gastric branches to the augmentation segment intact. In order that the eventual pedicle would be long enough to reach the bladder, the appropriate segment may be higher on the greater curvature if the right vessel is used as a pedicle, or lower if based on the left.

The vascular pedicle, with omentum, should not be free-floating through the abdomen. The segment and pedicle may be passed through windows in the transverse mesocolon and mesentery of the distal ileum and carefully secured to the posterior peritoneum. Despite careful consideration for an adequate pedicle length, on occasion the gastric segment initially does not reach the bladder without tension. Either gastroepiploic artery may be mobilized closer to its origin for further length. The first few branches from the gastroepiploic artery to the isolated gastric segment may also be divided. Because of the rich submucosal arterial plexus in the stomach, devascularization of the isolated segment does not result. Rarely, it may be necessary to approximate some of the isolated gastric segment to itself in one corner. The gastric segment should be approximated to the native bladder with one or two layers of absorbable sutures, taking care to invert the mucosa. Usually the gastric wedge fits well with the bivalved bladder.

Raz and colleagues (1993) have described the use of a much longer, narrower segment of stomach based along the greater curvature. Use of this segment, which includes both body and antrum, somewhat narrows the lumen of the stomach in its entire length except at the fundus and pylorus [31] Raz and colleagues (1993) isolated this segment with the use of a gastrointestinal stapler so that the native stomach was never open. Histamine 2 receptor blockers are often given in the early postoperative period to promote healing [31].

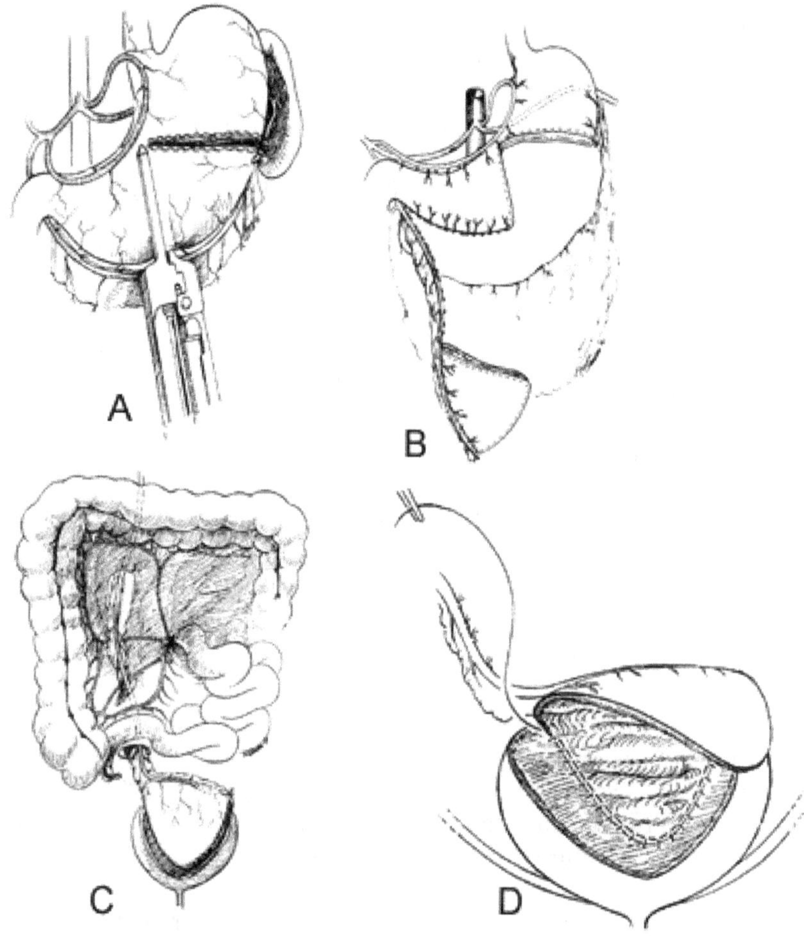

A). A wedge from the body of the stomach is harvested with a stapling device. B). The gastric wedge usually is based on the blood supply from the right gastroepiploic vessel. C). The gastric wedge is brought through the transverse colon and small bowel mesentery to reach the bladder. D). The gastric wedge is sutured to the bladder in two layers [1].

3.4.2 Patient selection for gastrocystoplasty

The stomach is unique with special physiologic and metabolic properties. Given the specific advantages and disadvantages that gastric segments exhibit in comparison to intestinal segments, gastrocystoplasty appears to be most appropriate for patients with renal insufficiency and for those with short intestines, as well as in patients with cloacal exstrophy. Also since the development of the hematuria dysuria syndrome is fairly common following gastrocystoplasty, this type of augmentation is most appropriate in patients who have minimal or no perineal and urethral sensation. If gastrocystoplasty is performed in patients that are sensate, it is important to ensure that patients are completely continent. Caution should be exercised when considering gastrocystoplasty in a patient with end stage renal disease in need of transplantation since ulcer formation and perforation of defunctionalized bladders have been reported [32]. In general, patients that fulfill the preoperative criteria for conventional enterocystoplasty can also be considered candidates for gastrocystoplasty.

3.4.3 Advantages

Surgically, the stomach is relatively thick and easy to work with. It is readily accessible and has a rich reliable vascular supply. The suppleness of the stomach and the well-defined submucosal plane makes it ideal for reimplantation of ureters and continent catheterizable stomas. Use of stomach for bladder augmentation has clear advantages in patients with renal insufficiency due to its ability to secrete acid. This allows for buffering of systemic acidosis and lessens the need for bicarbonate supplementation. The resultant acid urine also appears to decrease the incidence of bacteriuria.

In comparison to other intestinal segments, there is also decreased mucus production and stone formation. The inherent musculature of the gastric segment may also offer an additional advantage over small and large bowel in more often allowing for spontaneous voiding that can result in more efficient emptying, less residual urine, and decreased need for intermittent catheterization. [33, 34]. Lastly both gastrocystoplasty and ileocystoplasty can be accomplished laparoscopically which offers significant advantages in more rapid patient recovery following surgery [35].

3.4.4 Disadvantages

The main disadvantage of gastrocystoplasty that currently limits its widespread use in children with a neuropathic bladder is the high incidence of hematuria dysuria syndrome. This is most troublesome in patients that have a sensate urethra and perineum. Caution should be exercised in selecting patients who are sensate and are at risk for incontinence (i.e. bladder exstrophy) when other enteric segments are available.

3.4.5 Results

The urodynamic results of gastrocystoplasty are somewhat variable. Most authors report that it is useful in increasing capacity and compliance similar to large and small bowel [36]. In studies that have analyzed both pre- and postoperative urodynamics, gastrocystoplasty has been shown to increase bladder capacity by approximately 150 to 200 percent [37, 38]. However it should be noted that there is a wide range of results reported with regard to increased bladder capacity following gastrocystoplasty. In a recent series comparing the urodynamic findings and clinical outcomes following augmentation with stomach versus intestine, it was shown that both stomach and intestine are efficacious in improving compliance but that the use of ileum and colon results in a higher volume reservoir. Intestinal segments appear to expand more readily following augmentation than the stomach [39]. Some of the differences in the literature regarding improvements in capacity and compliance following gastrocystoplasty may be in part explained by variable amounts of stomach that are harvested in individual patients. However, less volume expansion seems inherent to gastric segments compared to ileum and colon.

3.4.6 Summary

Gastrocystoplasty is a useful procedure in the management of children with a neuropathic bladder. However, it has unique properties and potential complications from those seen with conventional enterocystoplasty. From the available experience, it appears that gastrocystoplasty is best suited for patients with renal insufficiency and metabolic acidosis, patients with a small amount of bowel available for augmentation, and patients with an insensate urethra and perineum. Despite some of the metabolic and physiologic advantages of gastrocystoplasty, potential disadvantages still make ileum the preferred intestinal segment for the majority of patients undergoing enterocystoplasty at this time [14].

3.5 Overall results of gastro-intestinal augmentation cystoplasty

The effect of cystoplasty on the patient should be considered in two main categories. First, the effect of removal of a relatively small portion of the gastrointestinal tract for use in urinary reconstruction must be considered. Any more than rare development of gastrointestinal problems would be prohibitive, even if the results were perfect from the standpoint of the urinary bladder. Second the effect of augmentation cystoplasty on the urinary bladder must be reviewed. The primary goal of augmentation is to provide a compliant urinary reservoir. Therefore the main consideration after augmentation is the storage pressure and capacity that are achieved. Any other effect in the urinary bladder is a side effect or complication that exists because bowel is not a perfect physiologic substitute for native bladder.

3.5.1 Bladder compliance after augmentation

An early lesson of past clinical experience with augmentation cystoplasty is the value of detubularization and reconfiguration of the bowel segment [16, 17]. Bowel in its native, tubular form continues to display peristalsis or mass contraction. The tubular form does not maximize the volume achieved for the surface area of bowel used. Hinman (1988) demonstrated with a mathematical model that the maximum volume achieved for a given surface area occurs when a sphere is created. No finished cystoplasty is a perfect sphere but, it should approach that shape as nearly as possible [16].

Many patients who historically underwent augmentation cystoplasty with a tubular segment of bowel have done well, but there have also been numerous failures caused by continued pressure in the bladder from the segment left in its native form. Some surgeons with extensive experience in augmentation cystoplasty and continent diversion have concluded that ileum is superior to other segments in terms of compliance after augmentation [40, 41, 42].Rare reports have suggested superior results with colon compared to ileum. These reports have involved longer colonic segments that were reconfigured in a U shape. Good results have been achieved with all segments in most cases, and it is more important to use a bowel segment well than to choose a particular bowel segment for every patient.

Lytton and Green (1989) demonstrated mass contractions generating pressures of 60 to 110 cm H_2O in right colon reservoirs despite detubularization (44). Such pressures approach those observed in native cecum (45). Hedlund and coworkers (1984) reported pressures of only 25 cm H_2O in detubularized cecal segments 1 year after reconstruction (46). Placement of an ileal patch on a cecal segment can be a more effective mean of decreasing mass contractions than simple reconfiguration (47).

Sidi and associates (1986) demonstrated early peak bladder pressures of 41 cm H2O after cup-patch sigmoid cystoplasty that improved with time (48). Goldwasser's review of enterocystoplasty using detubularized ileum and colon demonstrated contractions greater than 15 cm H_2O in 42% of patients after ileocystoplasty, compared with, 60% after colocystoplasty(18). Significant contractions, defined as those greater than 40 cm H_2O at a volume of less than 200 ml, were not noted in any of the ileal augmentations but did persist in 10% of cecal cystoplasties. In continent urinary diversion, ileal reservoirs have been noted to have lower basal pressures and less motor activity (24). Cecal reservoirs have been noted to generate more pressure per given volume than ileum despite detubularization and to exhibit more obvious uninhibited contractions (49).

Any problems with pressure after augmentation cystoplasty usually occur because of uninhibited contractions, apparently in the bowel segment. It is extremely rare not to achieve an adequate capacity or flat tonus limb unless a technical error has occurred with use of the bowel segment. Occasionally, a small, scarred pelvis prevents adequate expansion of the augmented bladder. When pressure contractions occur in the bladder after augmentation, they are often noted on a rhythmic or sinusoidal pattern, occasionally with increasing amplitude (15).

For most patients, the pressure contractions noted urodynamically are of theoretical interest only and have not affected the clinical result. Contractions that begin at low amplitude later in filling and progress only near capacity may be of no clinical significance at all. Early contractions of higher pressure may occasionally result in persistent incontinence, delayed perforation, hydronephrosis, or vesicoureteral reflux. If patients have such clinical problems after augmentation, repeat urodynamic testing is necessary.

One cannot assume that the bladder is compliant after augmentation. Rhythmic contractions have been noted postoperatively with all bowel segments, although ileum seems the least likely to demonstrate remarkable urodynamic abnormalities, and stomach the most. Rhythmic contractions after cystoplasty have been noted in up to 62% of patients (39, 50). The segment of stomach initially described for augmentation using the body was much smaller in size than segments of ileum or colon commonly used for cystoplasty. The use of a slightly larger gastric segment that is longer along the greater curvature results in improved urodynamics after augmentation, with less prominent contractions (38, 50). The antral segment of stomach is less likely to demonstrate such contractions (33).

In perhaps the largest experience with pediatric bladder augmentation, Rink and associates (1995) at Indiana University found that approximately 5% of several hundred patients had significant uninhibited contractions after augmentation cystoplasty causing clinical problems. Rink (1995) found that 6% of more than 300 patients required secondary augmentation of a previously augmented bladder for similar problems in long-term follow-up (51). These secondary augmentations represent true failures of the primary cystoplasty, not from any side effect or complication but from failure to achieve the objective capacity and compliance. In that series, sigmoid colon, followed by stomach and then ileum, was most likely to require reaugmentation. It should be noted that a colonic segment closed at the ends and not generally reconfigured otherwise was typically used in that experience. Other studies have suggested that stomach is more likely than colon to require secondary intervention [39].

Bowel Segment	Advantages	Disadvantages
Stomach	1. Previous radiation, short gut 2. Prevents systemic acidosis, salt retention 3. Facilitates tunnels for continence and antireflux 4. Reduces infection 5. May potentiate growth in children	1. Acid secretion salt loss, metabolic alkylosis 2. Hematuria-dysuria syndrome 3. More difficult to use
Jejunum	1. Few, not recommended	1. Salt and water loss, metabolic acidosis
Small Bowel	1. Availability 2. Good compliance 3. Less mucus	1. Metabolic acidosis salt resorption 2. Loss of resorption surface in GI tract (B12, folate) 3. Sometimes difficult to work with (no tunnels)
Cecum	1. Availability 2. Good compliance 3. Potential for tunnels and use of IC valve	1. Metabolic acidosis, salt and water resorption 2. Loss of IC valve may cause diarrhea
Sigmoid	1. Most available 2. Good compliance 3. Potential for tunnels	1. Not available in some patients (radiation, constipation) 2. Metabolic acidosis, salt and water resorption 3. Possible increased potential for rupture

GI, gastrointestinal.

Advantages and disadvantages of specific bowel segments [1]

4. Complications of gastrointestinal cystoplasty

4.1 Complications of bowel segment Isolation

4.1.1 Postoperative bowel obstruction

Postoperative bowel obstruction is uncommon after augmentation cystoplasty, occurring in approximately 3% of patients. The rate of obstruction is equivalent to that noted after conduit diversion or continent urinary diversion [51, 52]. Delicate handling of tissues, closure of mesenteric windows, and elimination of sites of internal herniation help to avoid obstruction. The incidence of bowel obstruction is low regardless of the gastrointestinal segment used and should not influence the choice of a particular segment for enterocystoplasty [15].

4.1.2 Malabsorption abnormalities and diarrhea

Loss of the distal ileum may result in fat malabsorption and decrease bile salt and fat soluble vitamin absorption. The distal ileum and ileocecal valve are important for reabsorption and regulation of bowel function. When fecal losses of bile acids exceed production from the liver, fat malabsorption occurs. Steatorrhea then occurs with possible impaired absorption of lipids and fat soluble vitamins (A, D, E & K).

The diarrhea associated with bile acid irritation of the colon can be severe. The secretary diarrhea is secondary to unabsorbed bile salts, causing active secretion of chloride and water in the colon. Reports of chronic diarrhea after bladder augmentation alone have been rare. Diarrhea can occur after removal of large segments of ileum from the gastrointestinal tract even with the preservation of the ileocecal valve (more than 100 cm). Although the length of the segments typically used for augmentation rarely are problematic unless other problems coexist [53, 54]. The use of a typical colonic segment for augmentation only rarely results in a change in bowel function and is less of a risk than the use of ileum.

Removal of a segment from the gastrointestinal tract that includes the ileocecal valve is the most likely procedure to cause diarrhea. Patients with neurogenic dysfunction have significant diarrhea after such displacement. Roth et al (1995) reported that 23% of patients in their experience had chronic diarrhea after ileocecal urinary diversion and 11% when ileum alone was used [53]. Some children with neurogenic impairment depend on controlled constipation for fecal continence. Removal of the ileocecal valve from the gastrointestinal tract may significantly decrease bowel transit time. Loss of the valve can also allow bacterial backflow into the ileum, and the organisms may interfere with metabolism of fat and vitamin B12.

Oral cholestyramine and a low fat diet can be used to treat the diarrhea. Diarrhea as a result of ileocecal valve resection with decreased transit time can be managed with codeine or lomotil. Some authors reported higher incidence of hypertriglyceridemia and gall stones [54].

4.1.3 Vitamin B12 deficiency

When portions of the alimentary tract are used for urinary reconstruction, nutritional deficiencies can occur. Resection of the terminal ileum can result in vitamin B12 deficiency. Vitamin B 12 (cyanocobalamin) cannot be synthesized by human tissues, so humans must receive their vitamin B12 supply from dietary sources. In the stomach, vitamin B 12 is released from food by hydrochloric acid and digestive enzymes. Intrinsic factor binds to vitamin B12 in the duodenum, and then attaches to receptors in the distal ileum. Vitamin B12 is then stored in the liver and supplies last up to three years.

Deficiency of vitamin B12 causes a megaloblastic anemia and neurologic changes including peripheral neuropathies, optic atrophy, degenerative changes of the spinal cord, and dementia in the late stages [54]. Several reports in the literature describe patients in whom the terminal ileum is resected for urinary diversion with a 3.3 to 20 percent incidence of vitamin B12 deficiency [55]. Fifty centimeters of ileum appear to be the critical length, with larger resections of small bowel placing the patient at risk for vitamin deficiency [56]. Neurological symptoms may occur before serum levels are depressed and without megaloblastic anemia. Pannek and associates recommend starting therapy with 100 mcg of hydroxycobalamin injected intramuscularly monthly one year after surgery for patients losing more than 50cm of terminal ileum (56).

4.2 Metabolic complications of gastrointestinal augmentation cystoplasty

To understand the potential complications of gastrointestinal cystoplasty, one must take into account many factors. These factors include the length and the type of intestinal segment, the general health of the patient, the time urine is in contact with bowel mucosa, and the basic underlying renal and hepatic function.

Serum electrolyte abnormalities are dependent upon the segment of bowel used. Other factors include the constituents of urine in the augmented bladder which depend on many factors including fluid intake, diet and intercurrent illness, gastroenteritis, and dehydration (57).

4.2.1 Hyperchloremic metabolic acidosis

Ileum and colon have similar solute transport properties. Normal urine has higher potassium and hydrogen ion concentration and a lower sodium concentration than normal intestinal contents.

Hydrogen ions in the urine must be excreted with a buffer. As a patient becomes acidotic, the kidneys initially excrete acid buffered with phosphates or sulfates, or titratable acids. As the acidosis becomes chronic however, the kidney generates ammonia (NH3) from the conversion of glutamine to alpha-ketoglutarate. Ammonia buffers the free hydrogen ion and becomes ammonium, NH_4^+. Ileal and colonic mucosa will therefore secrete sodium and bi-carbonate and absorb hydrogen, chloride, and ammonium upon exposure to urine, resulting in the development of a hyperchloremic metabolic acidosis (57). Patients with good underlying renal function can overcome this acid reabsorption by excreting even more urinary acid.

The majority of the acid load following augmentation cystoplasty is the result of the net ammonium absorption. Ammonia, ionized ammonium and chloride are absorbed when ileum or colon is exposed to urine, and the majority of the acid load is from the absorbed ammonium chloride. Ammonium and hydrogen are then transported with chloride to maintain electric neutrality (58).

In 1987, Mitchell and Piser noted that essentially every patient after augmentation with an intestinal segment had an increase in serum chloride and a decrease in serum bicarbonate level, although full acidosis was rare if renal function was normal (4). Mild metabolic acidosis is found in 15 percent of patients with ileal conduit diversions. As many as ten percent of patients with ileal conduits require therapy for persistent acidosis. Similarly, 10 to 15 percent of patients with colon conduits develop acidosis. Due to increased urine contact time, metabolic acidosis after bladder replacement with ileum is found in 50 percent of cases. Over 50 percent of colonic reservoirs also have some degree of hyperchloremic metabolic acidosis. Initial reports of ureterosigmoidostomy patients indicate that they have as much as an 80 percent incidence of metabolic acidosis. The risk of acidosis also appears to correlate directly with length of bowel used (54, 59).

The absorptive properties of the intestinal segment may diminish over time. Histological changes occur, including mucosal atrophy and decreased villous height. These histologic findings are believed to cause a reduced absorptive capacity of bowel, however, other studies demonstrate no change in absorptive capacity of the intestinal segment despite histological changes [60]. Most likely, the majority of individuals with metabolic derangement do not develop significant changes in electrolyte transport to protect them from untoward complications.

Patients may present with signs and symptoms of fatigue, diarrhea, weight loss, anorexia, and polydipsia. Laboratory studies demonstrate a significant non-anion gap acidosis with hyperchloremia and azotemia. Arterial blood gases values are more sensitive than serum bicarbonate or chloride levels for detection and early management of acidosis [61].

Acute management includes prompt drainage with treatment of any underlying urinary tract infection and correction of any electrolyte abnormalities. Treatment of mild and chronic forms of metabolic acidosis involves the use of alkalizing agents. Sodium bicarbonate and sodium citrate are useful in restoring acid-base balance. They, however, have untoward side effects, with sodium bicarbonate producing considerable gas and sodium citrate being very distasteful. To neutralize the acid load, supplementation of 1 -2 mEq kg/day of alkali is usually sufficient. In patients with refractory hyperchloremic metabolic acidosis, and those who cannot tolerate or have a contraindication to the alkalizing agents, chlorpromazine has been used successfully in an adult patient with refractory metabolic acidosis. Chlorpromazine and nicotinic acid inhibit cyclic adenosine monophosphate and thereby inhibit chloride transport and absorption in canine models [62]. The usefulness of these agents in humans has not been clinically validated.

4.2.2 Hypokalemia

Hypokalemia can occur in patients with augmentation cysloplasty. The depletion of potassium stores is likely due to the renal wasting of potassium and the chronic metabolic acidosis which causes intracellular potassium depletion. Compared to colon, ileal segments have been shown to have a greater ability to reabsorb potassium when exposed to high concentrations of the ion in urine. Chronic diarrhea may be also a contributing factor for hypokalemia.

The treatment is exogenous potassium replacement. Once the acidosis is corrected, there will be an influx of potassium into the cell because of the extracellular potassium shift. This can lead to profound hypokalemia if not recognized and treated promptly.

4.2.3 Hypocalcemia / Hypomagnesemia

Hypocalcemia and hypomagnesemia are uncommon complication of augmentation cysloplasty. Chronic metabolic acidosis causes loss of calcium from several mechanisms. Symptoms include tetany, tremors and irritability. Treatment consists of calcium replacement either enterally or parenterally depending on the severity. Hypomagnesemia, however uncommon, is due to malabsorption, renal loss, and decreased renal tubular absorption with acidosis. Symptoms are similar to hypocalcemia and the treatment again is exogenous replacement [57].

4.2.4 Ammioniagenic encephalopathy

Urinary ammonium excreted by the kidneys is reabsorbed by the intestinal segment, and then returned to the liver via the portal circulation. The liver metabolizes ammonium to urea via the ornithine cycle. The liver usually adapts to the excess ammonia in the portal circulation without difficulty and rapidly metabolizes it. In the setting of hepatic dysfunction, the hepatic reserve for ammonium metabolism may be exceeded, resulting in the rare complication of ammoniogenic coma. The syndrome also has been described in patients with normal hepatic function [63].

Systemic bacteremia, with endotoxin production, inhibits hepatic function and may precipitate this clinical entity. Urinary tract infections with urea-splitting organisms may also overload the ability of the liver to clear the ammonia. If this syndrome occurs in a patient suspected of having normal hepatic function, systemic bacteremia or obstruction of urinary drainage should be suspected.

Good urinary drainage and treatment of the offending urinary pathogens usually prevents development of the syndrome. Treatment consists of prompt drainage with a Foley catheter. Systemic antibiotics treat the possible underlying infection, and neomycin or lactulose is given to reduce absorption of ammonia in the gastrointestinal tract [54].

4.2.5 Bone disease and retarded growth

A potential long-term complication of intestinal diversion is bone demineralization. This clinical entity was initially found in children developing rickets after ureterosigmoidostomy, but has also been noted in adults with osteomalacia following ureterosigmoi-dostomy, ileal replacement of ureters, and coloplasty [64]. In rickets and osteomalacia, bone mineral loss is replaced with osteoid resulting in decreased bone strength. Fortunately, severe defects in bony demineralization are not common.

The cause of bone demineralization appears complex and multi-factorial, with changes in acid-base balance being the major contributing factor. In chronic acidosis, bone serves to buffer the excess acids. Bone minerals released into the circulation, including carbonate and phosphate, buffer the hydrogen ions, decreasing the axial skeleton calcium content. Systemic acidosis also appears to inhibit the conversionof of 25 hydroxycholecalciferol to 1,25 dihydroxycholecalciferol and appears to activate osteoclasts producing further bone resorption. Additionally, patients with urinary diversions have increased excretion of calcium and sulfate. Sulfate has been shown to cause increased excretion of calcium by the kidneys. The effect of sulfate is potentiated by acidosis. Chronic metabolic acidosis therefore results in negative calcium and phosphate balances [65].

Changes in acid-base status may be subtle with patients displaying only a minimal decrease or normal serum calcium and magnesium level and mild depression of serum bicarbonate level. Most patients who present are asymptomatic; however, they may have occult bone mineral defects that place the patient at higher risk for increased orthopedic morbidity.

The diagnosis can be particularly difficult to detect. Parathormone and vitamin D levels are typically normal, and radiologic examination is usually unremarkable. Post-menopausal women and children are at high risk for bone demineralization with several studies showing a reduction in growth potential for children following enterocystoplasty.

Patients presenting with rickets or osteomalacia should have correction of their acid-base disturbance first. Vitamin D and calcium supplements are then used if remineralization does not occur. Administration of vitamin C or oral alkalizing agents to children with urinary diversion may help reinforce normal bone development and prevent bone destruction [66].

4.2.6 Drug absorption toxicities

Absorption of drugs excreted in urine from bowel segments can cause toxicities. One must be aware of the potential toxicities that can result from absorption of active drug such as methotrexate or metabolites in patients with augmentation cystoplasty [54].

4.2.7 Hypochloremic alkalosis

Significant metabolic derangement can occur with gastric diversions. In contrast to ileum or colonic cystoplasty the stomach excretes chloride. This can lead to profound hypochloremic, hypokalemic alkalosis. It has been proposed that the alkalosis results from ongoing chloride loss from the gastric segment in the bladder in the face of decreased oral intake. The decreased ability to excrete bicarbonate from an impaired kidney may compound the problem. Gosalbez and associates (1993) demonstrated persistently increased traditional excretion of chloride despite profound hypochloremia, suggesting that inappropriate gastric secretion is probably the primary problem [39].

Patients may present with lethargy, mental status changes, intractable seizures, and respiratory compromise related to a compensatory respiratory acidosis [39]. Patients are prone to suffer from severe dehydration secondary to a loss of fluid, chloride, and potassium from the gastric segment. A simple viral gastroenteritis illness may trigger severe symptoms of dehydration and alkalosis.

Replacement with normal saline and correction of serum potassium abnormalities usually corrects the metabolic abnormalities. Patients should maintain good oral and normal salt intake. Additional oral salt and potassium supplementation may be needed. Histamine-2 blockers and anticholinergic therapy may also be needed in patients with low-grade alkalosis. Refractory episodes of hypokalemic, hypochloremic metabolic alkalosis may be treated with inhibiting K+/H+ exchange with such agents as omeprazole.

4.2.8 Hematuria-dysuria syndrome

Acid secretion by gastric mucosa may result in another unique problem after gastrocystoplasty, the hematuria-dysuria syndrome. Virtually all patients with normal sensation after gastrocystoplasty have occasional hematuria or dysuria with voiding or catheterization beyond that which is expected with other intestinal segments. All patients should be warned of this potential problem, although in most the symptoms are intermittent and mild and do not require treatment. Avoidance of gastrocystoplasty in patients with bladder exstrophy is recommended. The dysuria is certainly not a problem in patients with neurogenic dysfunction.

In the experience of Nguyen and coworkers (1993), 36% of patients developed signs or symptoms of the hematuria-dysuria syndrome after gastrocystoplasty; 14% required treatment with medications, 9% on a regular basis. They believed that patients who are incontinent or have decreased renal function are at increased risk [67]. The symptoms of the hematuria-dysuria syndrome respond well to administration of H_2 blockers and hydrogen ion pump blockers. Bladder irrigation with baking soda may also be effective. It has been demonstrated that urinary pH may decrease remarkably after meals in those who have undergone gastrocystoplasty.

The signs and symptoms of the hematuria-dysuria syndrome are most likely secondary to acid irritation. Acid in urine may cause external irritation and skin excoriation. Recent work has suggested that *Helicobacter pylori* may play a role in this complication, as it may increase acid complications in the native stomach [68]. Such problems are less frequent after antral cystoplasty, where there is a smaller load of parietal cells.

4.2.9 Mucus production

Intestinal segments continue to produce mucus after placement in the urinary tract. The proteinaceous material can potentially impede bladder drainage during voiding or CIC, particularly in pediatric patients who must use small-caliber catheters. Mucus may serve as a nidus for infection or stone formation when it remains in the bladder for long periods. Mucus production often increases after cystoplasty in the presence of cystitis. Colonic segments produce more mucus than ileum and gastric segments produce the least amount. Most patients do not require any routine bladder irrigations for mucus after gastrocystoplasty. Villous atrophy in the ileum has been documented after long-term placement in the urinary tract. It has been suggested that such atrophy may result in decreased mucus production

Hendren and Hendren (1990) noted a decrease in mucus production from colonic segments over years [3], however, others have not been impressed with such changes [51]. Glandular atrophy in colonic mucosa has not been noted histologically. Routine use of daily bladder irrigations to prevent mucus build up may minimize complications of enterocystoplasty such as urinary tract infection and calculi.

4.2.10 Urinary tract infection

Bacteriuria is very common after intestinal cystoplasty, particularly among patients requiring CIC. Recent experience with bowel neobladders has demonstrated that patients who are able to spontaneously void to completion frequently maintain sterile urine. It appears that the use of CIC is a prominent factor in the development of bacteriuria after augmentation cystoplasty; regardless of the segment considered [3, 25].

Bacteriuria has been noted even when patients are maintained on daily oral antibiotics or antibiotic irrigation. Persistent or recurrent bacteriuria occurs in 50% of patients augmented with sigmoid colon, compared with 25% of those undergoing ileocystoplasty. Recurrent episodes of symptomatic cystitis requiring treatment occurred in 23% of patients after cecocystoplasty, 17% after sigmoid cystoplasty, 13% after cecocystoplasty and 8% after gastrocystoplasty. Febrile attacks occurred in 13% [51].

Not every episode of asymptomatic bacteriuria requires treatment in patients performing CIC. Bacteriuria should be treated for significant symptoms such as incontinence or suprapubic pain and perhaps for hematuria, foul-smelling urine, or remarkably increased mucus production. Bacteriuria should be treated if the urine culture demonstrates growth of a urea-splitting organism that may lead to stone formation.

4.2.11 Calculus disease

Patients with augmentation cystoplasty are at risk for upper and lower urinary tract calculus disease. These patients are chronically dehydrated from water loss through the diversion producing concentrated urine which may be a nidus for stone disease. Additionally urinary stasis, mucous production from the intestinal segment and frequent colonization with urea-spitting organisms places the patient at risk [3]. Patients in whom large segments of ileum have been removed may develop enteric hyperoxaluria which places the patient at risk for calcium oxalate stone formation. Hypocitraturia a risk factor for stone disease may be found in patient with chronic metabolic acidosis and malabsorption abnormalities. Hypercalciuria is a result of the acidosis, and can lead to mobilization of calcium from bone and impaired reabsorption from acid renal tubule fluid.

Several series reported calculi in 18% of patients after augmentation cystoplasty [3, 43]. Patients catheterizing through an abdominal wall stoma had the highest risk, probably because of incomplete emptying. Palmer and associates (1993) noted urolithiasis in 52% of patients after augmentation cystoplasty. Rink and colleagues (1995) noted only an 8% rate of bladder stone formation in 231 patients with long-term follow-up after enterocystoplasty [(51)]. The reasons for these remarkable differences are not clear. Stones have been noted after the use of all intestinal segments, with no significant difference noted between small and large intestine. Struvite stones are less likely after gastrocystoplasty probably because of decreased mucus production and acid that minimizes bacteriuria. Uric acid calculi have rarely been noted in the bladder after gastrocystoplasty [(37)].

Patients should be instructed to keep adequately hydrated. Staples and nonabsorbable sutures should be avoided in the urinary diversion. Infection with urea-splitting organisms should be treated promptly. Patients should be instructed in the importance of regular reservoir catheterizing. Irrigation may be needed if one produces excessive amounts of mucous. Foods high in oxalate should be avoided in patients with enteric hyperoxaluria. Calcium citrate may be given to bind oxalate in the gut reducing its absorption. A low fat diet may reduce calcium saponification and increase the amount of calcium available to bind oxalate.

4.3 Long-term complications

4.3.1 Tumor formation

A well recognized complication of ureterosigmoidostomy has been the development of tumors, primarily adenocarcinoma, at the ureterocolonic anastomotic site. The latency for development of such tumors averaged 26 years and ranged from 3 to 53 years. Adenocarcinomas were the prominent tumors that developed, but benign polyps and other types of carcinoma were also found [(15)]. The exact basis for the increased risk is unknown; however, N-nitroso compounds thought to originate from a mixture of urine and faces may be carcinogenic. These compounds have been noted in the urine of patients with conduit diversion and augmentation [(69)]. Husmann and Spence (1990) suggested that those compounds are more likely enhancing agents rather than a lone cause for tumor development.

It has been proposed that inflammatory reaction at the anastomotic site may induce growth factor production, which, in turn, increases cellular proliferation [(68)]. Filmer and Spencer (1990) identified 14 patients who developed adenocarcinoma in an augmented bladder, and several more have been reported since then. Nine of those tumors occurred after ileocystoplasty and five after colocystoplasty [(70)].

Experimental work in the rat demonstrated hyperplastic growth in the augmented bladder with all intestinal segments, with no segment showing any particularly increased risk [(71)]. The applicability of such findings to humans is uncertain. The long latency period noted for tumor development after ureterosigmoidostomy suggests that short-term follow-up after augmentation cystoplasty is not adequate to evaluate tumor formation.

Patients undergoing augmentation cystoplasty should be made aware of a potentially increased risk for tumor development. Yearly surveillance of the augmented bladder with endoscopy should eventually be performed; the latency period until such procedures are necessary is not well defined. The earliest reported tumor after augmentation was found only 4 years after cystoplasty [(72)]. Transitional cell carcinoma, hyperplasia, and dysplasia have also been noted near the anastomoses in humans. Urine cytology or flow cystometry may ultimately become useful in surveillance [(73)].

4.3.2 Delayed spontaneous bladder perforation

Perhaps the most disturbing complication of augmentation cystoplasty is delayed bladder perforation. Patients presenting with spontaneous perforation after augmentation cystoplasty are usually quite ill with abdominal pain, distention and fever. Sepsis has been common. Nausea, decreased urine output, and shoulder pain from diaphragmatic irritation have also been noted. Perforations have been found in the evaluation of virtually asymptomatic pelvic masses Patients with neurogenic dysfunction often have impaired lower abdominal sensation and present later in the course of the illness; severe sepsis and death have occurred. Patients with perforation after gastrocystoplasty often present promptly because of acid irritation.

A high index of suspicion for perforation is necessary. Contrast cystography is diagnostic in most cases. Thorough technique is important to identify as many true-positive cases as possible with cystography. Some reports of perforations have noted a significant false-negative rate on cystography and suggested that ultrasonography and CT improve diagnostic accuracy. They recommended that one of those studies be done in any child with suspected perforation if the initial cystogram is negative [74, 75].

The cause of delayed perforations within a bowel segment is unknown. It has been suggested that perforation might be secondary to traumatic catheterization in some cases. It seems unlikely that catheterization trauma is the lone cause in most patients. The location of the perforations has been variable among patients and even in a single patient with multiple perforations. Perforations have occurred after augmentation in patients who did not catheterize at all. Others have suggested that trauma to the bowel caused by fixed adhesions that result in sheering forces with emptying and filling may result in perforation [15]. Chronic, transmural infection of the bladder wall has also been proposed as a cause. Histologic examination of bowel segments adjacent to areas of perforation has revealed necrosis, vascular congestion, hemorrhage, and hemosiderin deposition compatible with chronic bowel wall ischemia. Chronic overdistention of the bladder might result in such ischemia. Chronic ischemia may thus play a significant role in at least some delayed bladder perforations.

Pope and associates (1998) reported perforations occurring in bladders with significant uninhibited contractions after augmentation. High outflow resistance may maintain bladder pressure rather than allowing urinary leakage and venting of the pressure, potentially increasing ischemia. Hyperreflexia alone is unlikely as a solitary cause of perforation, because the complication was essentially never recognized in the era before bowel detubularization and reconfiguration, when persistent pressure contractions were more common after augmentation cystoplasty. Once bowel is reconfigured, however, it may be more prone to ischemia if high pressure does persist.

Once spontaneous perforation has occurred, the chance of recurrence is significant. One third of patients with rupture in one series had a recurrence [74]. Consideration must eventually be given to removal of the original segment and replacement by another after repeated perforation.

This problem has been noted with increasing frequency after augmentation cystoplasty and may involve all segments. There may be no particular increased risk of one intestinal segment over another. With the inconsistent differences across multiple large series, it is unlikely that any given enteric segment is at significantly increased risk for perforation and probable that multiple factors influence the risk for the complication [15, 20, 48].

The standard treatment for spontaneous perforation of the augmented bladder is surgical repair, as it is for intraperitoneal rupture of the bladder after trauma. There are reported series of conservative management for suspected perforation consisting of catheter drainage, antibiotics and serial abdominal examinations. It was successful in 87% of patients, although only 2 of 13 patients with suspected rupture had x-ray documentation unequivocally identifying a perforation (74). Even patients who do well with conservative management during the acute episode often require surgical intervention eventually. Such management may be a consideration in a stable patient with sterile urine. The surgeon should certainly have a low threshold for surgical exploration and repair.

Problem	Stomach	Ileum	Colon
Segment loss from GI tract	1. Early satiety 2. Decreased stomach-acid production 3. Increased gastrin production	1. Decreased absorption of B12, folate, and iron 2. Short-gut syndrome	1. Diarrhea 2. Water loss
Acid-base balance	1. Alkalosis 2. Hematuria/dysuria	1. Chronic metabolic acidosis 2. Ammonium and chloride resorption	1. Acidosis 2. Bicarbonate loss 3. Ammonium chloride resorption
Salt balance	1. Sodium and potassium loss	1. Sodium and chloride resorption	1. Sodium and chloride resorption
Mucus	1. More soluble, less apparent	1. Problem with catheter obstruction, irrigation necessary	1. Problem with catheter obstruction, irrigation necessary
Stone formation	1. Rare problem (low pH)	1. Can be a major problem, irrigations recommended	1. Can be a major problem, irrigations recommended
Infection	1. Moderate	1. Common	1. Common
Tumor	1. None documented but too early to tell	1. Reported	1. Significant in ureterosigmoidostomy
Perforation	1. Reported with potential for ulcer formation in anuric or diverted patient	1. Reported, major problem because of potential for infection	1. Reported, major problem because of potential for infection

Metabolic consequences of bladder reconstruction with bowel

5. Alternatives to gastrointestinal cystoplasty

Currently, gastrointestinal segments are commonly used as tissues for bladder replacement or repair. However, gastrointestinal tissues are designed to absorb specific solutes, whereas bladder tissue is designed for the excretion of solutes. As mentioned, when gastrointestinal tissue is in contact with the urinary tract, multiple complications may ensue.

Because of the problems encountered with the use of gastrointestinal segments, numerous investigators have attempted alternative methods, materials, and tissues for bladder replacement or repair. These include autoaugmentation, ureterocystoplasty, methods for tissue expansion, seromuscular grafts, matrices for tissue regeneration and tissue engineering with cell transplantation. Some of these alternatives appear to hold promise, but none has stood the test of time for true comparison to intestinal cystoplasty.

An ideal tissue for increasing capacity and improving compliance would have transitional epithelium so as to be relatively impermeable and avoid metabolic changes. The lining would also prevent mucus production and, probably the increased potential for tumor development. The ability to augment the bladder without violation of the peritoneal cavity would also decrease morbidity. Two such alternative procedures are ureterocystoplasty and autoaugmentation. With ureterocystoplasty, there is good muscle backing of transitional epithelium, whereas collagen eventually backs the transitional mucosa of an autoaugmentation.

5.1 Autoaugmentation

5.1.1 Techniques and results

Cartwright and Snow (1989) described an ingenious method to improve bladder compliance and capacity using native urothelial tissue. In their procedure, known as autoaugmentation they excised detrusor muscle over the dome of the bladder leaving the mucosa intact to protrude as a wide-mouth diverticulum. Initially they made a midline incision through the bladder muscle with the bladder distended with saline so that mucosa bulged from the incision. The muscle was mobilized and excised laterally in each direction. The lateral edges of the detrusor muscle were then secured to the psoas muscle bilaterally to prevent collapse of the diverticulum. Their early experience with a small group of patients resulted in improved compliance in most, with increasing capacity in some [(78)].

This producer has since been modified by a number of surgeons, particularly in adult patients, each providing a different name for the procedure depending on whether the detrusor muscle was simply incised (vesicomyotomy) or excised (vesicomyomectomy) to create the diverticulum. In an effort to determine whether incision or excision provided superior results, Johnson and colleagues (1994) performed 16 vesicomyotomies and 16 vesicomyomectomies in rabbits after previously reducing the bladder capacity. Functional bladder capacity in the animals increased by 43.5%, and there was no statistical difference between the two techniques. They then performed vesicomyotomies (incision) in 12 patients with neurogenic bladder dysfunction and demonstrated a mean increase in capacity of 40% and a mean decrease in leak point pressure of 33% [(78, 80)]. They concluded that detrusor excision offered no advantage over incision. All patients demonstrated some increase in capacity (15% to 70%), and no patient in early follow-up clinically deteriorated and required enterocystoplasty.

Detrusorectomy, leaving a small cap of muscle at the dome through which a suprapubic tube can be placed, was proposed by Landa and Moorhead (1994). They have been concerned that, although these procedures usually improve compliance, the increase in volume is "modest" at best [81].

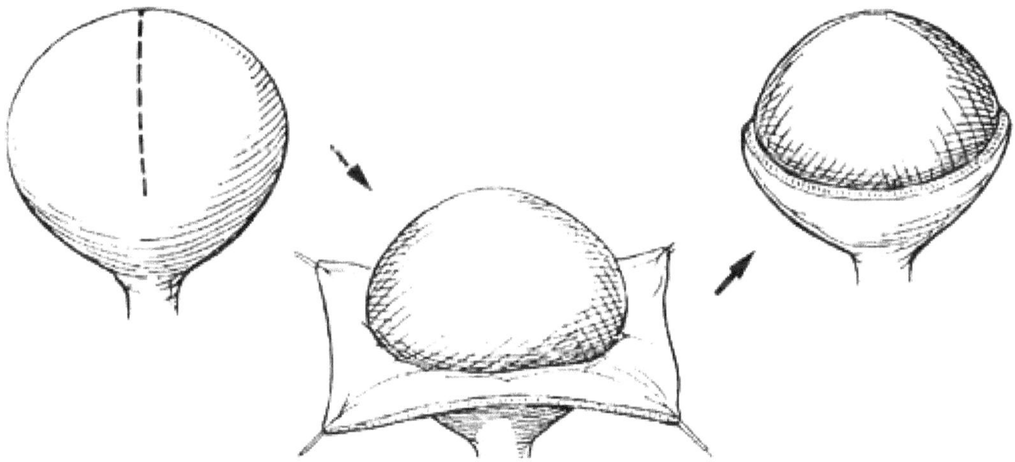

In autoaugmentation, the detrusor is excised leaving the urothelium to act as a diverticulum [1].

The efficacy of autoaugmentation in improving bladder capacity and compliance has been varied. Snow and Cartwright (1999) have follow-up of greater than one year in thirty patients. Nineteen of thirty patients had a neuropathic bladder secondary to spina bifida. All patients had preoperative urodynamic evidence of reduced bladder compliance and detrusor hyperreflexia. While clinical success has been dramatic in some, the overall results have been less impressive. One third of the patients had a significant increase in bladder capacity, an additional third were unchanged, while one third had actual loss of capacity. Evaluation of bladder compliance revealed that 60 percent had an improvement in compliance by greater than 50 percent in comparison to preoperative measurements, 20 percent had a 20 to 50 percent improvement, and the remaining did not change significantly. Overall fourteen patients (47%) had excellent results, showing a significant improvement in compliance, capacity, and dryness. Seven patients (23%) had fair results, described as stability or improvement of the upper tracts without scant improvement in the urodynamic parameters. Nine patients (30%) had poor results, remaining wet or with worsening hydronephrosis [82].

Following autoaugmentation, the majority of patients remained on intermittent catheterization, although 20 percent demonstrated the ability to void spontaneously. Seven patients have required secondary enterocystoplasty following the initial autoaugmentation. Reoperative enterocystoplasty was not hampered by the prior detruseroctomy. The urothelial diverticulum at the time of augmentation cystoplasty was noted to be thick and fibrous similar to a leather bag [82].

5.1.2 Advantages

The primary advantage that autoaugmentation has over conventional enterocystoplasty is that it preserves the patient's native urothelium in the augmented segment. This avoids the complications associated with enterocystoplasty related to the presence of heterotopic epithelium in contact with the urine including electrolyte disturbances, mucus, bladder calculi, hematuria dysuria syndrome, and later tumor occurrences. Technically, autoaugmentation is an extraperitoneal procedure that can be performed through a Pfannestiel incision and avoids the complications of bowel surgery including the development of intraperitoneal adhesions and postoperative bowel obstruction. Although autoaugmentation is performed without a formal cystotomy; other bladder procedures such as ureteral reimplantation and appendicovesicostomy can be performed (intravesically or extravesically) at the same time. Lastly, it is important to note that autoaugmentation does not preclude further augmentation procedures if unsuccessful.

5.1.3 Disadvantages

The major drawback of autoaugmentation is that clinical experience has failed thus far to identify the most appropriate patients for this procedure. Mixed results have been obtained clinically with regard to symptomatic and postoperative urodynamic improvement in the autoaugmented bladder. Evaluations of the available data indicate that there is no direct correlation between preoperative urodynamic findings and future success. It works well in some patients while it fails in others. It is of note that many patients have demonstrated clinical improvement after these procedures without a significant change in urodynamics. The exact reasons for the improvement are unknown.

Another drawbacks of autoaugmentation is a limited increase in bladder capacity. Landa and Moorhead (1994) noted that if the maximum capacity and the volume of urine held at 40 cm H_2O are similar, the patient may be better served by immediate intestinal cysloplasty.. The patient and surgeon must be prepared for such an event on occasion. Even if adequate expansion is achieved initially, there is concern that any improvement may not last in the long term. In animals, the surface area of the autoaugmentation site was observed to decrease by approximately 50% at 12 weeks. Progressive thickening and contractor of the site because of collagenous infiltrate was noted. Almost one-half of is adult patients with hyperreflexia who early on had a good result after autoaugmentation failed with longer follow-up [79].

An additional concern with autoaugmentation is the theoretical increased risk of bladder rupture that has been demonstrated in animal studies. Although perforation of the autoaugmented bladder has been reported in one patient, the overall increased risk of bladder rupture as compared to other types of bladder augmentation has yet to be defined [83].

Inadvertent opening of the mucosa during the procedure can make subsequent mobilization more difficult and may promote prolonged postoperative extravasation. Such extravasation usually stops with bladder drainage. Prolonged drainage, however, may lead to compromised results due to collapse of the diverticulum. If concomitant ureteral reimplantation or bladder neck surgery is necessary, various authors have recommended that such procedures should be done first with the bladder then closed before detrusorectomy.

5.1.4 Patient selection for autoaugmentation

Leng and associates (1999), reported good results with the technique among patients with hyperreflexia[85]. Adequate preoperative volume may be the most important predictor of success. *Autoaugmentation probably should be considered only in patients who have reasonable capacity but poor compliance due to uninhibited contractions*[82]. If a remarkable increase in capacity is needed, autoaugmentation is unlikely to be as definitive as other techniques. However, it should be noted that autoaugmentation has been successful in some patients with a small capacity, poorly compliant bladder.

5.2 Seromuscular grafts and de-epithelialized bowel segments

5.2.1 Technical considerations

Seromuscular grafts and de-epithelialized bowel segments, either alone or over a native urothelium have been attempted [24, 86]. The concept of demucosalizing organs is not new to urologists. More than four decades ago, in 1961, Blandy proposed the removal of submucosa from intestinal segments used for augmentation cystoplasty to ensure that mucosal regrowth would not occur [13].

Hypothetically, this would avoid the complications associated with use of bowel in continuity with the urinary tract. Since Blandy's initial report, 25 years transpired before there was a renewed interest in demucosalizing intestinal segments for urinary reconstruction [87].

Several other investigators have pursued this line of research [24, 86, 88]. These investigative efforts have emphasized the complexity of both the anatomic and cellular interactions present when tissues with different functional parameters are combined. The complexity of these interactions is emphasized by the observation that the use of demucosalized intestinal segments for augmentation cystoplasty is limited by either mucosal regrowth or contraction of the intestinal patch [88].

It has been noted that removal of only the mucosa may lead to mucosal regrowth, whereas removal of the mucosa and submucosa may lead to retraction of the intestinal patch [89].

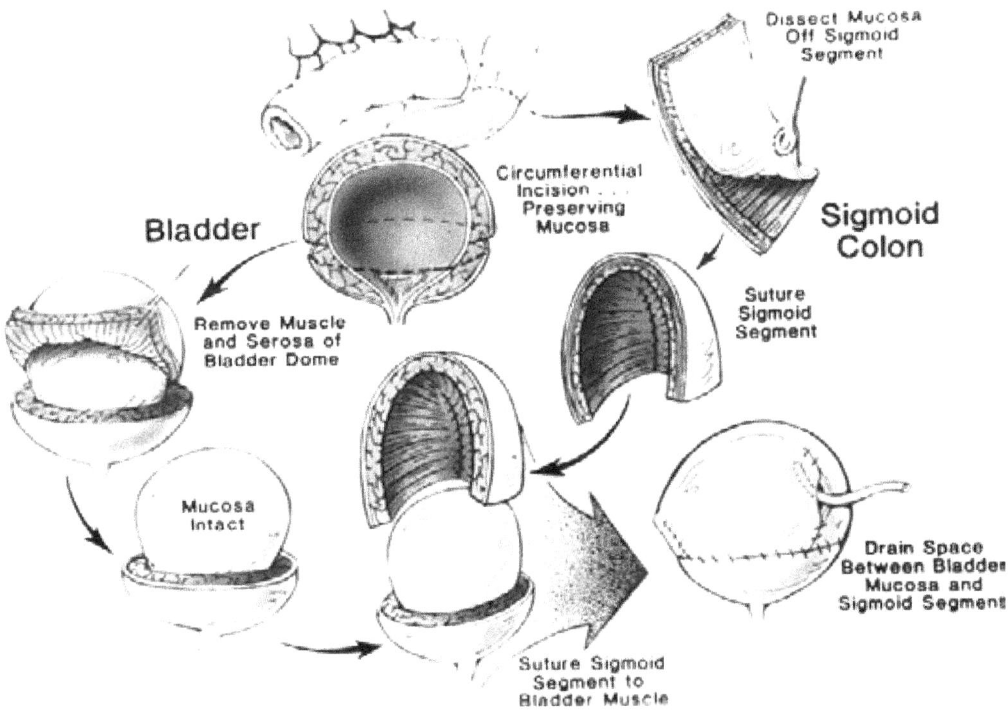

Seromuscular enterocystoplasty using sigmoid colon (SCLU). Detrusor incision is performed similar to autoaugmentation; however, the bulging mucosa is covered with a demucosalized segment of sigmoid colon. (From Buson H, Manivel JC, Dayanc M, et al: Seromuscular colocystoplasty lined with urothelium: Experimental study. Urology 1994;44:745.

Seromuscular enterocystoplasty combines autoaugmentation with a demucosalized flap of colon or stomach. The removal of the gastrointestinal mucosa results in a denuded seromuscular flap that can be placed over the exposed bladder mucosa of an autoaugmented bladder to avoid collagen deposition and contraction. This combination has been done to potentially preserve the advantages of both procedures.

5.2.2 Results

The clinical results of seromuscular enterocystoplasty have been mixed and unpredictable. Initial reports by Dewan and Gonzales in both animal models and humans have been encouraging [24, 86]. In the Gonzales et al series of 16 patients undergoing seromuscular colocystoplasty utilizing sigmoid colon, bladder capacity was increased to almost two and one half times the preoperative volume and end filling-pressures decreased by approximately 50 percent in 14 patients. Two patients failed and required ileocystoplasty their urodynamic data were excluded. Two other patients developed an hourglass deformity [24]. Endoscopic biopsy of the segments was interesting: of 10 biopsies in the series, 1 revealed urothelium with islands of colonic mucosa, and 2 others found only colon mucosa. Removal of all of the enteric mucosa is important when using sigmoid to prevent mucoceles or overgrowth of intestinal mucosa [24].

Dewan and associates (1997) reported on five patients undergoing seromuscular gastrocystoplasty. Four of the five patients have had urodynamic evidence of improved bladder capacity and compliance during the first postoperative year. They believed that preservation of the submucosa eventually promoted regrowth of bowel mucosa. The interaction of the two different tissues will be interesting to follow. The long-term effects on the urothelium by the seromuscular segment and vice versa are unknown. Work has shown that persistent transitional lining will protect from metabolic problems and mucus production [24, 86].

Despite these initial encouraging results, it is important to note that the follow-up in these series has been relatively short and approximately 25 percent of patients have eventually required a secondary operation due to either complication related to the seromuscular flap (contracture) and/or failure to adequately improve bladder capacity and/or compliance [86].

A more recent report of long-term follow-up of 13 patients after seromuscular gastrocystoplasty by Carr et al (1999) describes variable results, at best. The mean follow-up was 50 months. Five patients had a good outcome with regard to objective urodynamic and subjective clinical improvement. Four patients were found to have a "fair" outcome in that they had some objective improvement, while the remaining four patients had a poor result and required re-augmentation [90]. Evaluation of preoperative urodynamic and radiographic data in these patients again demonstrated that it was not possible to predict preoperatively which patients would do well after seromuscular gastrocystoplasty. These procedures are technically more demanding than simple augmentation or autoaugmentation and are associated with more blood loss and a longer operative time [24]. Increased bleeding is particularly likely when using stomach.

These urothelium-lined, seromuscular augmentations are theoretically attractive. Thus far, the failure and reoperation rate after such procedures remains higher than that noted for standard enterocystoplasty [90]. The best results have been reported with the use of colon. Those results may be partially attributed to the learning curve with a new, complex procedure. Longer follow-up and more experience arc necessary to determine whether the complication rate will decrease with experience or increase because of problems with the combination.

In summary, seromuscular enterocystoplasty appears to parallel autoaugmentation that is technically feasible and useful in many patients. However, it has significant shortcomings. It is not possible at this time to define which patients will succeed and which ones will fail. Advantages beyond autoaugmentation appear to be minimal. Further long-term studies are required to determine the true efficacy of this technique. Also, additional studies are needed to determine if there are significant functional differences between seromuscular colocystoplasty and seromuscular gastrocystoplasty.

5.3 Ureterocystoplasty

The use of ureteral tissue for bladder augmentation purposes was first described in 1992 [91]. Native ureter is for many reasons the best tissue available for augmentation cystoplasty. It is autologous, lined with urothelium, backed by muscle, distensible, and complaint [92, 93]. However, not all patients in need of bladder augmentation have dilated ureteral tissue available for use. Patients that are candidates for ureterocystoplasty should have either i) a nonfunctional renal unit that can be removed making the ureter and renal pelvis available, or ii) a functional renal unit that is associated with a massively dilated, tortuous, and elongated ureter. The lower ureter can then be used for augmentation, while kidney drainage is re-established by reimplantation of the straightened upper ureter into the bladder or by transureteroureterostomy.

An example of an ideal candidate is one with vesicoureteral reflux and dysplasia (VURD) syndrome from posterior urethral valves. In patients with posterior urethral valves, unilateral reflux may behave as a "pop-off" valve to lower intravesical pressures and protect the contralateral upper tract. In many of these patients, the refluxing ureter is massively dilated, draining a poorly functioning or nonfunctioning kidney. It was a logical extension to use this ureteral tissue to augment the bladder. Ureterocystoplasty is also appropriate in patients on dialysis with end-stage renal failure who are awaiting transplantation and are in need of augmentation due to bladder dysfunction.

More recently, the use of ureterocystoplasty has been expanded in an attempt to take advantage of this valuable tissue and make it available to more surgical candidates. Its use has been reported in patients with a duplex system in which either the upper or lower pole is nonfunctioning [96]. In patients with a duplex system and a dilated ureter in conjunction with a functioning renal segment, drainage of that segment can be accomplished with an ipsilateral ureteroureterostomy with preservation of the lower portion of the ureter for augmentation. Ahmed et al have also described the "tandem" use of bilateral megaureters for ureterocystoplasty [97].

5.4 Technical considerations

Ureterocystoplasty can be performed through a midline, intraperitoneal incision. This incision provides access to the intestine should mobilization of the ureter be unsatisfactory. Ureterocystoplasty may also be done through two incisions, remaining completely extraperitoneal. The general technique is the same. A standard nephrectomy is performed with great care to preserve the renal pelvic and upper ureteral blood supply. All adventitia and periureteral tissue is swept from the peritoneum toward the ureter during mobilization to protect the ureteral blood supply. Proximally, this blood supply typically arises medially. As the ureter enters the true pelvis, the blood supply arises posteriorly and laterally.

After mobilization of the ureter into the pelvis, the bladder is opened in the sagittal plane. Posteriorly, this incision has typically been carried offcenter directly into and through the ureteral orifice of the ureter used for cystoplasty. The ureter is not detached from the bladder but is opened longitudinally along its entire length, with care taken to avoid its main blood supply. The incision in the bladder and distal ureter should avoid branches of the superior vesical artery, which serves as an important blood supply to the mobilized ureter. The ureter is folded on itself, and the ureter-to-ureter and ureter-to-bladder anastomoses are performed with running absorbable suture.

Alternatively, the bladder incision can be stopped approximately 2 cm from the orifice, with a similar length of distal ureter left in situ and intact without incision. The resulting small loop of intact ureter does not create clinical problems or adversely affect the end volume in a significant manner [20]. This modification of technique is easier and may be safer in that, it avoids potential injury to the blood supply of the mobilized ureter near the ureterovesical junction.

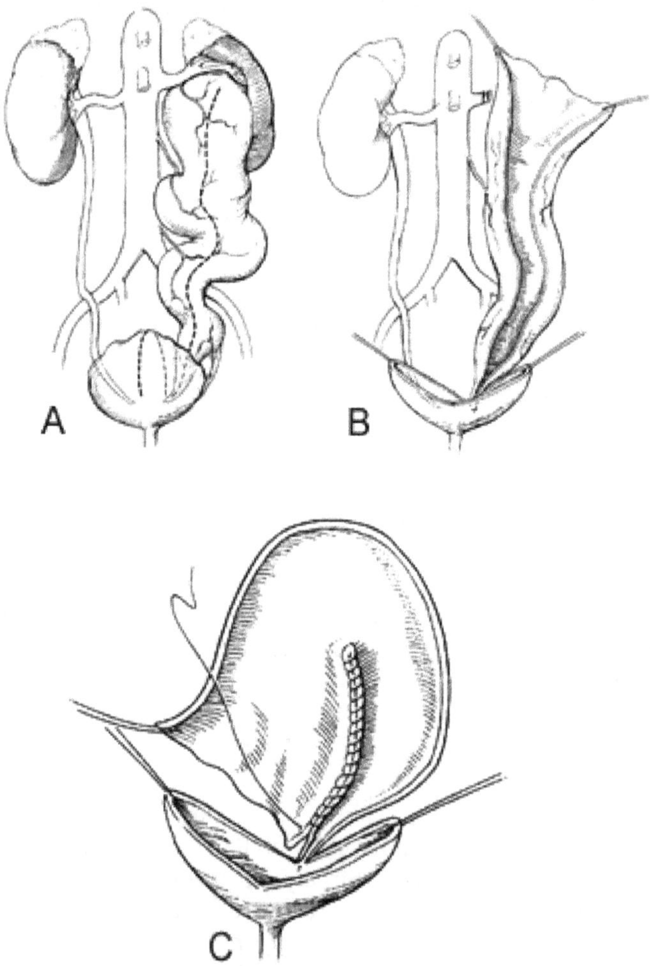

A) A megaureter and poorly functioning kidney are required for ureterocystoplasty.
B) After nephrectomy, the dilated ureter is detubularized, taking care to preserve the blood supply. C) The detubularized ureter is reconfigured before being anastomosed to the bladder [1].

5.4.1 Results

Numerous series have reported good results after augmentation using ureter, some with follow-up as long as 8 years. The upper tracts have remained stable or improved in virtually all patients. Complications have been uncommon, with only a rare early extravasation of urine reported [(92)].

The largest published series is that of Churchill et al (1993) in which ureterocystoplasty was performed in 16 patients. Thirteen patients had enough urodynamic data available postoperatively for adequate evaluation. Twelve out of thirteen patients had excellent results. As a group, there was a 218 percent increase in bladder capacity, a 284 percent increase in pressure specific bladder capacity, and a 227 percent increase in bladder compliance.

Landau and colleagues (1994), compared age-matched and diagnosis-matched children who underwent ureterocystoplasty or ileocystoplasty. The total mean bladder capacity was 470 ml in the ureterocystoplasty group and 381 ml in the ileocystoplasty group. Bladder volumes at 30 cm H_2O were 413 ml and 380 ml after ureterocystoplasty and ileocystoplasty, respectively. Ureter effectively enhanced both volume and compliance. They reported no significant differences in the postoperative mean increase in bladder capacity and pressure specific bladder volume. Both procedures resulted in excellent functional results [(94)].

Hitchcock et al (1994) has described similar excellent short-term results in eight patients [(95)].

5.4.2 Advantages

There are several advantages of using the ureter for augmentation. As is the case with autoaugmentation, the major advantage of ureterocystoplasty is that the native urothelium is preserved, thereby avoiding the specific potential problems associated with the use of bowel. Unlike some cases following autoaugmention, the full thickness opened ureter does not tend to shrink with time, unless the vascular supply is compromised. In patients with end-stage renal disease, the procedure can be performed extraperitoneally, thus, preserving the peritoneum for future peritoneal dialysis. When necessary, concomitant procedures in the bladder may also be performed. It seems likely that the risk of tumor formation will be avoided, and perforation of the augmented bladder may be less probable. However, long-term follow-up will be needed to confirm these notions [(92)]. Lastly, there is increased potential for spontaneous voiding postoperatively in patients who are able to empty their bladders adequately preoperatively.

5.4.3 Disadvantages

The main disadvantage of ureterocystoplasty is that it is only applicable in a minority of patients. Surgical candidates for ureterocystoplasty include patients with either a nonfunctioning renal unit or a megaureter long enough that ipsilateral renal drainage can be re-established following use of the lower ureter for augmentation [(92)].

6. To the future: Tissue expansion for bladder augmentation

6.1 The experiments

In an attempt to make ureterocystoplasty available to make to patients with non-dilated ureters, some have developed methods of producing a dilated ureter. Lailas et al (1996) have demonstrated in a rabbit model that a temporary cutaneous ureterostomy can be used to perform hydrostatic distention of the ureter with subsequent successful ureterocystoplasty. In this study, the ureteral units were dilated at least 10 fold, as measured by radiography, after daily injection of a saline-antibiotic solution for 1 month. Augmentation cystoplasty was performed with the reconfigured dilated uretral segment. Repeated cystography and cystometry showed an increased bladder capacity ranging from 190 % to 380% (98). In a similar system, a dilating catheter was used to dilate tissue in pigs (99).

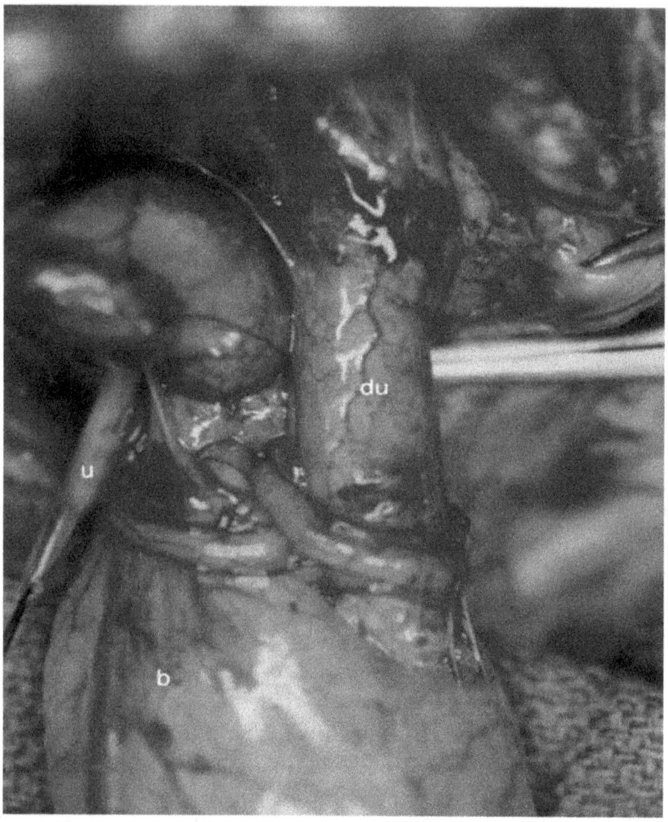

Progressive dilation can be performed in a normal-caliber ureter, which can be subsequently used for ureterocystoplasty. After placement of a ureteral dilation device, comparison is made of progressively dilated ureter (du) and native undilated ureter (u) coming off the bladder (b) (13).

A system for the progressive expansion of native bladder tissue has also been used for augmenting bladder volumes (Satar et al, 1999). Beagle dogs underwent urodynamic studies and the bladders were divided horizontally into two segments: a superior bladder neoreservoir, and an intact smaller bladder inferiorly with both ureters left intact and draining. A silastic catheter was threaded into the newly formed, superiorly located neoreservoir, and connected to an injection port, which was secured subcutaneously. Four weeks after surgery, a saline-antibiotic solution was injected daily into the palpable injection port. Dilating the neoreservoir through the silastic catheter within 30 days after progressive dilation, the neoreservoir volume was expanded at least 10-fold, as measured by radiography and cystometrography. Urodynamic studies of the dilated neoreservoirs showed normal compliance in all animals. Microscopic examination of the expanded neoreservoir tissue showed a normal histology (100).

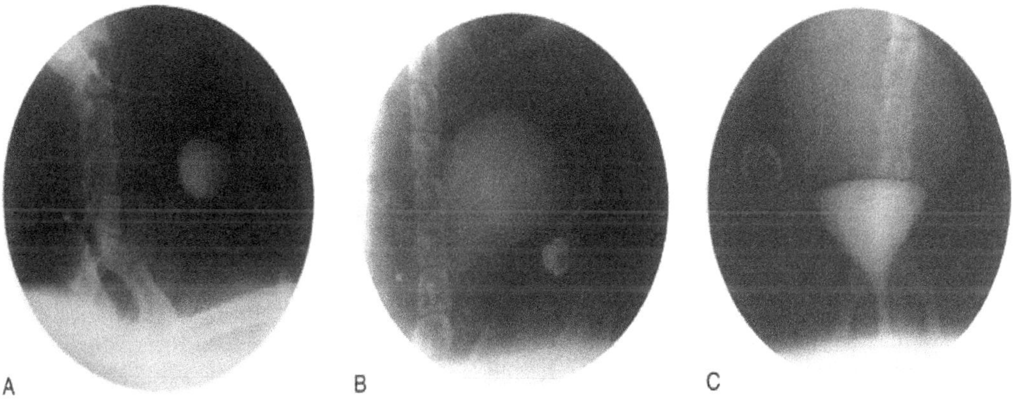

A B C

Progressive bladder dilation can be performed with adequate increases in capacity. Cystography of bladder neoreservoir before progressive dilation *(A)* is compared with cystography results after progressive dilation *(B)* and with cystogram showing dilated neoreservoir and intact bladder segment *(C)* [13]

6.2 The expectations

Ideally, bladder tissue expansion could be performed with an indwelling dilation catheter, similar to a Foley catheter with a large balloon. In the future, one could foresee placing a dilating catheter intravesically in a patient who either requires augmentation, in an intermittent fashion (e.g. four times daily) or left indwelling. An expanding balloon within the catheter could then be filled progressively, with either continuous or intermittent filling until the desired bladder volume is achieved. Studies associated with this concept are currently being conducted in the laboratory. Clinical application of these interesting ideas has yet to be undertaken [13].

7. Tissue engineered bladder

The complications that are associated with using various portions of the gastrointestinal tract for genitourinary reconstruction in both adults and children have stimulated the development of tissue engineering techniques for bladder reconstruction through bladder regeneration. Current research efforts are focused on the development of biodegradable materials which are well-characterized with predictable behavior that can be used as alternatives to gastrointestinal segments for bladder reconstruction.

Tissue engineering follows the principles of cell transplantation, materials science, and engineering toward the development of biologic substitutes that can restore and maintain normal function. Bladder reconstruction via tissue engineering and bladder regeneration involve the use of a *biomaterial graft (matrix)*, either permanent or biodegradable, that will function as a suitable scaffold to allow the body's ability of regeneration and growth to occur either naturally (matrices alone unseeded) or with the addition of cultured cells (matrices with cell - seeded) [3, 101].

The ideal graft material is one that would be replaced by the host tissue, provide a low-pressure reservoir, and serve as a scaffold for regeneration of the bladder wall with normal function characteristics. If a suitable graft material can be developed, the need for autogenous tissue and the associated complications of intestinal segments could be eliminated. Currently, there are two types of tissue engineering technologies that have preliminarily been shown to induce bladder regeneration. These are the unseeded and seeded technologies (14).

7.1 Biomaterials

7.1.1 Functions

Biomaterials in genitourinary tissue engineering function as an artificial extracellular matrix (ECM) and elicit biologic and mechanical functions of native ECM found in tissues in the body. Native ECM brings cells together into tissue, controls the tissue structure, and regulates the cell phenotype. Biomaterials facilitate the localization and delivery of cells and/or bioactive factors (e.g. cell adhesion peptides, growth factors) to desired sites in the body; define a three dimensional space for the formation of new tissues with appropriate function. The configuration of the biomaterials can guide the structure of an engineered tissue. The biomaterials provide mechanical support against in-vivo forces of tissue development. The biomaterials can be loaded with bioactive signals, such as cell-adhesion peptides and growth factors, which can regulate cellular function (102).

7.1.2 Design and selection

The design and selection of the biomaterial is critical in the development of engineered genitourinary tissues. The biomaterial must be capable of controlling the structure and function of the engineered tissue in a predesigned manner by interacting with transplanted cells and/or host cells. Generally, the ideal biomaterial should be biocompatible, promote cellular interaction and tissue development, and possess proper mechanical and physical properties.

The selected biomaterial should be biodegradable and bioresorbable to support the reconstruction of a completely normal tissue without inflammation. Such behavior of the biomaterials avoids the risk of inflammatory or foreign body responses that may be associated with the permanent presence of a foreign material in the body. The degradation products should not provoke inflammation or toxicity, and must be removed from the body via metabolic pathways. The degradation rate and the concentration of degradation products in the tissue surrounding the implant must be at a tolerable level (103).

The biomaterials need to be processed into specific configuration. A large ratio of surface area to volume is often desirable to allow the delivery of a high density of cells. A high-porosity, interconnected pore structure, with specific pore sizes promotes tissue ingrowth from the surrounding host tissue. Several techniques have been developed that readily control porosity, pore size, and pore structure (13).

7.1.3 Types of biomaterials

Generally, three classes of biomaterials have been used for engineering of genitourinary tissue: ***synthetic polymers***, such as polyglycolic acid (PGA), polylactic acid (PLA), and poly-lactic-co-glycolic acid) (PLGA), ***naturally derived materials***, such as collagen and alginate; and ***cellular tissue matrices***, such as bladder submucosa and small-intestinal submucosa. These classes of biomaterials have been tested in regard to their biocompatibility with primary human urothelial and bladder muscle cells. Naturally, derived materials and cellular tissue matrices have the potential advantage of biologic recognition. Synthetic polymers can be produced reproducibly on a large scale with controlled properties of strength, degradation rate, and microstructure (105).

7.2 Matrices for bladder regeneration

A. Unseeded matrices (Acellular)

The first technique currently being investigated for bladder regeneration is the unseeded technology. This technology involves placement of matrix graft into the wall of the host-bladder. The body then provides the needed environment for subsequent cell growth and tissue regeneration. This represents an unseeded bladder regenerating process.
Thus far, the major obstacle to unseeded tissue engineering technology has been the inability to develop an optimal biomaterial that will act as a suitable scaffold for the "natural" process of regeneration.

7.2.1 Synthetic non-biodegradable biomaterials

Synthetic non-biodegradable biomaterials such as silicon, Teflon, rubber, polytetrafluoroethylene, and polypropylene have been tried with unsuccessful results because of host foreign body reactions. Most of these attempts have failed because of mechanical, structural, functional, or biocompatibility problems. Usually, permanent synthetic materials used for bladder reconstruction succumb to mechanical failure and urinary stone formation, and use of degradable materials leads to fibroblast deposition, scarring, graft contracture, and a reduced reservoir volume over time.

7.2.2 Synthetic biodegradable biomaterials

As a consequence of these failures with non biodegradable materials, synthetic biodegradable material e.g. collagen and Vicryl (PGA) matrices were developed in the hope that these grafts would allow the host bladder adequate time for regeneration but dissolve prior to sever foreign body reaction. These materials have been used experimentally and have shown less graft encrustation and infectious complications compared to non-biodegradable materials. However, graft shrinkage still limited potential clinical utility of these materials.
Collagen/Vicryl composite membranes were used as a scaffold for tissue ingrowth to repair a full thickness defect in the bladder of rabbits. The collagen membranes were reinforced with meshes of Vicryl, a biodegradable polimer composed of PLGA, to strengthen the collagen membranes, which are too soft to suture reliably. The results of the initial study were not encouraging because of the occurrence of sever infection (Monsour et al, 1987). However, a later study obtained a high success rate when the experiments were repeated using purification and γ irradiation of collagen and postoperative administration of antibiotics. At 3 weeks, a normal urothelium was noted. At 6 weeks, no implanted biomaterial was identified. At 35 weeks, smooth muscle regeneration was evident. During this period, there was no evidence of urinary leakage, infection, or bladder calculi (Scott et al, 1988).

7.2.3 Natural biodegradable materials

Collagen based matrices for tissue regeneration such as placenta, amnion and pericardium have been investigated in dogs and have shown clear evidence of bladder regeneration [106, 107, 108]. Functionally, the implanted bladders showed adequate capacity for up to 36 months. Nevertheless, they were observed grossly to undergo graft shrinkage. Histologically, the epithelial layer was present, but the muscular layer was absent.
However, despite initial encouraging results, none of these materials has been found to be suitable for clinical use. The reasons for this are not entirely clear. It can only be speculated

from the available literature that long-term experimental results with these biodegradable materials did not recapitulate the initial results and therefore clinical trials were not undertaken.

7.2.4 Acellular Extracellular Matrix (ECM) grafts

Recently there has been the development of new types of biodegradable materials that have shown tremendous potential for the induction of bladder regeneration with unseeded tissue engineering technology. These materials are acellular extracellular matrix (ECM) grafts that are derived from various different organs. The graft is made acellular by a mechanical process that lyses the cells and/or by detergent and enzymatic extraction. These types of ECM grafts may be xenogenic or allogenic and have been derived from full thickness bladder, stomach, and the submucosal layer of small intestine (109).

7.2.5 Xeogenic acellular matrix grafts

Small Intestinal Submucosa (SIS)

The most thoroughly studied collagen based ECM graft for bladder augmentation and urinary reconstruction utilizing unseeded technology is small intestinal submucosa (SIS) (109). SIS is a xenogentic membrane derived from pig small intestine in which the mucosa is mechanically removed from the inner surface and the serosa and muscularies are mechanically removed from the outer surface. This result in a thin, translucent membrane (0.1 mm wall thickness) composed mainly of the submucosal layer of the intestinal wall. Production of SIS is reminiscent of the manufacturing of sausage casing. This unique material has been shown to function well as an arterial or venous graft with rapid replacement by native tissues and evidence of tissue specific regeneration (101).

SIS grafts have been shown to promote full thickness bladder regeneration in both rat and canine animal models. The regenerated bladder tissue is composed of all three layers of the normal bladder wall (urothelium, smooth muscle, and serosa). In addition, the regenerated segment is contractile, compliant, and functionally innervated. Urodynamic studies in a long-term canine augmentation model have demonstrated that the SIS augmented bladder maintains normal bladder capacity and compliance that persist for at least 15 months postoperatively. In vitro muscle strip studies on the regenerated portions of the bladders also demonstrate contractility and compliance that is similar to normal bladder (110).

SIS has been shown to be non-immunogenic with over 1000 cross species transplants and direct challenge testing elucidating no response. In addition, SIS is unique from other biomaterials that have been studied thus far in that it contains a combination of active intrinsic growth factors, cytokines, structural proteins, glyeoproteins, and proteoglycans that may assist in cell migration, cell-to-cell interaction, as well as cell growth and differentiation during the regenerative process. These inherent elements within SIS may prove to be vital to the regenerative process. Further research is needed to identify the functional importance of each of these elements and factors (101).

7.2.6 Allogenic acellular matrix grafts

Bladder Acellular Matrix Grafts (BAMG)

Similar types of cellular ECM grafts to SIS have also been shown to induce bladder regeneration in vivo. Preliminary works have demonstrated that successful morphologic and functional regeneration of the rat urinary bladder can be accomplished with homologous bladder acellular matrix grafts (BAMG).

The allogeneic acellular bladder matrix has served as a scaffold for the ingrowth of host bladder wall components in rats. The matrix was prepared by mechanically and chemically removing all cellular components from bladder tissue. Partial cystectomy (25% to 50%) was performed, followed by augmentation cystoplasty using acellular bladder matrices. The mucosal lining was complete within 10 days. After 4 weeks, muscular and vascular regeneration was completed. Nerve regeneration continued to improve until week 20. The grafted bladders had significantly better capacity and compliance than the autoregenterated bladders after partial cystectomy alone. The bladders regenerated with acellular matrix grafts exhibited contractile activity to electric and carbachol stimulation. Clinically relevant antigenicity was not evident. However, there was a 26% to 36% incidence of bladder stone formation [111, 112].

B. Seeded matrices

Allogenic Cellular Matrix Grafts

In multiple studies using various materials as acellular grafts for cystoplasty, the urothelial layer was able to regenerate normally, but the muscle layer, although present, was not fully developed [111, 112, 113].

Allogenic bladder submucosa preloaded with cells was used as a biomaterial for bladder augmentation in dogs [113]. The regenerated bladder tissues contained a normal cellular organization consisting of urothelium and smooth muscle and exhibited a normal compliance. Biomaterials preloaded with cells before their implantation showed better tissue regeneration compared with biomaterials implanted with no cells, in which tissue regeneration depended on ingrowth of the surrounding tissue. The bladders showed a significant increase (100%) in capacity when augmented with scaffolds seeded with cells, compared to scaffolds without cells (30%).

7.2.7 Summary

Studies involving acellular matrices that may provide the necessary environment to promote cell migration, growth, and differentiation are being conducted, and demonstrate that bladder regeneration using unseeded tissue engineering technology is feasible without the complications of graft shrinkage, incrustation, and infection. These observations have obvious and significant clinical ramifications. The ability to augment the bladder without the use of bowel or other native host tissue would eliminate many of the complications of conventional enterocystoplasty and would simplify the technical aspects of this operation. Further research into the individual composition of the various biomaterials, the cell-to-cell interaction, and the growth factors that are involved in the bladder regenerative process will be required prior to clinical use of these grafts.

7.3 Bladder tissue engineering with selective cell transplantation (seeded technology)

The second type of tissue engineering technology, the seeded technique, involves the use of *biodegradable materials* that act as cell delivery vehicles for *cultured cells* from the patient. This technique has been applied to the urinary bladder. Initially, this process is begun by harvesting native bladder tissue for the establishment and expansion of primary cultures of

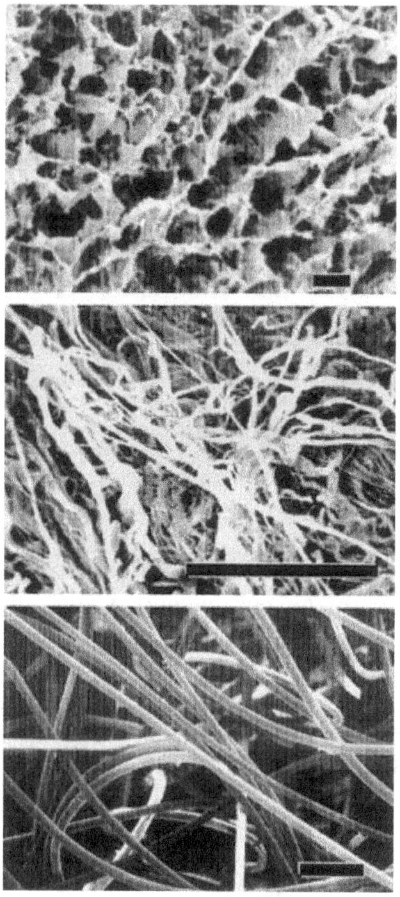

Scanning electron micrographs of biomaterials: collagen sponge *(top)*, acellular matrix prepared from pig bladder submucosa *(center)*, and polyglycolic acid fiber-based matrix *(bottom)*. (Size bars = 100 µm.) [13].

both bladder smooth muscle and epithelial sells. It is possible to expand a bladder epithelial cell culture from a single biopsy specimen such that the cultured cells could cover a surface area of over 400 m within eight weeks [14]. Once the cells are grown, they are seeded on a biodegradable membrane in vitro and then transplanted back into the host for continuation of the regenerative process.

In 1992, 1993 Atala and associates demonstrated the successful use of non-woven polyglycolic acid polymers sheets, which allow the in-vitro growth of rabbit and human bladder epithelium and smooth muscle cells [114, 115]. Further work demonstrated that these cell-polymer constructs could be implanted into athymic mice with the subequent formation of organized layers of bladder epithelial and smooth muscle cells.

In these studies, urothelial and muscle cells were expanded in-vitro, seeded onto a polymer scaffold (non-wonen polygycolic acid), and allowed to attach and form sheet of cells. The cell-polymer scaffold was then implanted in-vivo. A series of in vivo urologic associated cell-polymer experiments were then performed. Histologic analysis of human urothelial, bladder muscle, and composite urothelial and bladder muscle polymer scaffold, implanted in athymic mice and retrieved at different time points, indicated that viable cells were evident in all three experimental groups (115). Implanted cells oriented themselves spatially along the polymer surfaces. The cell populations appeared to expand from one layer to several layers of thickness with progressive cell organization over extended implantation times. Cell-polymer composite implants of urothelial and muscle cells, retrieved at extended times (50 days), showed extensive formation of multilayered, sheet-like structures and well defined muscle layers. Polymers seeded with cells and manipulated into a tubular configuration showed layers of muscle cells lining the multilayered epithelial sheets. Cell polymers implanted with human bladder muscle cells alone showed almost complete replacement of the polymer with sheets of smooth muscle at 520 days. This experiment demonstrated that composite tissue-engineered structures could be created de novo.

Recently, Yoo et al (1998) and Oberpenning et al (1999), reported on the feasibility of dog bladder augmentation using allogenic bladder submucosa or polyglycolic acid polymers seeded with urothelial and smooth muscle cells (113, 116). Organized bladder histology was noted in the regenerated bladder tissue. More importantly, the regenerated bladder tissue was found to increase bladder capacity and was urodynamically compliant.

In order to determine the effect of implanting engineered tissues in continuity with the urinary tract, Yoo and associates (1998), used an animal model of bladder augmentation. Partial cystectomies, which involved removal of approximately 50% of the native bladder, were performed in 10 dogs. In five, the retrieved bladder tissue was micro dissected and the mucosal and muscular layers separated. The bladder urothelial and muscle cells were cultured. Urothelial and smooth muscle cells were harvested and expanded separately. A collagen-based matrix, derived from allogenic bladder submucosa, was used for cell delivery. This material was chosen for these experiments because of its native elasticity.

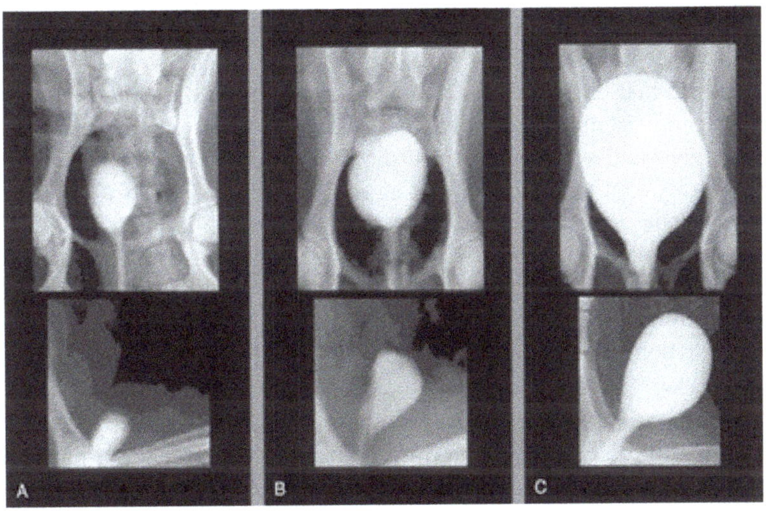

Radiographic cystograms in beagles 11 months after subtotal cystectomy without reconstruction *(A)*; with reconstruction using a polymer without cells *(B)*; and with reconstruction with a polymer and cell-seeded tissue-engineered organ *(C)*. Organs after trigone-sparing cystectomy retained a small-sized reservoir. Tissue-engineered neobladders showed a normal configuration and a larger capacity than the trigones grafted with polymer only (13).

Within 6 weeks, the expanded urothelial cells were collected as a pellet. The cells were seeded on the luminal surface of the allogenic bladder submucosa and incubated for five days. Muscle cells were seeded on the opposite side of the bladder submucosa. Augmentation cystoplasty was performed with the matrix including cells in one group and the matrix without cells in the second group. The augmented bladders were covered with omentum to facilitate angiogenesis to the implant. Bladders augmented with the matrix seeded with cells showed a 99% increase in capacity compared with bladders augmented with the cell-free matrix, which showed only a 30% increase in capacity. Functionally, all animals showed normal bladder compliance as evidenced by urodynamic studies; however, the remaining native bladder tissue may have accounted for these results. Histologically, the retrieved engineered bladders contained a cellular organization consisting of a urothelium-lined lumen surrounded by submucosal tissue and smooth muscle. However, the muscular layer was markedly more prominent in the cell-reconstituted scaffold (113).

7.3.1 Histologic Parameters of Tissue-Engeneered Bladders

It has been well established for decades that the bladder is able to regenerate generously over free grafts. Urothelium is associated with a high reparative capacity. Bladder muscle tissue is less likely to regenerate in a normal fashion. Most of the free grafts (without cells) used for bladder replacement in the past were able to show adequate histology in terms of a well-developed urothelial layer, but they were associated with an abnormal muscular layer that varied in terms of its full development. Because native muscle cells are less likely to regenerate over the free grafts, presence of both urothelial and muscle cells on the matrices used for bladder replacement is important for successful tissue bioengineering.

Both urothelial and muscle ingrowth are believed to be initiated from the edges of the normal bladder toward the region of the free graft. Usually, however, contracture or resorption of the graft has been evident. The inflammatory response toward the matrix may contribute to the resorption of the free graft (89,104).

It was hypothesized that building the three-dimensional structure constructs in vitro, before implantation, would facilitate the eventual terminal differentiation of the cells after implantation in vivo and would minimize the inflammatory response toward the matrix, thus, avoiding graft contractor and shrinkage. The study by Yoo and associates (1998) demonstrated a major difference between matrices used with autologous cells (tissue-engineered matrices) and those used without cells as regards the graft diameter (113). Matrices implanted with cells for bladder augmentation retained most of their implanted diameter, as opposed to matrices implanted without cells for bladder augmentation, in which graft contraction and shrinkage occurs.

7.3.2 Functional parameters of tissue-engeneered bladders

The results of initial studies showed that the creation of artificial bladder may be achieved in vivo; however, it could not be determined whether the functional parameters noted were caused by the augmented segment or by the intact native bladder tissue. To better, address the functional parameters of tissue-engineered bladders; an animal model was designed that required a cystectomy with subsequent replacement organ (116).

A total of 14 dogs underwent a trigone-sparing cystectomy. The animals were randomly assigned to one of three groups. Group A (n= 2) underwent closure of the trigone without a reconstructive procedure. Group B (n= 6) underwent reconstruction with a cell- free bladder

shaped biodegradable polymer. Group C (n=6) underwent reconstruction using a bladder-shaped biodegradation polymer that delivered autologous urothelial cells and smooth muscle cells harvested from autologous bladder biopsy and expanded.
The cystectomy -only controls and polymer-only grafts maintained average capacities of 22% and 46% of preoperative values, respectively. An average bladder capacity of 95% of the original precystectomy volume was achieved in the tissue-engineered bladder replacements.
The subtotal cystectomy reservoirs that were not reconstructed and the polymer-only reconstructed bladder showed a marked decrease in bladder compliance (10% and 42% total compliance). The compliance of tissue-engineered bladders showed almost no difference from preoperative values. Histologically, the polymer-only bladder presented a pattern of normal urothelial cells with a thickened fibrotic submucosa and a thin layer of muscle fibers. The retrieved tissue- engineered bladders showed a normal cellular organization, consisting of a trilayer of urothelium, submucosa, and muscle. The results from this study showed that it is possible to tissue - engineer bladders that are anatomically and functionally normal [116].
Clinical trials for the application of this technology are currently being arranged [116].
Progressive bladder dilation can be performed with adequate increases in capacity. Cystography of bladder neoreservoir before progressive dilation *(A)* is compared with cystography results after progressive dilation *(B)* and with cystogram showing dilated neoreservoir and intact bladder segment *(C)*

7.3.3 In summary

It is clear that bladder regeneration is possible utilizing both unseeded and seeded tissue-engineering technologies. Further advances in our current techniques will eventually revolutionize urologic reconstructive surgery, as we know it today. It is important to note that all of the animal studies performed thus far have been in animals with a normal bladder. It is not known whether normal or abnormal bladder regeneration can be achieved with either unseeded or seeded technology in an animal or patient with a neuropathic bladder. Active research is currently investigating this vital question. Additionally, studies are needed to better understand the differences that exist between the unseeded and seeded approaches and the resultant regenerated bladder, so that unseeded and aspect approaches and the resultant regenerated bladder so that the best aspects of each technology may be utilized to achieve a superior result. It is the authors' opinion that future chapters on bladder augmentation will discuss the use of intestinal segments as historical footnote while the major focus will be on the indications and methods for various types of tissue engineering technology.

8. Laparoscopic augmentation cystoplasty

8.1 Laparoscopic enterocystoplasty

8.1.1 Patient selection

Laparoscopy has distinct advantages when compared with open surgical procedures, such as decreased postoperative pain and morbidity, improved cosmoses, a shorter hospital stay, and decreased convalescence. Recent studies have indicated that postoperative intra-abdominal adhesions are reduced significantly after laparoscopic surgery when compared with open surgery [117].

Alternative	Advantages	Disadvantages
Ureter	1. Urinary epithelium, no mucus 2. Good compliance	1. Only applicable if the patient has a dilated ureter 2. Ureter may be scarred (reflux, infection)
Autoaugmentation (bladder myomectomy)	1. Urinary epithelium, no mucus 2. Relatively easy, no bowel resection	1. Inconsistent results can result in bladder scarring 2. Sometimes difficult (bladder scarring or diverticula)
Demucosalized intestinal flap on urothelium (colon, DAWG)	1. Urinary epithelium, decreased mucus 2. More physiologic	1. Difficult procedure 2. Inconsistent results
Bladder regeneration on substrate (SIS)	1. No bowel resection 2. Easily performed	1. Unproven in children 2. Dependent on native bladder potential for regeneration
Tissue engineering	1. Bladder regrowth in laboratory 2. Potentially unlimited capacity, no mucus	1. Unproven in children 2. Dependent on vascular and nerve ingrowth

DAWG, demucosalized augmentation with gastric segment.

Alternatives to intestinocystoplasty

Despite the established role of laparoscopy in diagnostic and ablative urologic surgery, the use of laparoscopic techniques in reconstruction has been limited because of the technical complexity of the procedures involved. The technical steps in performing laparoscopic bladder augmentation are designed to emulate the open surgical counterpart in every aspect, thereby producing similar functional results with an improved recovery.

A relative contraindication specific to laparoscopic bladder augmentation is the presence of extensive intra-abdominal and pelvic adhesions that would preclude laparoscopic dissection. Patients with ventriculo-peritoneal shunts, as noted in cases of myelomeningocele, have increased abdominal adhesions that may preclude a successful laparoscopic approach [(117)].

8.1.2 Technical considerations

Important elements of the operation include:

- Cystoscopic placement of ureteric catheters (optional).
- Transperitoneal placement of 4 to 5 redially arranged trocars.

- Identification of the cecum and ileocecal junction.
- A 5-mm laparoscope can be introduced through the lower left port to transilluminate the mesentery and identify its vascular pedicle.
- Bowel segment selection and mobilization sufficient for pelvic placement.
- Exteriorizing the bowel loop outside the abdomen through a 2-cm extension of the umbilical port site, preventing twisting of the mesenteric vessels;
- Using traditional open surgical techniques, the bowel segment is isolated, bowel continuity is re-established, mesenteric window is closed, the bowel segment is detubularized along its antimesenteric border and reconfigured (117,118).
- Alternatively, bowel division and side-to-side anastomosis may be done intracorporeally using endoscopic gastrointestinal stapling device with detubularization and freehand intracorporeal suturing to reconfigure the bowel (119).
- Incising the peritoneum, entering the space of Retzius, mobilization of the bladder.
- Vertical incision creating a large cystotomy (bivalving).
- Mobilization of the bowel patch, and fixing it at 6 and 12-o'clock positions.
- Circumferential completion of enterovesical anastomsis in quadrants intracorporeally with running sutures.

8.1.3 Results

Hedican and associates (1999) performed laparoscopic assisted bladder augmentation in eight patients. In addition to using a bowel segment for augmentation, in many of these cases they were also able to laparoscopically mobilize the appendix to perform a Mitrofanoff continent catheterizable stoma. They described using both ileum and cecum as the enteric patch for the bladder. The bladder augmentation was done through a low Pfannenstiel incision. Many of these patients were children and this allowed a rapid recovery with decreased pain as well as a good cosmetic result (120).

Gill and associates (2000) underwent laparoscopic enterocystoplasty for three patients with functionally reduced bladder capacities due to neurogenic causes: ileocystoplasty (n=1), sigmoidocystoplasty (n=1), and cystoplasty with cecum and proximal ascending colon (n=1). In all patients, bowel reanastomosis was performed by exteriorizing the bowel loop outside the abdomen. All three laparoscopic enterovesical anastomoses were water tight without postoperative urinary extravasation. The operative times were 5.3, 8, and 7 hours. The hospital stay was 7, 5, and 4 days (118).

Rackley and associates (2001) performed laparoscopic enterocystoplasty in 12 patients with functionally reduced bladder capacities owing to neurogenic causes. Procedures included ileocystoplasty (2), sigmoidocystoplasty (2), colocystoplasty (1), and cecocolocystoplasty with continent catheterizable ileal stoma (7). Total surgical time ranged from 5.3 to 8 hours (average 7.0 hours). The time of laparoscopic suturing ranged from 1.7 to 3.1 hours (average 2.4 hours). Blood loss was minimal and did not exceed 250 ml during any of the procedures (average 175 ml). The only intra-operative complication was a trocar-induced rectus sheath hematoma. Oral feeding was resumed by 24 hours in 11 of the 12 patients. The average hospital stay was 5.7 days and ranged from 3 to 7 days (117).

Unlike the previously published reports, where portions of the procedure were performed extracorporeally, Elliott and associates (2002) reported their technique of complete laparoscopic ileocystoplasty (119).

8.2 Laparoscopic autoaugmentation

Ehrlich and Gershman (1993), reported the first laparoscopic autoaugmentation in an 8-years-old child with a neurogenic bladder. In this case, the procedure required 70 min, follow-up of the patient at 1 year, documented improvement in his symptoms with rare incontinence (121).

In 1995, McDougall and colleagues described the initial laparoscopic retropubic autoaugmentation of the bladder in an adult (12). In this case, the extraperitoneal approach was used and the incision was made in the detrusor muscle leaving the mucosa intact. There was a significant drop in bladder pressure. At the 6-month follow-up, the bladder capacity increased from 85-350 ml. However, in a second case, while the procedure could be successfully completed, the long-term result was unsatisfactory.

Due to the success of enteric augmentation and the variable results with autoaugmentation, this procedure has largely fallen into disuse (122). Nevertheless, laparoscopic retropubic autoaugmentation allows a brief hospital stay and minor postoperative discomfort. Moreover, the laparoscopic approach should not complicate or preclude subsequent enterocystoplasty if necessary (123).

9. Conclusion

Laparoscopic enterocystoplasty is technically feasible and successfully emulates the established principles of open enterocystoplasty while minimizing operative morbidity. As is true in open surgery, various bowel segments can be fashioned and anastomosed to the bladder laparoscopically. The increased costs associated with laparoscopy and weight minimally invasive surgery in general have been a significant disadvantage; however, a pervious report on the costs of laparoscopic procedures concluded that increased surgical experience reduces the surgical time and length of hospital stay, thereby decreasing costs. Furthermore, the increased use of reusable instruments results in considerable economic benefits. Implementation of appropriate cost-saving strategies ultimately will result in decreased expenses associated with laparoscopy. Although laparoscopic enterocystoplasty is currently a lengthy procedure lasting twice as long as open surgery, further technical modifications and increasing experience will continue to reduce the surgical time involved. For patients with complex co-morbid illness who desire the improved quality of life associated with traditional augmentation cystoplasty, the reduced morbidity observed in the authors' series of patients undergoing a laparoscopic procedure makes this approach an attractive option to consider. The authors' initial experience suggests that laparoscopic enterocystoplasty has the potential to become a viable alternative to open enterocystoplasty.

10. References

Mitchell ME, Plaire JC: Augmentation cystoplasty. In Gillenwater JY, Grayback JT, Howards SS, Mitchell ME (eds): Adult and Pediatric Urology. Philadelphia, Lippincot Williams and Wilkins, 2002, P. 2445.

Lapides J, Diokno Ac, Gould FR, et al. Further observations of self – catheterization. J Urol 1976; 116: 169.

Hendren WH, Hendren RB. Bladder augmentation: experience with 129 children and young adults. J Urol 1990; 144: 445.

Mitchell ME, Piser JA. Intestinocystoplasty and total bladder replacement in children and young adults: follow-up in 129 cases. J Urol 1987; 138: 579.

Nguyen DH, Mitchell ME. Gastric bladder reconstruction. Urol Clin North Am 1991; 18: 649.

Bellinger MF. Urterocystoplasty. Curr Surg Tech Urol 1995; 8: 2.

Cartwright PC, Snow BW. Bladder augmentation: early clinical experience. J Urol 1989; 142: 505.

Cartwright Pc, Snow BW. Bladder augmentation: partial detrusor excision to augment the bladder without use of bowel.l J Urol 1989; 142: 1050.

Dewan PA, Nicholls EA, Goth DW. Ureterocystoplasty: an extraperitoneal urothelial bladder augmentation technique. Eur Urol 1994; 2685.

Ikeguchi HW, Stifelman MD, Hensle TW. Ureteral tissue expansion for bladder augmentation. J Urol 1998; 159: 1665.

Kropp BP, Sawyer BD, Shannon HE, et al. characterization of small intestine submucosa regenerated canine detrusor: assessment of reinnervation in vitro compliance and contractility. J Urol 1996; 156: 599.

Pope JC, Davis MM, Smith ER, et al. ontogeny of canine small intestine submucosa regenerated bladder. J Urol 1997; 158: 105.

Atala A: Tissue Engineering Perspectives for reconstructive surgery. In Walsh PC, Retick AB, Vaughan ED, Jr, Wein AJ (eds); Campbell's Urology. Philadelphia, WB Sauders, 2002, P. 2523.

Colvert JR, Kropp BP, Cheng EY: Bladder augmentation: Current and future techniques. AUA update series 2003: 22 (32) - 250.

DeMarco RT, Koch MO: Metabolic complications of continent urinary diversion AUA update series: 22 (15) - 114.

Hinman F Jr. Selection of intestinal segments for bladder substitution: physical and physiological characteristics. J Urol 1988; 139: 519.

Koff SA. Guidelines to determine the size and shape of intestinal segments used for reconstruction. J Urol 1988; 140: 1150.

Goldwasser B. Barrett DM, Webster GD, et al: Cystometric properties of ileum and right colon after bladder augmentation. Substitution or replacement. J Urol 1987: 138: 1007.

Adams MC, Mitchell ME, Rink RC. Gastrocystoplasty: An alternative solution to the problem of urological reconstruction in the severely compromised patient. J Urol 1988; 140: 1152.

Adams MC, Brock JW, Pope JC, et al. Ureterocystoplasy: is it necessary to detubularize the distal ureter? J Urol 1998; 160: 851.

Gonzalez R, Cabral BHP. Rectal continence after enterocystoplasty. Dialysis Pediatr Urol 1987; 10 (12): 3.

Abol-Enein H, Ghoneim MA: A novel uretero-ileal reimplantation technique: the serous lined extramural tunnel. A preliminary report. J Urol 1994; 151: 1193.

Mitchell ME: Use of Bowel in undiversion. Urol Clin North Am 1986; 13: 349.

Gonzalez R. Buson H. Reid C, Reinbert Y: Sermoucular colocystoplasty lined with urothelium: experience with 16 patients. Urology 1994; 45: 124-129.

King LR: Cystoplasty in children. In King LR, Stone AR, Webster GD (eds): Bladder Reconstruction and Continent Urinary Diversion, 2nd ed. St. Louis, Mosby - Year Book, 1991, 115-125.

Cain MP, Husmann DA: Cecal bladder augmentation with a tapered catheterizable stoma: A modification of the Indiana pouch. Presented at the Urology Section Meeting. American Academy of Pediatrics. Dallas. TX, 1994.

Cain MP, Casale AJ, King SJ, Rink RC: Appendicoversicostomy and newer alternatives for the Mitrofanoff procedure: Results in the last 100 patients at Riley children's Hosptial. J Urol 1999; 54: 909-912.

Leong CH: The use of gastrocystoplasty. Dialog Pediatr Urol 1988; 11: 3-5.

Adams MC, Mitchell ME, Rink PC: Gastrocystoplasty: An alternative solutioni to the problem of urological reconstruction in the severely compromised patient. J Urol 1988; 140: 1152-1156.

Mitchell ME, Rinck RC, Adams MC: Augmentation cystoplasty, implantation of artificial urinary sphincter in men and women, and reconstruction of the dysfunction urinary tract. In Walsh PC, Retik AB. Stamey TZ, Vaughn ED, (eds): Campbell's Urology, 6th ed. Philadelphia. WB Saunders, 1992, pp 2630-2653.

Raz S, Ehrilich RM, Babiarz JW, et al: Gastrocystoplasty without opening the stomach. J Urol 1993; 150: 713-715.

Reinberg Y, Manivel JC, Froemming C, et al: Perforation of the gastric segment of an augmented bladder secondary to peptic ulcer disease. J Urol 1992: 148 (2 pt 1). 369- 371.

Sheldon CA, Gibert A, Wacksman J, et al: Gastrocystoplasty: Technical and metabolic characteristics of the post versatile childhood bladder augmentation modality [see comments]. J Pediatr Surg 1995: 30 (2): 283-287: discussion 287-288.

Kajbafzadeh AM, Quinr. FM, Duffy PG, et al: Augmentation cystoplasty in boys with posterior urethral values. J Urol 1995: 154 (2 pt 2): 874-877.

Docimo SG, Moore RG, Adams J, et al: Laparoscopic bladder augmentation using stomach. Urol 1995: 46 (4): 565-569.

Kurzock EA, Baskin LS, Kogaa Ba: Gastocystoplasty: Is there a consensus? World Urol 1998: 16 (4): 242-250

Kurzrock EA, Baskin LS. Kogan BA: Gastrocystoplasty: long–term follow up. J Urol 1998. 160 (6 pt 1): 2182-2166.

Atala A, Bauer SB, Hendren WH, et al: The effect of gastric augmentation on bladder function. J Urol 1993: 149: 1099-1102.

Gosalbez R, Woodard JR, Broecher BH, et al: The use of stomach in pediatric urinary reconstruction. J Urol 1993. 150 (2 pt 1): 438-440.

Goldwasser B, Webster GD: Augmentation and substitution enterocystoplasty. J Urol 1986; 138, 215-224.

Rink RC, Mclaughlin KP: Indication for enterocystoplasty and choice of bowel segment. Probl Urol 1994; 8: 389-403.

Studer UE, Zingg EJ: Ileal orthotopic bladder substitutes: What we have learned from 12 years, experience with 200 patients. Urol Clin North Am 1997; 24: 781-793.

Shekarriz B, Upadhyay J, Demirbilek S, et al: Surgical complications of bladder augmentation: Comparison between various enterocystoplasties in 133 patients. Urology 2000; 55: 123-128.

Lytton B, Green DF: Urodynamic studies in patients undergoing bladder replacement surgery. J Urol 1989; 141: 1984.

Jakobsen H, Steven K, Stigsby B, et al: Pathogensis of nocturnal urinary incontinence after ileocecal bladder replacement: continuous measurement of urethral closure pressure during sleep. Br J Urol 1987; 59: 148-152.

Hedlund H, Lindstrom K, Mansson W: Dynamics of a continent Cecal reservoir for urinary diversion. Br J Urol 1984; 56: 366-372.

Thuroff JW, Alken P, Reidmiller H, et al: 100 cases of Mainz pouch: Continuing Experience and evolution. J Urol 1988: 140: 283.

Sidi AA, Reinberg Y, Gonzalez R: Influence of intestinal segment and configuration on the outcome of augmentation enterocystoplasty. J Urol 1986b; 136: 1201-1204.

Berglund B, Kock NG, Norlen L, Philipson BM: Volume capacity and pressure characteristics of the continent ileal reservoir used for urinary diversion. J Urol 1987; 137: 29.

Adams MC, Bihrle R, Rink RC: The use of stomach in urologic reconstruction. AUA Update Series 1995; 27: 218-223.

Rink RC, Hollensbe D, Adams MC: complications of augmentation in children and comparison of gastrointestinal segments. Americal Urological association Update series 1995: 14: 122-128.

Mitchell ME, Piser JA: Intestinocystoplasty and total bladder replacement in children and young adults: Follow-up in 129 cases. J Urol 1987; 138: 579-584.

Roth S, Semjonow A, Waldner M, Hertle L: Risk of Bowel dysfunction with diarrhea after continent urinary diversion with ileal and ileocecal segments. J Urol 1995; 154: 1696-1699.

Smith RB, Can Cangh P, Skinner DG, et al. Augmentation enterocystoplasty: a critical review. J Urol 1977; 118: 799.

Rogers E, Scardino PT: A simple ileal substitute bladder after cystectomy: Experience with a modification of the Studer pouch. J Urol 1995; 153: 1432-1438

Pannek J, Haupt G, Schulze H, et al: Influence of continent ileal urinary diversion on vitamin B12 absorption. J Urol 1996; 155: 1206-1208.

Mills RD, Studer UE: Metabolic consequences of continent urinary diversion. J Urol 1999; 161: 1057-1066.

Koch MO, McDougal WS, Thomson CO: Mechanisms of solute transport following urinary diversion through intestinal segments: An experimental study with rats. J Urol 1991; 146: 1390-1397.

Poulsen AL, Steven K: Acid – base metabolism following bladder substitution with the ileal urethral Kock reservoir. Brit J Urol 1996; 78: 47-53.

Hall MC, Koch MO, Halter SA, et al: Morphologic and functional alterations of intestinal segments following urinary diversion. J Urol 1993; 149: 664-666.

Stein R. Fisch M, Ermert A, et al: Urinary diversion and orthotopic bladder substitution in children and young adults with neurogenic bladder: A safe option for treatment? J Urol 2000; 163: 568-573.

Kock MO, McDougal WS, Reddy PK, et al: Metabolic alterations following continent urinary diversion through colonic segments. J Urol 1991; 145: 270-273.

Kavaggia FF,Thompson JS, Schaefer EC, et al: Hyperammonemic encephalopathy in urinary diversion with urea-splitting urinary tract infection. Arch intern Med 1990; 150 (11): 2389-2392.

Hessain M: The osteomalaica syndrome after colocystoplasty: A cure with sodium bicarbonate alone. Brit J Urol 1970; 42: 243-245.

Wagstaff KE, Woodhouse CRJ, Rose GA, et al: Blood and urine analysis in patients with intestinal bladders. Brit J URol 1991; 68: 311-316.

Mundy AR, Nurse DE: Calcium balance, growth and skeletal mineralizatin in patients with cystoplasties. Brit J Urol 1992; 69: 257-259.

Palmer LS, Franco I, Koan SJ, et al: Urolithiasis in children following augmentation cystoplasty. J Urol 1993; 150: 726.

Husman DA, Spence HM: Current status of tumor of the bowel following ureterosigmoidostomy: A review. J Urol 1990; 144: 607.

Teriger BFG, Marshall FF: Carcinogenesis and the use of intestinal segments in the urinary tract. Urol Clin North Am 1991; 18: 737.

Filmer RB, Spencer JR: Malignancies in bladder augmentations and intestinal conduits. J Urol 1990: 143: 671.

Little JS, Klee LW, Hoover DM, Rink. RC: long-term histopathologic changes observed in rats subjected to augmentation cystoplasty. J Urol 1994; 152: 720-724.

Carr LK, Herschorn S: Early development of adenocarcinoma in a young woman following augmentation cystoplasty for undiversion. J Urol 1997; 157: 2255-2256.

Barrington JW, Fulford S, Griffiths D, Stephenson TP: Tumors in bladder remnant after augmentation enterocystoplasty. J Urol 1997; 157: 482-486.

Pope JC, 4th, Albers P, Rink RC, Cain MP, et al: Spontaneous rupture of the augmented bladder from silence to chaos. Presented at the European Society of Pediatric Urologists Meeting, Istanbul, Turkey. 1999.

Sheiner JR, Kaplan GW: Spontaneous bladder rupture following enterocystoplasty. J Urol 1988: 140: 1157-1158.

Bauer SB, Hendren WH, Kozakewich H. et al: Perforation of the augmented bladder. J Urol 1992; 148: 699.

Slaton JW, Kropp KA: Conservative management of suspected bladder rupture after augmentation enterocystoplasty. J Urol 1994; 152: 713-715.

Cartwright PC, Snow BW: Bladder augmentation: Partial detrusor excision to augment to bladder without use of bowel. J Urol 1989; 142: 1050.

Johnson HW, Nigro MK, Stothers L, et al: Laboratory variables of autoaugmentation in an animal model. Urology 1994; 44: 260-263.

Stohrer M, Goepel M, Krmaer G, et al: Detrusor myectomy (auto augmentation) in the treatment of hyper-reflexive low compliance bladder. Urology 1999; 38: 30-37.

Landa HM, Moorhead JD: Detrusorectomy. Probl Pediatr Urol 1994; 8: 204-209.

Snow BW, Cartwright P: Why bladder autoaugmentation is a good choice for detrusor instability or bladder hyperreflexia. Contemp Urol 1999:11:96-100.

Ahmed S, Sripathi V, Sen S: Perforation of an autoaugmented bladder autougmentation. New Urol Urdyn 1996 15 (3): 223-233.

Landman J, et al: Laparascopic autoaugmentation of the urinary bladder: Literature review and state of the art. Ped Endo Inno Tech 2000; 4(3): 213-221.

Leng WW, Blalock HJ, Fredriksson WH, et al: Enterocystoplasty or detrusor myectomy? Comparison of indications and outcomes for bladder augmentation. J Urol 1999; 161: 758-763.

Dewan PA: Autoaugmentation demucosalized enterocystoplasty. World J Urol 1998: 16: 255-261.

Salle JL, Fraga JC, Lucib A, et al: Seromuscular enterocystoplasty in dogs. J Urol 1990; 144: 454-456.
Cheng E, Rento R, Grayhack TJ, et al: Reversed seromuscular flaps in the urinary tract in dogs. J Urol 1994; 152: 2252.
Atala A: Commentary on the replacement of urologic associated mucosa. J Urol 1995: 156:338.
Carr MC, Docimo SG, Mitchell ME: Bladder augmentation with urothelial preservation. J Urol (in press) 1999.
Wolf JS Jr, Turzan CW: Augmentation urelerocystoplasty. J Urol 1993: 149(5): 1095-1098.
Churchill BM, Aliabadi H, landau EH, et al: Ureteral bladder augmentation. J Urol 1993. 150 (2 pt 2): 716-720.
Bellinger MF: Urelerocystoplasty update. World J Urol 1998: 16 (4): 251-254.
Landau EH, Jayanthi VR, Khoury AE, et al: Bladder agumentation: Ureterocystoplasty versus ilcocystoplasty. J Urol 1994: 152 (2 pt 2): 716-719.
Hitchcock RJ, Duffy PG, Malone PW: Ureterocystoplasty: The bladder augmentation of choice. Br J Urol 1994: 73(5):575-579.
Ben-Chaim J, Partin AW, Jeffs RD: Ureteral bladder augmentation using the lower pole ureter of a duplicated system. Urol 1996: 47 (1): 135-137.
Ahmed S, Neel KF, Sen S: Tandem Ureterocystoplasty. Aust N Z J Surg 1998: 68(3): 203-205.
Lailas NG, Cilento B, Atala A: Progressive ureteral dilation for subsequent ureterocystoplasty. J Urol 1996: 156 (3): 1151-1153.
Ikeguchi EF, Stifelman MD, Hensle IW: Ureteral tissue expansion for bladder augmentation. J Urol 1998: 159 (5): 1665-1668.
Satar N, Yoo J, Atala A: Progressive bladder dilation for subsequent augmentation cystoplasty. J Urol 1999: 162: 829-831.
Atala A: New methods of bladder augmentation. BJU international (2000), 85, suppl. 3, 24-34.
Kim BS, Mooney DK: Development of biocompatible synthetic extracellular matrices for tissue engineering. Trends Biotechnol 1998: 16:224-230.
Atala A: Future perspectives in reconstructive surgery using tissue engineering. Urol Clin North Am 1999; 26:157-165, ix-x.
Atala A: Autologous cell transplantation for urologic reconstruction. J Urol 1998; 159: 2.
Pariente JL, Kim BS, Atala A: In vitro biocompatibility assessment of naturally derived and synthetic biomaterials using normal human urothelial cells. J Biomed Mater Res 2001: 55: 33-39.
Fishman U, flores En, Scott B, et al: Use of fresh placental membranes for bladder reconstruction. J Urol 1987: 138: 1291.
Kambic H, Kay R, Chen JF, et al: Biodegradable pericardial implants for bladder augmentation: a 2.5 year study in dogs. J Urol 1992; 539-543.
Scott R, Mohammed R, Gorham SD, et al: The evolution of a biodegradable membrane for use in urological surgery: A summary of 109 in vivo experiments. Br J Urol 1988: 62(1): 26-31.
Kropp BP: Small-intestinal submucosa for bladder augmentation. A review of preclinical studies. World J Urol 1998: 16 (4): 262-267.
Kropp BR, Rippy MK, Badylak SF, et al: Regenerative urinary bladder augmentation

using small intestinal submucosa: Urodynamic and histopathologic assessment in long-term canine bladder augmentations. J Urol 1996: 155 (6): 2098-2104.

Piechota HJ, Dahms SE, Nunes LS, et al: In vitro functional properties of the rat bladder regenerated by the bladder acellular matrix graft. J Urol 1998: 159(5): 1717- 1724.

Probst M, Dahiya R, Garrier S, tanagho EA: Reproduction of functional smooth muscle tissue and partial bladder replacement. Br J Urol 1997; 79: 505-515.

Yoo JJ, Men J, Oberpenning F: A bladder augmentation using allogenic bladder submucosal seeded with cells. Urol 1998: 51(2): 221-225.

Atala A, Vacanti JP, Peters CA, et al: Formation of urothelial structures in vivo from dissociated cells attached to biodegradable polymer scaffolds in vitro. J Urol 1992b; 148:658.

Atala A, Freeman MR, Vacanti JP, et al: Implantation in vivo and retrieval of artificial structures consisting of rabbit and human urothelium and human bladder muscle. J Urol 1993b; 150:608-612.

Oberpenning F. Meng J, Yoo JJ, et al: De novo reconstitution of a functional mammalian urinary bladder by tissue engineering [see comments]. Nat Biotechnol 1999; 17(2): 149-155.

Rackley RR, Abdelmalak JB: Laparoscopic augmentation cystoplasty: surgical technique; Urol Clin Nor Am (2001); 28 (3): 663.

Gill IS, Rackley RR, Merancy AM, et al.: Laparoscopic enterocystoplasty. Urology (2000); 55(2): 178 - 81.

Elliolt SP, Meng MV, Anwar HP, et al.: Complete laparoscopic ileal cystoplasty. Urology (2002); 59(6): 939 - 43.

Hedican SP, Schulam PG, Docimo SG (1999): Laparoscopic assisted reconstructive surgery: J Urol 161(1): 267- 270.

Ehrlich RM, Gershman A (1993): Laparoscopic seromyotomy (auto-augmentation) for non-neurogenic neurogenic bladder in a child: initial case report. Urology 42(2): 175 - 178.

McDougall EM, Clayman RV, Figenshau RS, Pearle MS (1995): Laparoscopic Retropubic autoaugmentation of the bladder. J Urol 153: 123– 126.

Baren V, Bishop MR: Laparosopic bladder autoaugmentation in children. Urol. Clin. N. Am. (1998); 25 (3): 533 – 40.

Permissions

All chapters in this book were first published by InTech Open; hereby published with permission under the Creative Commons Attribution License or equivalent. Every chapter published in this book has been scrutinized by our experts. Their significance has been extensively debated. The topics covered herein carry significant findings which will fuel the growth of the discipline. They may even be implemented as practical applications or may be referred to as a beginning point for another development.

The contributors of this book come from diverse backgrounds, making this book a truly international effort. This book will bring forth new frontiers with its revolutionizing research information and detailed analysis of the nascent developments around the world.

We would like to thank all the contributing authors for lending their expertise to make the book truly unique. They have played a crucial role in the development of this book. Without their invaluable contributions this book wouldn't have been possible. They have made vital efforts to compile up to date information on the varied aspects of this subject to make this book a valuable addition to the collection of many professionals and students.

This book was conceptualized with the vision of imparting up-to-date information and advanced data in this field. To ensure the same, a matchless editorial board was set up. Every individual on the board went through rigorous rounds of assessment to prove their worth. After which they invested a large part of their time researching and compiling the most relevant data for our readers.

The editorial board has been involved in producing this book since its inception. They have spent rigorous hours researching and exploring the diverse topics which have resulted in the successful publishing of this book. They have passed on their knowledge of decades through this book. To expedite this challenging task, the publisher supported the team at every step. A small team of assistant editors was also appointed to further simplify the editing procedure and attain best results for the readers.

Apart from the editorial board, the designing team has also invested a significant amount of their time in understanding the subject and creating the most relevant covers. They scrutinized every image to scout for the most suitable representation of the subject and create an appropriate cover for the book.

The publishing team has been an ardent support to the editorial, designing and production team. Their endless efforts to recruit the best for this project, has resulted in the accomplishment of this book. They are a veteran in the field of academics and their pool of knowledge is as vast as their experience in printing. Their expertise and guidance has proved useful at every step. Their uncompromising quality standards have made this book an exceptional effort. Their encouragement from time to time has been an inspiration for everyone.

The publisher and the editorial board hope that this book will prove to be a valuable piece of knowledge for researchers, students, practitioners and scholars across the globe.

List of Contributors

Quirino Lai, Francesco Nudo, Vincenzo Morabito, Giovanni Battista Levi Sandri, Fabio Melandro, Lucia Parlati, Nicola Guglielmo, Marco Di Laudo, Manuela Garofalo, Luca Poli, Renzo Pretagostini and Pasquale B Berloco
Department of General surgery and Organ transplantation, Sapienza University of Rome, Rome, Italy

Mina Hur, Hee-Won Moon and Seog-Woon Kwon
Konkuk University and University of Ulsan, Korea

Jorge Ortiz, Jason Andre, Kamran Khanmoradi and Victor Araya
Albert Einstein Medical Center, Philadelphia PA, USA

Saman Nikeghbalian
Shiraz University of Medical Sciences, Iran

Cláudia Fagundes and Mónica Guevara
Liver Unit/Hospital Clinic Barcelona, Spain

Robles Piedras Ana Luisa and Monroy Funes Manuel Alejandro
Universidad Autónoma del Estado de Hidalgo, México

Farzad Kakaei
Tabriz University of Medical Sciences, Iran

Juana Margarita Rufino Hernández and José Manuel González-Posada Delgado
Nephrology Section, Hospital Universitario de Canarias, Tenerife, Spain

Domingo Hernández Marrero
Nephrology Section, Hospital Universitario Carlos Haya, Málaga, Spain

Giuseppe Cavallari, Flavia Neri and Bruno Nardo
Department of General Surgery and Transplantation University of Bologna, Italy

Junjie Zhao, Zhenli Gao and Ke Wang
Yantai YuHuangDing Hospital, China

Burak Sayin
Baskent University Faculty of Medicine, Ankara, Turkey

Ashraf Abou-Elela
Cairo University, Egypt

Index

www.ingramcontent.com/pod-product-compliance
Lightning Source LLC
LaVergne TN
LVHW062234200926
848484LV00006B/1542
* 9 7 9 8 8 8 7 4 0 2 2 7 7 *